FOOD ALERT!

The Ultimate
Sourcebook
For Food Safety
Second Edition

FOOD ALERT!

The Ultimate
Sourcebook
For Food Safety
Second Edition

by Morton Satin

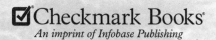

Checkmark Books®
An imprint of Infobase Publishing

Checkmark Books
An imprint of Infobase Publishing
132 West 31st Street
New York NY 10001

Library of Congress Cataloging-in-Publication Data

Satin, Morton.
  Food alert! : the ultimate sourcebook for food safety / by Morton Satin.—2nd ed.
    p.; cm.
  Includes bibliographical references and index.
  ISBN-13: 978-0-8160-6968-2 (hardcover : alk. paper)
  ISBN-10: 0-8160-6968-9 (hardcover : alk. paper)
  ISBN-13: 978-0-8160-6969-9 (pbk. : alk. paper)
  ISBN-10: 0-8160-6969-7 (pbk. : alk. paper) 1. Foodborne diseases—Prevention.
I. Title. II. Title: Ultimate sourcebook for food safety.
  [DNLM: 1. Food Poisoning—prevention & control. 2. Food Contamination—prevention & control. 3. Food Handling. 4. Food Technology. WC 268 S253f 2008]

RA601.5.S28 2008
615.9′54—dc22   2008011038

Checkmark Books are available at special discounts when purchased in bulk quantities for businesses, associations, institutions, or sales promotions. Please call our Special Sales Department in New York at (212) 967-8800 or (800) 322-8755.

You can find Facts On File on the World Wide Web at http://www.factsonfile.com

Text design by Evelyn Horovicz
Cover design by Salvatore Luongo

All illustrations, unless otherwise credited, are courtesy the author's collection or copyright Infobase Publishing.

Printed in the United States of America

MP MSRF 10 9 8 7 6 5 4 3 2 1

This book is printed on acid-free paper and contains 30 percent postconsumer recycled content.

For Bella

and

Abe Faierstein

CONTENTS

Appendix III

PREFACE TO THE FIRST EDITION

I don't care how long I live, I will never believe that my son died from eating a cheeseburger. Never.

—Michael Nole

During the last few days of 1992 at the height of the Christmas holiday period, several people on the U.S. West Coast began to succumb to a lethal food-borne infection. Most of the unfortunate victims were children who had eaten hamburgers at one of the many Jack-in-the-Box fast-food restaurants so popular in that part of the country. Toddlers who came in close contact with other children who had eaten the hamburgers were also affected. By the time the outbreak was finally under control, almost 700 people in the states of Washington, Idaho, California and Nevada had been stricken with the disease. Tragically, several of the youngest victims died an unusually cruel and agonizing death.

It seems inconceivable that this devastating episode and all the grief and anguish that accompanied it resulted from the simple and innocent act of eating a hamburger. Hamburgers are the quintessential icons of American fast food. Nearly everyone eats hamburgers. Hamburger advertising is everywhere. In some downtown areas, you can find four different hamburger restaurants on one intersection! Who has not seen the signs declaring the billions of hamburgers sold annually? No wonder that Michael Nole, the father of a two-year-old victim, could not believe that a plain cheeseburger was responsible for his son's death. However, it was. The particular strain of Escherichia coli bacteria concealed by those contaminated hamburgers is a fierce and deadly killer. A significant number of those children that survived had to undergo repeated intestinal surgery and extended kidney dialysis. Many of them will be affected for the rest of their lives.

Unfortunately, hamburgers are not the only offenders. Almost every form of food we eat has the potential to be a hidden reservoir of disease-causing organisms. The problem exists whether we eat foods inside or outside of the home. Food-borne diseases are certainly not limited to restaurants, cafeterias or fast-food outlets. Improper handling or cooking of foods in the home can be equally fatal and very often is. Both the frequency and the severity of food-borne disease outbreaks are on the rise—trends that will most probably continue because of the proportionate increase in the population of older and immunocompromised consumers. These projections are neither exaggerations nor any sort of doomsday prognoses—they are simply facts of life—authoritative, quantifiable, recorded and indisputable facts of life!

More than 600 food-borne diseases are known today. Reliable estimates by health professionals place the annual number of cases of intestinal infectious diseases in the United States as high as 99 million with related costs in excess of 25 billion dollars. Even though this may seem like an enormous amount of money, it is really only the tip of the iceberg. The value of lost opportunities and ruined reputations is very difficult to calculate. How can one place a price on the grief and anguish due to sickness and death with any real meaning, particularly for the victims and their families?

Not surprisingly, food-borne diseases have become an issue of growing concern for most adult consumers. On a daily basis, we are confronted with alarming newspaper and television reports of food-poisoning outbreaks involving many of the foods we regularly eat. Hardly a form of food is exempt from this danger. Often, the implicated products are associated with brand names and corporations that are so familiar they seem like second nature to most of us. The threat of illness or death resulting from nothing more than the mere act of eating common foods is a new and frightening prospect for consumers who have for so long taken the safety of their food supply for granted.

Throughout history, we have been confronted with the invisible threat of disease-causing organisms. Although infinitesimally small and fragile, these creatures have killed more humans than all the wars and natural disasters combined. These microorganisms constitute some of the earth's most basic forms of life—that is precisely the problem! In order to stay alive and breed, they have no options—they must infect us! The terrible harm and tragedy they cause are of no concern to their survival. The tiny organisms responsible for food-borne diseases have no conscience and no religious beliefs or political inclinations. They neither care for social ideals nor for bottom-line profitability. Disease-causing microorganisms merely want to survive and, through their astonishing evolutionary adaptability, have managed to do so rather skillfully from the dawn of time.

In the beginning, the greatest ally these disease-causing organisms had in their battle for survival was humankind's complete innocence. Although our ancestors were bitterly aware of the painful consequences of intestinal diseases, they simply knew nothing of their origins. As time went on, a vague connection began to develop between certain foods and corresponding illnesses. Literally thousands of years of careful observation, study and speculation went by before we clearly understood what the connection actually was. Now that we understand the causes of most food-borne diseases and have ready access to the technologies that can completely control them, we can no longer claim innocence as our excuse. Our conflict with infective and toxic microorganisms is a never-ending battle. History has clearly demonstrated that our intelligence and our wits are the greatest weapons in our arsenal against these microscopic enemies. Yet, on a daily basis, we see examples where our superstitions and ignorance outrank intelligence. The primary reason for the continued, malignant influence of food-borne disease microorganisms on all of us is little more than our callous disregard for each other tempered with a healthy dose of greed and self-interest.

Aside from poor eating habits, food-borne diseases are the greatest food-related risk we face. Our individual, innate abilities to overcome their symptoms are our only defense against them. The young, the old and all the other individuals whose immune systems are compromised in some way exceed 40 million people in America today. They do not have an equal chance to ward off the misery, discomfort and tragic consequences resulting from these diseases. Even the strongest among us become susceptible the moment our defenses are down. Food-borne diseases are not inevitable, they are preventable. It is simply not acceptable for a country that boasts of its modern technological prowess and "can-do" spirit to allow this national scandal to continue. This is the reason I decided to write this book.

—Morton Satin
Rome, Italy

PREFACE TO THE
SECOND EDITION

Since the publication of the first edition of *Food Alert!* there have been many significant developments in the field of food safety. These have come in the wake of greater consumer awareness of the scope and significance of food-borne illnesses, as well as other landmark events that have made us realize just how vulnerable our current industrialized food system is to new challenges—be they from nature, terrorists or inadequate regulatory procedures. In addition to updating all of the data in the original edition, *Food Alert!, Second Edition,* addresses the new issues and challenges that have arisen in the intervening years and provides a glimpse into the future impact of food-borne diseases upon consumers.

I have added a new section on the latest large-scale multistate food-borne disease outbreaks that spread to the population through vegetable products infected with animal pathogens in order to stress the growing susceptibility of our highly integrated industrial food and agriculture system. We continue to face the risks resulting from a regulatory system that refuses to recognize the needs of a growing population of immuno-compromised people, a complex food labeling and information system that seems to provide limitless information, but often leaves consumers confused, and the growing threat of bioterrorism to our food supply.

Two interesting new additions are a section on new government, industry and consumer advocacy initiatives that are designed to reduce the risk of food-borne diseases and another on the results of a CBS News/ New York Times Poll that presents an interesting perspective on just how low the levels of reporting of food-borne disease incidents really are.

—Morton Satin
Rockville, Maryland

ACKNOWLEDGMENTS

I would like to thank Mr. Ed Knappman of New England Publishing Associates, who originally suggested this book and provided helpful guidance throughout its preparation. I would also like to express my sincere appreciation to Dr. Jocelyne Rocourt of the Pasteur Institute and Dr. Yasmine Motarjemi of the World Health Organization in Geneva for reviewing the original manuscript and providing valuable technical advice. I am particularly grateful to Mr. James Chambers and Ms. Jane Hickok of Facts On File, Inc., who put so much effort into turning the manuscript into a finished product. Finally, I would like to thank my wife, Miriam, for her patience, understanding and support throughout the course of this work.

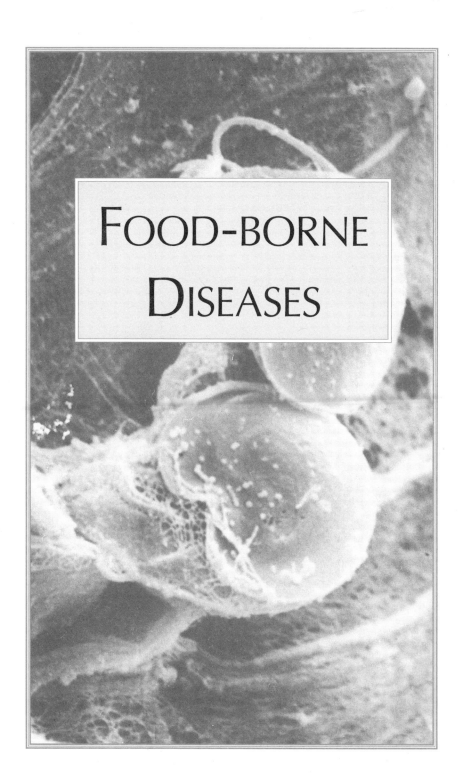

FOOD-BORNE
DISEASES

HISTORICAL BACKGROUND

Roast Beef, Medium, is not only a food. It is a philosophy. Seated at Life's Dining Table, with the menu of Morals before you, your eye wanders a bit over the entrées, the hors d'oeuvres, and the things à la though you know that Roast Beef, Medium, is safe and sane, and sure.

Edna Ferber (U.S. author 1897–1911)
Roast Beef, Medium, Foreword (1911)*

Gastrointestinal disorders and the miserable consequences that so often accompany them have always been a feature of human existence. Throughout history, our ancestors went to great lengths to try and interpret all the reasons for the multitude of gastric ailments that afflicted them. Much of the rationale behind those ancient theories and taboos has been lost in history. However, they undoubtedly served the very useful purpose of advising future generations about the careful selection and preparation of certain foods and cautioned against the consumption of others.

Interestingly, the very first law given by God to man, as recorded in the Bible, was a dietary law. "Of every tree of the garden thou mayest freely eat; but of the tree of knowledge of good and evil, thou shalt not eat of it" (Gen. 2:16, 17). According to the Bible, humans were originally intended to be strict vegetarians, "And God said, 'Behold, I have given you every herb yielding seed, which is upon the face of the earth, and every tree, on which is the fruit of a tree yielding food—to you it shall be for food . . .'" (Gen. 1:29, 30). Only after the great flood did God relent and permit Noah and his descendants to partake of meat, of animal flesh, "Every moving thing that liveth shall be food for you, as the green herb have I given you all" (Gen. 9:3). People have often debated and rationalized from both secular and religious viewpoints the reasons for this sudden shift to allow for meat. However, any conclusive interpretation for the motives of Divine Law is, almost by definition, beyond us mortals. This concession to the animal nature of humans was not without conditions, however. The verse immediately following expressly forbids the consumption of the blood (representing the life) of animals. This particular restriction was to distinguish humankind from all the other beasts.

The earliest recorded detailed references regarding the consumption of specific types of foods were the prohibitions that formed the basis of the

---

ancient Jewish dietary laws. Despite much that has been written to the contrary, the kosher laws were not formulated as health laws per se. With little doubt, they made good hygienic sense at the time, and many still do. However, the sovereign and only purpose for the kosher laws was to aspire to holiness—the perfection of humankind. The laws served as a set of practical commands governing the decrees articulated by God. In reality, they had far more to do with morals and ethics than the pursuit of a healthy diet.

An interesting example of this is the case of leavened products—foods such as bread that have risen through the action of yeast. Throughout the book of Leviticus, prohibitions are leveled against the consumption of leavened products. Not only were the ancient Jews forbidden to eat leavened bread on the religious festival of Passover, but they were not even allowed to present it as a sacrifice in the temple nor give it as a contribution to the priests. Leviticus 2:11 states, "No meal offering which ye shall bring unto the Lord, shall be made with leaven." Why is this? What sort of moral, ethical or hygienic principle do leavened foods contravene? We now know that the English word *leaven* is a mistaken translation of the Hebrew word *hametz*. In fact, *hametz* does not mean "to rise," it means "to sour." Even a soured relationship between two people is referred to in this way in modern Hebrew. The real meaning of *hametz* in the context of the Bible passages is therefore spoiled, corrupted or unhealthy. When using the proper translation, both religious and secular considerations fall rather neatly into place.

Needless to say, incorporating all the available wisdom about the safety of foods into the prevailing laws governing religion and ethics would make practical sense. However, no evidence shows that such knowledge existed at the time when the dietary laws were originally promulgated. Indeed, considerable doubt has been expressed that the health benefits of dietary prohibitions could possibly have been known at the time.[1] Although a relationship was implied between spoiled food and ill health, any direct connection between the two was not well understood. Certainly, microorganisms were completely unknown. Even the tiny worms or maggots that inevitably appeared on spoiled foods were the subject of pure philosophical speculation. (Modern knowledge and accessibility to a far greater number of foods have made interpretation of the kosher laws more difficult. Vegetables are not only a basic staple in our diet, but current understanding of the importance of their nutritious phytochemicals and antioxidants means they will play an increasingly important role. Unfortunately, certain vegetables provide a safe haven for insects and, as kosher law strictly prohibits the consumption of insects, this has made the kosher certification of vegetables highly challenging.)

The Greek philosopher Anaximander (610–547 B.C.) spent a good part of his life teaching students that certain animals were miraculously formed out of pure moisture. Aristotle (384–322 B.C.) continued to pursue this line of thinking and proposed that animals spontaneously arose out of soil, plants or even other species of animals.

So with animals, some spring from parent animals according to their kind, whilst others grow spontaneously and not from kindred stock; and of these instances of spontaneous generation some come from putrefying earth or vegetable matter, as is the case with a number of insects, while others are spontaneously generated in the inside of animals out of the secretions of their several organs.

Aristotle
History of Animals (350 B.C.)

The influence of these and other classical Greek philosophers was so overwhelming that their simple hypotheses were almost taken as if they were divine edicts. As a consequence, the theory of the "spontaneous generation" of life was firmly established very early in recorded history and became a constant source of intellectual and scientific debate until the Middle Ages and beyond. During the Renaissance period, Girolamo Cardano (1501–76) stated that water gave rise to fish. Even Jan Baptista van Helmont (1578–1644), the famous Belgian physician and chemist, gave out detailed recipes for the preparation of spontaneously generated mice.[2] For 2,000 years, polemics were the only means of dealing with this issue, for never once in the history of the debate had anyone ever thought of carrying out experiments to prove or disprove the validity of their theories. Because of our physical inability to see microorganisms, all the discussions about their existence were confined to the realm of pure speculation. Fortunately, the times were ripe for change.

In the meantime, the Italian physician Gerolamo Fracastoro (1484–1553), of Verona, published a work containing the very first statements about the true nature of contagious disease organisms and the ways in which they were transmitted.[3] He speculated that these disease particles, which he called *Seminaria*, were too small to be seen. However, they were capable of reproducing in the appropriate nutrient media and became infective through the action of what he mysteriously labeled "animal heat." It was all speculation, of course, but was remarkably close to the truth. He was so close, in fact, that Fracastoro was accorded the ultimate honor of all great scientists of his particular time—his theory was abruptly and totally ignored for almost two centuries.

The 17th century saw a new breed of thinker arise to question seriously the conventional, but unproven, dogmas about the nature of things. Francis Bacon (1561–1626) could not help questioning every traditional doctrine of nature that did not make sense. He insisted that only careful experimentation and precise observation would lead to the truth. He thought little of Aristotle's theories and even less of the man himself as can be seen from the following quote:

He [Aristotle] is the greater and deeper politician, that can make other men the instruments of his will and ends, and yet never acquaint them with his purpose, so as they shall do it, and yet not know what they do.[4]

Bacon's powerful role in English politics and the sheer volume of his writings made him an extremely influential figure in the overall development of science and technology. He became the period's most eloquent and persistent proponent of methodical experimentation and has often been referred to as the Father of the Scientific Method.

The Italian scholar Francisco Redi (1626–98) followed Bacon's advice. He carried out several experiments to prove that tiny maggots did not arise spontaneously in meat, as everyone generally believed, but were able to develop only when flies were first given an opportunity to lay their eggs on that meat. The experiment could not have been more elementary. He simply protected the freshly cut meat by placing it into a jar covered with a fine gauze, thus preventing flies from depositing their eggs on it (see figure 1). It may have been a modest beginning. However, at last, the first penetrating cracks began to appear in the spontaneous generation theory that had dominated human understanding for more than two millennia.

While studying organisms visible to the naked eye was possible, true microorganisms were well beyond our physical ability to observe. The eye can barely perceive objects that have a diameter of less than 0.1 mm

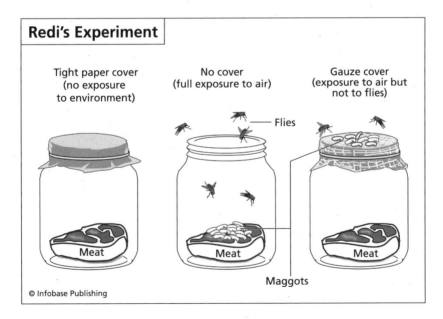

Figure 1. **Redi's Experiment**

(1/250 in.). The technology for grinding small lenses, which might greatly magnify objects, gradually improved to a point where the first double lens or compound microscopes (see figure 2) were devised in the town of Middleburg, Holland, by Hans Zansz and his son in 1590. Although the quality of the optics was not quite good enough to observe microorganisms, technology was steadily progressing. The drive to explain all natural phenomena systematically began to be pursued in earnest. It became a career for some and a respectable pastime for others.

The title First of the Great Microbe Hunters[5] goes to a rather unlikely character by the name of Antoni van Leeuwenhoek (lay-ven-hook) (see figure 3). Born in the prosperous city of Delft, Holland, in 1632, he spent his professional career in the drapery business. He was also appointed to the honorary post of caretaker of the Delft City Hall. Despite his heavy workload, van Leeuwenhoek still found the time to indulge in his favorite pastime of grinding miniature lenses and making simple microscopes. Even though his microscopes (see figure 4) were much more elementary than the compound models designed almost a century before, the superb quality of his lenses allowed him to see things accurately no one had ever seen before.

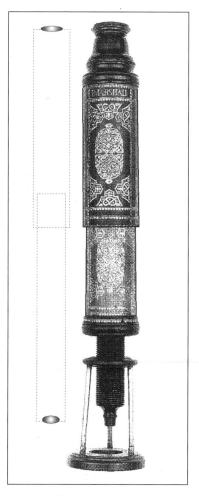

Figure 2. **The Compound Microscope**

He set about carefully observing everything he could find. He looked at the barbed stings of bees and the hairy legs of common lice. He dissected worms and flies, and he squinted for hours at the tartar material he scraped from his own teeth. In one of those serendipitous quirks of fate that have so often accompanied great scientific discoveries, a local acquaintance of his, Regnier de Graaf, happened to be a corresponding member of the prestigious Royal Society of London. After seeing what van Leeuwenhoek was able to observe with his fantastic lenses, de Graaf urged the Royal Society to request formally that

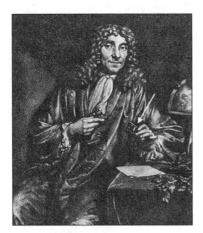

Figure 3. **Antoni van Leeuwenhoek**

van Leeuwenhoek carefully describe his discoveries to them, which they did. This fortunate turn of events assured van Leeuwenhoek's unique and honored place in the historic annals of science. Left to his own devices, it is unlikely that he would have ever published his findings. As it turned out, however, he eventually became one of the Royal Society's most famous members, second only to Sir Isaac Newton. During the 50 years from 1673 to 1723, van Leeuwenhoek managed to send the Royal Society a staggering 112 papers, complete with accurate drawings describing all the things he had observed with his remarkable little microscopes.

On one fateful day, van Leeuwenhoek filled a tiny glass tube with a drop of rain-water he got from an old bucket and peered at it with his microscope. Suddenly, he began to make out infinitesimally tiny forms swimming about in the water—they were alive! At that precise moment, Antoni van Leeuwenhoek flung open the doors to the fascinating world of microscopic life. He had accidentally intruded upon an incredible universe of creatures that lived, fought and died right before the eyes of everyone yet had always remained invisible.

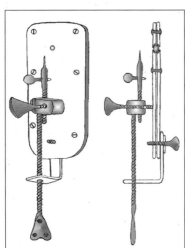

Figure 4. **van Leeuwenhoek's Microscope**

He then peered at droplets of water in which particles of pepper had been steeped and once more saw the little moving creatures. He called them "animalcules" and wasted no time in letting the Royal Society of London know of his fantastic new discoveries (see figure 5).[6] At first, the Royal Society simply could not believe what he had written. The Society asked their most illustrious microscopist, Robert Hooke, to verify van Leeuwenhoek's findings. On November 15, 1677, he did! The Royal Society proudly announced that, as a result of the splendid labors of that distinguished Delft City Hall janitor Antoni van Leeuwenhoek, microorganisms

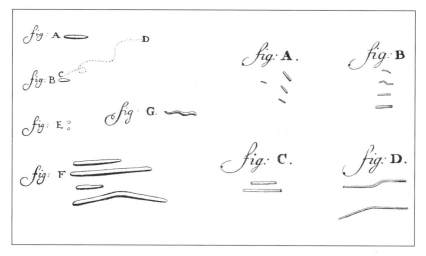

Figure 5. **van Leeuwenhoek's Animalcules**

were formally and officially declared to be an integral part of the natural order of things in the world.

The famous Dutch painter Jan Vermeer (1632–75), who happened to be born in Delft on the same day as van Leeuwenhoek, was a close friend of his throughout life. When he first saw the animalcules, he swore they reminded him of the fantastic creatures in Hieronymus Bosch's nightmarish paintings. He feared that van Leeuwenhoek was embarking on a dangerous journey that might ultimately bring humanity more harm than good. By reflecting the fear of the unknown that always accompanies new breakthroughs, he likened his friend's discoveries to erecting a Tower of Babel.[7]

During his lifetime, the Dutch draper made countless, accurate descriptions of the microorganisms he encountered in an incredibly wide variety of circumstances. He studied the parasites that killed shellfish and the bacteria that dwelt inside his mouth. Van Leeuwenhoek was the first person in the world to observe sperm cells and the concave red cells of blood. He studied the intestinal inhabitants of various animals, fish and birds. He was even able to detect the organisms in his own discharges when "he was troubled with a looseness," making him the first individual to examine the organisms responsible for food-borne diseases. Nothing escaped his magnified observations. Van Leeuwenhoek continued his investigations up until the grand old age of 91. On his deathbed, his last request was that his final two reports be safely delivered to the Royal Society of London. Thus, the science of microbiology began in earnest.

With little doubt, the contribution of this simple man was the greatest in all of microbiology. Van Leeuwenhoek described almost every major type of unicellular microorganism known today—yeast, algae, bacteria and protozoa. Of course, many that followed may have been more intellectually creative or scientifically sophisticated. However, this man's earnest and determined observations put the visible face of reality on the nature of microscopic life. Indeed, within a few years of van Leeuwenhoek's death, his efforts received supreme recognition from the world's foremost classifier of nature's many forms. In his book *Systema Naturae* (1635), Carolus Linnaeus, the Swedish botanist universally considered to be the founder of modern classification systems for plants and animals, officially placed van Leeuwenhoek's animalcules together with various agents of disease, putrefaction and fermentation into a separate category of life he cryptically labeled "chaos."

The modern scientific world was stunned in 1981 when biologist Brian Ford discovered the original letters of van Leeuwenhoek deep in the historical archives of the Royal Society of London. Attached to these letters were several samples of the very specimens that van Leeuwenhoek had carefully studied, described and sent in as proof of his discoveries more than three centuries earlier. These materials had been so well prepared that it was possible to study them once more under the microscope but this time using the most modern, state-of-the-art technology. Much to his credit, the three-century-old samples showed that van Leeuwenhoek's methods and techniques were very exacting and every bit as sound as those used today. Indeed, the most modern light microscopes revealed little more than had van Leeuwenhoek's amazing little lenses.[8, 9]

Once the existence of microorganisms was firmly established and the means to observe them was readily available, the pace of progress in the field of microbiology began to increase. Although the first elementary hypotheses regarding the possible role of microorganisms in disease and spoilage began to surface, the main intellectual preoccupation regarding microorganisms lay elsewhere. From the middle of the 18th to the middle of the 19th centuries, the history of microbiology appeared to be little more than the bitter controversy between the age-old concept of spontaneous generation and the idea that all life came from preexisting life—*omne vivum ex vivo.*

Once again, the sagacious Italians, this time led by Lazzaro Spallanzani (1729–99), led the way. Through careful experiments designed to exclude all forms of contamination, he conclusively proved in 1769 that all living things, large and small, had parents—they simply could not generate spontaneously. He executed his studies so flawlessly that no one had the skill or patience to duplicate them. During the course of his work, he developed many of the basic techniques used for microscopic observation until today and was the first person to observe the organisms responsible for fermentation. Unfortunately, few people paid much attention to him at the time. Almost 70 years passed before the German scientist Max Schultze fully confirmed his results. Even then, the spontaneous generation theory still had many tenacious and influential supporters.

The growing body of knowledge about the nature of microorganisms, the passion of the ongoing spontaneous generation debate and the visible, tragic effects of disease set the stage for an outburst of scientific discovery in the infant field of microbiology. The scholarly endeavors of many scientists began to establish a foundation of understanding that has survived to the present day. In this crowd of intellectual giants, however, one individual stands out as an icon representing the potential that science holds for the benefit of humankind's existence on this planet. While most other scientists practiced objective, dispassionate, cold-blooded research in their quest for knowledge, this person could not help but suffer the intense anguish of his fellow persons in his crusade to make life better. Whereas other scientists became associated with specific discoveries in their respective fields, this man became the compelling symbol of all humankind's efforts to live without fear of the afflictions that have plagued us all from the dawn of time. The drive, the passion, the charisma of this man gave hope to all humanity, from street sweepers to the privileged nobility, that disease and pestilence were not a necessary condition of our existence—they could finally be conquered.

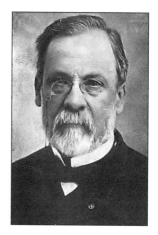

Figure 6. **Louis Pasteur**

Louis Pasteur (1822–95) (see figure 6)[10] was originally trained as a chemist and spent the first years of his professional life studying the basic problems of chemistry and physics. In 1856, while he was dean of the faculty of sciences at Lille University, he was asked to look into the alcohol fermentation problems with which some local entrepreneurs were having serious difficulties. In this case, necessity was not only the mother of invention but also the back door through which Pasteur stepped into the field of microbiology. He had a burning desire to fight the good fight, and the plight of his commercial neighbors in Lille allowed him to enter the fray. He began by reconfirming the 20-year-old observation by fellow French scientist, Cagniard de la Tour, that microscopic yeasts were responsible for the production of alcohol from sugar beets. In record time, he determined that pure yeast cultures resulted in good fermentation, while a variety of other microorganisms were responsible for spoilage. Not only did he work to uncover the causes of the problem, but he gave practical recommendations to eliminate them effectively. Shortly after he got involved in the microscopic world, Pasteur destroyed the age-old concept of spontaneous generation so convincingly that, a full century later, biophysicists working on the spontaneous origin of primordial life malevolently cursed him as

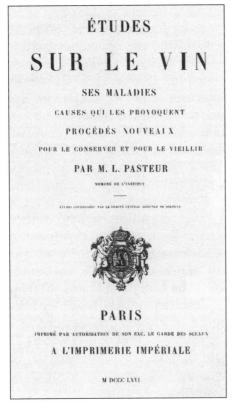

ÉTUDES

SUR LE VIN

SES MALADIES

CAUSES QUI LES PROVOQUENT

PROCÉDÉS NOUVEAUX

POUR LE CONSERVER ET POUR LE VIEILLIR

PAR M. L. PASTEUR

MEMBRE DE L'INSTITUT

ÉTUDES COURONNÉES PAR LE COMITÉ CENTRAL AGRICOLE DE SOLOGNE

PARIS

IMPRIMÉ PAR AUTORISATION DE SON EXC. LE GARDE DES SCEAUX

A L'IMPRIMERIE IMPÉRIALE

M DCCC LXVI

Figure 7. **Pasteur's Classic**

the primary reason why they could not get anyone to believe in their new theories.

From general problems in the field of fermentation, Pasteur shifted his focus toward the difficulties faced by France's silk, beer and wine industries (see figures 7 and 8).[11] In a series of stunning technical successes, he defined the problems and set out remedial measures to remove them. The ubiquitous term "pasteurization" describes his process for heating wine to prevent unwanted spoilage from undesirable microorganisms. While this process became a major commercial success, it realized its greatest impact when later applied by others to the treatment of milk. The resulting process of milk pasteurization has saved innumerable lives and provided us with exceptional social and economic benefits.

Pasteur firmly established the relationship between spoilage, disease and microorganisms. Always controversial and often spellbinding, Pasteur brought the issue of microbes and disease to the attention of the masses. His tireless devotion to the eradication of disease and the spectacular public demonstrations of his work convinced everyone that living in a world free of the ravages of illness would one day be possible.

Countless others made technical contributions to microbiology and control of disease that equaled or even exceeded those of Pasteur. The most notable of these was Robert Koch (1843–1910) who discovered the anthrax and tuberculosis bacteria. The second half of the 19th century was the golden age of microbiological science. The list of scientists and their discoveries is a veritable Who's Who of infectious disease.

The first important landmark in the microbiological investigation of food poisoning was the isolation of *Bacillus enteritidis* (salmonella) from a fatal case of food poisoning by the German scientist August Gärtner in 1888.[12] Very early in the study of food-borne disease, it became clear that two well-recognized factors caused food poisoning. "Food-borne infections" were caused by the development and growth of disease-causing microorganisms in the victim's intestine. "Food-borne intoxications" resulted from toxins formed in the food before it was consumed.

Thus, the basis of modern microbiology was well established before the turn of this century. Of course, the level of sophistication was not comparable to the advanced techniques employed today. However, the conceptual foundation of the

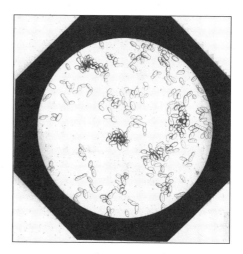

Figure 8. **Microorganisms in Wine**

science was firmly rooted in the burst of brilliant work carried out in the second half of the last century. The historical parade of events ranged from philosophical speculations through myth and superstition to the observation and gradual understanding of microscopic life. The science of microbiology, like so many other disciplines, evolved through a torturous ride that reflected the strength, the genius and the pigheadedness of humankind. By the turn of the 19th century, the consuming pastime of the janitor of Delft City Hall had blossomed into the most important area of scientific understanding to be applied to the fight against disease.

BASIC CONCEPTS

Before proceeding further, a few basic concepts and definitions must be reviewed. Unfortunately, a certain amount of technical jargon is unavoidable, but it will be kept to a minimum.

Volume of Cell Type μm^3		
CELL TYPE	NORMAL RANGE	EXTREME LIMITS
Protozoa	10,000–50,000	20–150,000,000
Molds	Highly variable	—
Yeasts	20–50	15–75
Bacteria	0.01–10	0.01–5,000
Viruses	0.00001–0.01	0.00001–0.01

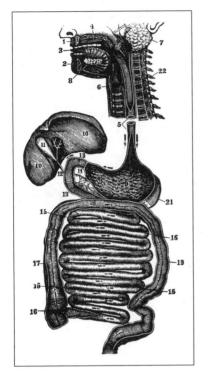

Figure 9. **The Digestive Tract**

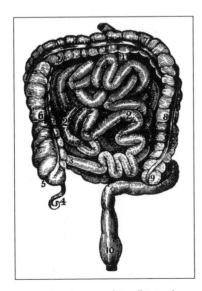

Figure 10. **Large and Small Intestine**

RELATIVE SIZES OF DIFFERENT MICROORGANISMS

The term "microorganism" refers to those organisms that are so small (0.1 μ–100 μ)* they are totally invisible to the naked eye. In order of decreasing size, they are made up of protozoa, molds, yeasts, bacteria and, the tiniest of all, viruses. Considerable overlap in size (which is best measured as volume) between the various groups occurs, as shown in the table "Relative Sizes of Different Microorganisms." Although only bacteria, yeasts and molds can produce toxins, all classes of microorganisms are capable of causing infections. Some, as we shall see later, can be virulent killers. The term "pathogenic" is commonly used and simply means capable of causing disease. In other words, those microorganisms responsible for making people sick are referred to as pathogenic microorganisms or just pathogens.

THE DIGESTIVE TRACT

In order to understand how food-borne diseases affect us, we must first picture the digestive tract and how it works. The entire gastrointestinal tract is a complex, twisted tube open at both ends—the mouth and the anus. All along this convoluted tube are organs that allow us to take in and digest our foods, absorb the nutrients and finally eliminate the waste products. It is like a production line (see figures 9 and 10).[13]

Food enters the mouth where it is mixed with saliva, ground up and swallowed. (Digestion actually starts in the mouth because saliva contains

---

* 1 μ (micron) = 1/25,000 of an inch = 1/10,000 of a centimeter

some digestive enzymes.) The moist mass of food, which is now called a "bolus," passes from the mouth down through the esophagus and into the stomach. Each day, the stomach routinely secretes about three full quarts of gastric juices containing high concentrations of hydrochloric acid and enzymes that begin to break down the bolus. From the stomach, the partially digested food, now called "chyme," is conveyed into the front end of the small intestine, called the duodenum. Here is where the liver, the pancreas and the gallbladder inject about two quarts of fluid into the digestive tract. This fluid (bile and pancreatic juice) contains salts and enzymes that neutralize the acid and break down all those components that the stomach was not able to digest.

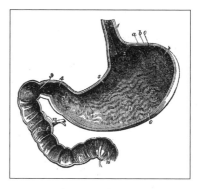

Figure 11. **The Stomach and Duodenum**

Although the remaining section of small intestine also produces secretions to aid digestion, it is here in the duodenum where the critical process of nutrient absorption begins in earnest. The small intestine is approximately 20 feet long. It has an extremely complex surface that is able to assimilate the nutrients from the digested food very efficiently. These nutrients are quickly picked up by the circulatory system and carried to those organs of the body that require them. The residual material then passes on to the last part of the gastrointestinal tract, the large intestine, which is considerably wider but much shorter than the small intestine. Here, all of the excess water and salts used in the digestion process are absorbed so they can be recycled for the body's reuse. Finally, the remaining indigestible waste products are discharged.

The gastrointestinal tract of a newborn baby is sterile. Within a very short period, though, it starts to become colonized by friendly, helpful bacteria. Within a year, the gastrointestinal tract contains over 100 trillion such bacteria from over 400 different species.[14] These beneficial bacteria help us digest our food and also help defend us against pathogenic microorganisms, which are not at all friendly.

WHAT IS FOOD POISONING?

"Food poisoning" is a rather general term that includes almost all forms of serious injury from food resulting in "gastroenteritis." This word refers to the irritation and inflammation of the digestive tract. Gastroenteritis generally results from eating foods that contain toxins or pathogenic microorganisms. "Toxin" is simply another word for poison. As explained previously, a pathogen is any microorganism capable of producing a disease or sickness. The term "food-borne disease" is slightly broader and also includes allergic reactions to foods and other conditions where food acts as the carrier of infections or toxins. Although some people refer to food poisoning as the act of ingesting a toxin, in everyday practice, the terms food poisoning and food-borne diseases are used interchangeably. Food-borne diseases are generally classified into three categories.[15]

"Food-borne infections" are caused by the consumption of foods or beverages that contain sufficient numbers of pathogenic microorganisms to colonize and multiply in the victim's gastrointestinal tract and cause the sorts of symptoms and consequences typical of that organism. The actual number of organisms required to cause a disease incident (referred to as the "infective dose") will often vary with the particular strain of microorganism involved as well as with the state of health of the consumer. When examining the actual rate of incidents, food-borne infections are the most frequent forms of food-borne diseases. Typical examples of food-borne infectious diseases are salmonellosis, shigellosis and campylobacteriosis gastroenteritis. In other words, these diseases are an irritation and inflammation of the gastrointestinal tract resulting from its infection by certain pathogenic organisms. Also remember that such infections are by no means an easy feat. The microorganisms must be able to survive through all the digestive enzymes and all the acid produced by the digestive system before they can begin to infect their victims. To our great discomfort and regret, this is a marvelous example of biological evolution and adaptability—a subject that will come up time and again throughout this book.

"Food-borne intoxications," as their title suggests, result from the straightforward ingestion of toxins or poisons. The most common forms of toxins involved develop from the growth of microorganisms in heavily contaminated foods. These toxins are actually normal by-products of the microbes' metabolism and are usually produced in foods long before people consume them. Some of these toxins are very heat resistant and, once formed, are not destroyed by the cooking process. The most well-known examples of food intoxication are staphylococcal food poisoning and botulism. Biochemical toxins (the majority of which are from natural plant and animal sources) account for a relatively minor percentage of food-borne disease cases.[16] The last and least common form of food-borne intoxication results from chemicals or pesticides that accidentally find their way into food products.

"Food-borne toxicoinfections" are, as their name implies, an amalgam of the previous two characteristics. The ingested food contains sufficient numbers of pathogenic microorganisms to infect the victim's intestinal tract heavily. Once the infection is established, the microbes then start to produce toxins that result in symptoms of the disease. In other words, the toxins are actually produced in the gastrointestinal tract itself, rather than in the food. Toxicoinfections are among the most serious forms of food-borne diseases, because they are not a one-time ingestion of toxin—the infecting bacteria produce toxin continually. Examples of typical microorganisms involved in toxicoinfections are *Clostridium perfringens, Escherichia coli* and *Vibrio cholerae.*

HOW DOES FOOD POISONING AFFECT US?

The most common symptoms of food poisoning are abdominal pain, diarrhea and vomiting. They all result from various degrees of irritation and inflammation of the digestive tract. Gastroenteritis also occurs when we are infected by certain communicable virus infections such as the 24-hour stomach flu. It can also result from a major change in the population of friendly bacteria in the digestive tract following antibiotic treatment, for instance.

"Diarrhea" occurs when the digestive tract (mainly the large intestine) is affected to the extent that it cannot properly reabsorb the water and salts used throughout the digestive process. The natural consequence is the frequent evacuation of very watery and occasionally bloody stools. This condition can result from infections or toxins that damage or disturb the intestinal tract. Although diarrhea may simply seem to be an uncomfortable or even an embarrassing situation, its physiological effects are far more serious. If the large volumes of water that the body uses in the routine digestive process cannot be recovered and recycled, the risk of severe dehydration and its complications such as shock from an insufficient blood supply become very real.

"Vomiting," as everyone is familiar with, means the sudden and powerful expelling of stomach and intestinal contents up through the mouth. It is one of those unpleasant experiences we have all faced at one time or another. Once the process starts, we are virtually helpless to do anything about it until it is over. Strong nausea, sweating and a feeling of faintness often precede it. The brain, which receives signals from nerves situated along the stomach or intestines, controls the vomiting reaction itself. These nerves are particularly stimulated by toxins and immediately elicit the vomiting reaction in a defensive attempt to rid the body of poisonous materials. Unpleasant as it is, vomiting is an effective natural defense process, and most people usually benefit from its consequences.

The range of other symptoms associated with food poisoning is very broad in terms of effects and severity. High fevers, internal hemorrhaging, kidney failure and death are just a few of the numerous repercussions and complications of food poisoning. Secondary, after-effect illnesses, many of which can have very serious long-term and life-threatening consequences, are also a major consideration of food poisoning and food-borne diseases.

THE EXTENT OF THE PROBLEM

Health professionals place the estimated annual number of cases of intestinal infectious diseases in the United States at 76 million,[17] although previous estimates project figures as high as 99 million.[18] This means that more than one in three Americans suffer at least once from some form of gastroenteritis every year—the major cause being food-borne diseases. Since the food system in the United States is technically advanced and regulations are strictly enforced, the rate of food poisoning in other countries is very likely considerably higher. If the global figures for food-borne diseases were estimated on an annual basis, they would be staggering.

The more recent appreciation of the seriousness of various food-poisoning problems does not necessarily mean that they are an entirely new phenomena. In many cases, it simply means that they were not well identified previously. In the case of food-borne diseases, several new and improved methods for the detection of microorganisms and their toxins have recently uncovered problems that were formerly hidden from us. The picture we now have indicates that the problem of food-borne diseases is serious, widespread and growing in both size and complexity. Changes in our lifestyles seem to have aggravated the problem.[19] Demand is growing for foods that are more natural or less processed, a far greater number of meals are being consumed outside the home, and the market for imported exotic foods has skyrocketed. Fortunately, the technology and hygienic practices currently available can considerably reduce the incidence of food-borne diseases. Unfortunately, the public has limited awareness of the problem and expresses insufficient public pressure to implement these technological and hygienic practices.

The average consumer's knowledge about food-borne diseases is very limited. Despite their significant implications on the general health of people the world over, food-borne diseases have never been an issue of major public concern in the past. This is no longer the case. The United States Food and Drug Administration has ranked food-borne diseases first in importance among all the food-related risks.[20]

THE RANKING OF FOOD-RELATED RISKS
1—Food-borne diseases 2—Malnutrition 3—Environmental contaminants 4—Naturally occurring toxicants 5—Pesticide residues 6—Food additives

Most public health and related agencies around the world generally agree upon this ranking. Consumers, on the other hand, traditionally place food additives and pesticide residues at the top of the list and food-borne diseases way down near the bottom. This totally opposing view between public health professionals and consumers is most likely due to the negative image that food additives and pesticides have with many consumer advocacy groups. However, as a consequence of the rash of highly publicized food-borne disease incidents, this perception is beginning to change. Research indicates that consumers are indeed showing a greater concern over microbiological hazards in foods. In fact, food-borne diseases are expected to be in the spotlight for years to come, particularly if little is done to control the major causes of outbreaks.

A more recent survey carried out in Europe provides additional insights on consumers' perceptions of health risks, particularly those related to food safety.[21] This survey was jointly commissioned by the European Food Safety Authority and the European Commission on Health and Consumer Protection. When consumers were asked about food risks, only 20 percent mentioned health. When they were further probed to cite specific problems or risks associated with food, no single issue emerged. Major food crises from the recent past such as that surrounding BSE (bovine spongiform encephalopathy) seem to have been forgotten. Among the problems cited by the 20 percent who did feel there were problems, food poisoning came to mind most often, followed by chemicals, pesticides, toxic substances and obesity.

Consumers tended to worry most about risks caused by external factors over which they had no control. At the top end of the worry scale (over 60 percent of respondents), there were concerns regarding pesticide residues, new viruses (such as avian flu), residues in meats, food hygiene (in restaurants or the food plant) and contamination of food by bacteria. Consumers were far less worried about risks associated with their own hygiene or practices.

Public opinion remains divided regarding food safety improvements over the last 10 years. The largest group (38 percent) of respondents felt that the situation has improved, while 29 percent said that nothing has changed and 28 percent were convinced that they were worse off than before. Strangely, more than 40 percent of people either ignore stories they hear in the media about a type of food being unsafe or worry about it and do nothing.

The undeniable fact is that most incidents of food-borne disease are totally avoidable both by the consumer as well as by the food provider. The majority of outbreaks occur in food-catering establishments, street kitchens and the home. Yet, a little understanding and appreciation of the subject would eliminate much of the grief, discomfort and misery for so many of us. We can no longer take so many stomachaches, bouts of nausea, cramps and diarrhea for granted. They result from wholly preventable diseases. Only a lack of definitive action allows them to continue plaguing us.

Some of the more infamous outbreaks of food poisoning have involved thousands of people and many deaths. The only recorded grounding of the famous Concorde supersonic transatlantic flight service was due to an incident of food poisoning. In 1996, more than 10,000 people were struck by a particularly virulent form of E. coli bacteria in Japan. A national outbreak of Salmonella enteritidis from ice cream was estimated to have affected almost a quarter of a million people in an area covering six midwestern states in the United States.[22, 23] Several other large outbreaks have occurred in Canada, the Netherlands, Sweden, France and other countries. In a famous incident in Scotland, a single can of corned beef resulted in the infection of more than 500 people. A meat slicer was first contaminated by the infected corned beef and then continued to be used for many other meats that were consumed, and thus the infection spread everywhere. Salmonella poisoning in chocolate affected over 200 people in Canada[24] and resulted in the ultimate demise of the company involved.

A reported outbreak of salmonella poisoning among the delegates of a medical conference demonstrates that all strata of society can be equally affected. Approximately 200 out of the 266 physicians who attended the gala conference buffet were seriously poisoned.[25] Infected along with the physicians were the numerous waiters, busboys and kitchen staff who all tasted the buffet food. In fact, the problem of salmonella in poultry is so widespread and has become so common that many hospitals have stopped bringing in raw chicken altogether for fear of cross contaminating the entire kitchen and food preparation area.[26]

The short-term impact of food-borne diseases on our overall well-being and its impact on the economy are both immense. When the longer-term complications (sequelae), such as Guillain-Barré syndrome (discussed later), are factored into this dilemma, the situation becomes even more critical. More recently, researchers have discovered that certain food-borne pathogenic microorganisms, such as Staphylococcus, Listeria and Clostridium perfringens, are capable of producing toxins that can trigger such massive immune responses that they have been menacingly classified as "superantigens."[27] These superantigens have been implicated in encephalomyelitis (brain and spinal chord inflammation), Crohn's disease and a variety of other autoimmune diseases.[28, 29] More often than not, however, the relationship between these medical conditions and food-borne microorganisms is never made. As a consequence, food-borne diseases are beginning to provide us with a frightening panorama of wide-spread health hazards previously hidden from sight.

Food-borne diseases cannot be considered as minor inconveniences. They are not. They are real diseases, and they are hazardous. People must regard them with the attention and seriousness they deserve. In the majority of instances, their symptoms do not last too long. However, in many cases, they can result in permanent crippling effects and even death as a result of long-term complications. Although the symptoms of vomiting and diarrhea are embarrassing and occasionally made the subject of humor, food-borne diseases and their effects are definitely not a joke.

ANTIBIOTIC RESISTANCE

Throughout our history, disease organisms have been responsible for more deaths, suffering and human misery than all the wars and natural disasters combined. Despite our remarkable advances in the arts, sciences and engineering, lessening the effects of these invisible enemies was not within our power. On a number of occasions in the past, lethal forces that were unseen, unheard and untouched completely decimated the populations of cities, countries and even continents. Plagues came and went as if by magic. Little wonder that the only recourse was to consult priests and magicians who could summon mystical powers that might match this evil magic with an even greater magic. Nothing really worked.

With Pasteur's illuminating discoveries about the nature of spoilage and disease, a practical understanding of microbes began to develop. Together with this knowledge came an awareness that these organisms were centrally involved in many critical diseases of humankind. Continued research and observation slowly began to reveal that several different means could control microbes. Pasteur discovered that in some cases, certain bacteria could not exist in the presence of others. Other researchers found that some bacteria produced metabolic end products toxic to other bacteria, but they did not fully understand the significance of all this. In 1928, Sir Alexander Fleming discovered penicillin totally by accident. He found that the by-products of the green penicillium mold (growing on some old bread) were capable of arresting the growth of many well-known pathogenic bacteria. However, he performed no clinical trials with this material on animals or human subjects, and further progress in this area was regrettably delayed.

The first time an antibiotic was used to treat human diseases was in 1939 when microbiologist René Dubos used a form of gramicidin isolated from the cultivation of soil bacteria. During the war-torn winter of 1940, penicillin was first used on humans by the British scientists Sir Howard Florey and Ernst Chain. The practical significance of this new field took a giant leap forward when Selman Waksman of Rutgers University discovered and started to produce streptomycin in 1944. The fledgling science of antibiotics was firmly established along with the rudimentary knowledge and technology required to produce them on a large scale.

For the first time in our history, physicians had a simple means with which to fight the invisible enemy that had afflicted humanity since the dawn of time. We no longer had to accept the horrendous death rates so commonplace during periods of hospitalization. Infant mortality rates began to plummet as hospital infections became a phenomenon of the past. Ear infections became easily treatable and no longer required eardrum lancing to drain the inevitable buildup of fluids and pus. Wound infections, tonsillitis, scarlet fever, cholera, tetanus, gonorrhea and all the other infectious diseases that had previously struck fear and anxiety into the hearts of everyone became routinely managed with an air of casual informality. Even dentists began using antibiotics to reduce pretreatment and posttreatment pain and infection. Within a single decade, antibiotics became the most potent weapon in the physician's entire arsenal. Antibiotics were considered nothing less than the greatest single advance in the entire history of medicine.

Unfortunately, this situation did not last for a very long time. As often happens with new technologies, mismanagement and abuse soon began to compromise the impact and effectiveness of one of civilization's most valuable inventions. Within a short period of time, pathogenic organisms resistant to antibiotics began to appear. That the inappropriate application of antibiotics was a prime factor responsible for the evolution of these difficult organisms quickly became clear. Without a doubt, the improper use of antibiotics, which resulted in the development of this resistance, was initially due to a lack of knowledge about microbial evolution and adaptability. In fact, some time elapsed before physicians fully appreciated the significance of antibiotic resistance. The abuse that occurred largely resulted from innocence and inexperience. However, much of the same abuse continues today, and the excuse of naïveté can no longer apply.

Antibiotic resistance in bacteria has evolved through a number of different mechanisms. One major way in which bacteria resist antibiotics is simply by destroying them. Resistant bacteria can produce enzymes capable of specifically digesting, and thus rendering useless, the most sophisticated antibiotics. Another defense mechanism that the microbes have come up with is to alter their own cell wall properties in order to prevent the entry of antibiotics. Once locked out of the microbial cell, an antibiotic is unable to exert any useful therapeutic effects. Bacteria that do not have the ability to destroy antibiotics with specific enzymes or the ability to prevent antibiotics from entering the cells still have viable mechanisms with which to resist antibiotics. A third way for bacteria to avoid the effects of antibiotics is to modify the site in the cell that the antibiotic normally attacks. The antibiotic can still enter the cell, but once inside, it cannot find any familiar target to attack. While armed with these formidable defense mechanisms, more and more pathogenic bacteria are developing the capability of resisting the strongest weapon our scientists have come up with to combat them.

Bacteria can develop these various forms of resistance through random genetic mutation or through the exchange of genetic materials with other bacteria. This exchange of material can take place through the processes of transformation (the exchange of DNA among various bacteria's hereditary chromosomes), transduction (which employs viruses to interchange DNA between bacteria) or the exchange of nonchromosomal

DNA using cell components called "plasmids." Our recent knowledge about bacteria appears to indicate that plasmid transfer among bacteria commonly occurs. Yet another means of exchanging genetic material is through "transposons," which are specific sections of chromosomal DNA that can jump into plasmids or other chromosomes.

This ability to transfer the genetic material controlling antibiotic resistance to other bacteria freely, including those of different species, has extreme significance for our health. Most of us eat animal products. The digestive systems of the food animals we eat are veritable microbial production factories. Here, billions and billions of microorganisms live in intimate contact with each another. Bacteria necessary for digestion live side by side with organisms considered to be pathogens. Resistance developed in harmless organisms can be easily transferred to others that cause disease either in the animals or in the humans that consume them. Once a bacterium picks up the genetic material responsible for resistance, its chances for survival and reproduction improve tremendously.

By definition, resistance is developed by all those bacteria that have managed to survive a course of antibiotic treatment. Resistance may be very weak at first and continue to strengthen with increasing exposure to greater concentrations of antibiotics. Carelessness or ignorance in selecting proper dosages or courses of treatment may easily contribute to the sort of sublethal exposures of antibiotics that would foster the development of resistance. During the early days of their use, physicians commonly stopped giving antibiotics before ensuring that all the infective organisms were killed. Many patients themselves stopped taking antibiotics before the course of treatment was completed simply because they felt better and saw no need to continue.

Antibiotics are an extremely convenient medicine for physicians to administer, and it is not at all surprising that most are overprescribed. A North American survey revealed that antibiotic treatment was irrationally administered as often as it was rationally administered.[30] Another survey indicated that almost 60 percent of physicians incorrectly used antibiotics in the treatment of common colds.[31] Other studies have shown that the most frequent therapeutic abuse in hospitals is the unnecessary prescription of antibiotics.[32] At the slightest signs of a suspected infection, whether it be respiratory, urinary or otherwise, antibiotics are administered. Upon closer scrutiny, antibiotic treatments were unjustified almost half the time. Antibiotics are also administered as a preventative measure to reduce the risk of patients undergoing some type of surgical or analytic procedure. While largely legitimate, this application is carried out in some circumstances where it may not be necessary.

While the excessive or irrational use of antibiotics cannot be condoned, it has been justified on the basis of human cost/benefit factors. The argument is put forth that the medical benefits of antibiotics are so great that any negative effects of misuse are insignificant in comparison. When actually tallied, the tangible cost of antibiotic resistance is minuscule in comparison with the economic benefits of widespread antibiotic use.[33] While defensible, this argument does not foresee a time when antibiotic technology will no longer be able to treat any pathogens. It is also a difficult argument to put forth to the many victims who have suffered or died of antibiotic-resistant pathogens.

As one can guess from the way in which it evolves, antibiotic resistance is a natural consequence of all antibiotic applications. While abuse cannot be tolerated, no meaningful argument exists against the therapeutic use of antibiotics in medicine. However, only half of all the antibiotics produced are used for this purpose. The other half of all the antibiotics manufactured worldwide are destined for use in the food animals and plants we eat. These antibiotics are not used to cure the poor animals from life-threatening diseases, they are used to make them grow faster at a lower cost. The most potent weapon in the physicians' war against disease, the discovery that held the potential to free us from the diseases that plagued us for centuries, the technology that was arguably the greatest advance in the history of medicine can also be used to make meat cheap.

For more than 40 years, subtherapeutic doses of wide-spectrum antibiotics have been a standard component of animal feeds. After researchers first discovered that antibiotics promote growth in animals in a very cost-effective manner, everybody in the animal-rearing business got on the bandwagon and began using them. Currently, more than an estimated 25 million pounds of antibiotics are used for this purpose in the United States alone. These antibiotics are no different from the ones that a physician uses, except that they are much, much cheaper. They are also regarded differently from antibiotics destined for human use—they are simply a component of feed. Instead of being prescribed by a physician, a farmhand often doles them out.

If one were to sit back and dream up a set of conditions ideal for the development of antibiotic resistance in bacteria, of what would they consist? First of all, the doses applied should be low enough to ensure that some bacteria (those that develop resistance) would survive. The destruction of antibiotic-sensitive bacteria opens the way for antibiotic-resistant bacteria to flourish with relatively little competition. As it happens, the subtherapeutic doses of broad-spectrum antibiotics used in animal feeds fit this bill perfectly.

What about the spread of antibiotic resistance among bacteria? Ideally, you would have a setting where millions upon millions of bacteria live in intimate contact with one another to ensure that transformation, transduction and plasmid or transposon transfers can take place. What is a better environment than the digestive systems of chickens, pigs, sheep or cows? In one animal's gut you can find all forms of microbes, from those useful for digestion to harmless microbes that live symbiotically with the host (called commensals) to accidental visitors to the most deadly of pathogens. They all live, eat and reproduce in this microenvironment. The close proximity of these organisms to one another allows the exchange of resistance and virulence factors to occur within the same plasmid—in fact, it makes this exchange easy.[34]

If we now review these particular conditions, what do we have?

- Inexpensive antibiotics are perceived as growth-promoting feed additives rather than as therapeutic medicines.
- Nonmedical personnel (farm workers) regularly give subtherapeutic dosages.
- Animal recipients are routinely exposed to high levels of a wide range of barnyard bacteria.
- Antibiotic-resistant bacteria remain in intimate contact with millions of other bacteria, including human pathogens.

Voila! What we have is the recipe for an "antibiotic-resistance factory." This factory not only encourages the evolution of antibiotic resistance but effectively transfers the resistance to many other bacteria. In case any doubt remains about the possibilities of all this occurring, examples abound in all the authoritative medical literature. Reports detail the spread of antibiotic-resistant bacteria (and their transferable plasmids) from chicken to chicken and from chicken to human.[35] Many reports describe the widespread movement of pathogenic, antibiotic-resistant bacteria from other farm animals to humans[36–39] and from bacteria to bacteria.[40] Once antibiotic-resistant organisms are firmly established, the animals act as true reservoirs, shedding these bacteria in feces and quickly infecting other animals and humans.[41]

In addition to being used as an ingredient in animal feeds, antibiotics are also applied as aerosol sprays to fruit trees to prevent bacterial infections.[42] By their very nature, aerosols are dispersed in air and result in a highly variable strength dosage that depends upon the area sprayed and the distance traveled. It is another example of an antibiotic application that has not considered the overall repercussions for the consumer even if it does make fruit look nicer and cost a little less.

If we factor in the consequences of antibiotic resistance, then the use of antibiotics as an agricultural agent must take on an additional dimension—the increased risk to human health from resistant organisms and the added cost to the health care system. Although little doubt remains that antibiotic resistance is a natural consequence of antibiotic use in general, the poorly controlled use of antibiotics in feeds for food animals and sprays for fruit trees greatly accelerates this process and the attendant risks. Antibiotics are the greatest advance we have ever seen in the history of treating human disease—which is why they were invented. Somewhat ironically, the cost of antibiotics for a nonessential, nonmedical luxury in animal feeds or on fruit trees is much lower than the cost of antibiotics for essential human therapeutic uses. Perhaps we would not be facing the fearful dilemma of antibiotic resistance if the pricing situation were reversed.

EDIBLE VACCINES

While the situation may look bleak with antibiotics, considerable new developments have occurred in the area of vaccines. Perhaps the most interesting concerning food-borne diseases is the work about edible vaccines. These developments have taken excellent advantage of the new genetic engineering techniques that have accompanied the biotechnology revolution. Since the human body is capable of forming an immune response to the surface proteins of bacteria and viruses, the idea was simply to engineer plants genetically so they would produce and contain some of the surface proteins of these pathogens. In this way, merely eating the plant would produce an immune response to the protein without being subjected to infection from the organisms themselves.

These developments are particularly important for food-borne diseases. Edible vaccines have the particular ability to induce what is referred to as mucosal immunity—the production of antibodies in the saliva and the other secretions that coat the surfaces of the respiratory, gastrointestinal and urinary tracts. These secretions are the first level of defense the body mounts against organisms invading through open surfaces. This, of course, is the route of entry for all food-borne pathogens.

Thus far, proteins from bacteria that cause tooth decay and diarrhea as well as from the viruses that cause hepatitis have been produced in various plants such as bananas, tomatoes, alfalfa and potatoes. Technical developments in this area have been very positive, and a number of patents have already been issued. Clinical trials to determine the effectiveness of edible vaccines are under way. One of the newer developments is a genetically engineered potato that can deliver an edible vaccine that works against the food-borne Norwalk virus, which is notorious for causing diarrhea.[43] Once eaten by volunteers, the potatoes produce a significant number of antibodies that prevent the virus from attaching to the cells that line the intestine, completely preventing all disease symptoms. The Norwalk virus infects more than 23 million people in the United States every year causing diarrhea, nausea and stomach cramps, according to the Centers for Disease Control and Prevention.

In another development, scientists from Novosibirsk in Russia have created an edible vaccine that incorporates the HIV antigen into tomatoes.[44] While they have not fully developed a vaccine yet, they have managed to incorporate the critical gene into tomato plants and have demonstrated that the protein required for the vaccine is in both the leaves and the tomato itself.

These developments hold great promise for all consumers, particularly those in developing countries. On an annual basis, diarrheal diseases in developing countries result in approximately 10 million deaths. About one-third of these fatalities occur in children under the age of five years. The ability of bananas or some other food product to simulate an effective immune response against diarrheal diseases would indeed be a triumph of science. However, these developments will also benefit a great many people in advanced countries. While, on the one hand, we must employ technologies that destroy offending pathogens in our food supply, we must, at the same time, ensure that our bodies continue to maintain a high level of immune resistance to as many pathogens as possible. Edible vaccines may be just one of the technologies to meet this latter challenge.

EMERGING INFECTIOUS DISEASES

Little doubt exists that the greatest achievement in recent medical history has been the dramatic reduction in mortality from infectious diseases. However, despite all the major developments in medical science during the past century, infectious diseases continue to be the primary cause of death worldwide. To add to this crushing public health burden, several new or emerging infectious diseases have begun to appear that harbor the threat of significantly increased mortality. ("Emerging infectious diseases" are simply defined as those infectious diseases that have greatly proliferated during the last 20 years and threaten to increase in severity in the future.)

The term "emerging" almost conveys a sense of approaching doom and results from two unrelated circumstances. The first is our dismay that the world of nature is not as easy to conquer as we had originally thought. Not long ago, while flushed with the global victory over small-pox, the United Nations was predicting a virtual end to infectious diseases. The successes we experienced in treating and controlling major infectious diseases left most of us with the impression that the threat from microbial pathogens had all but disappeared. Now that this does not appear to be the case, many people have become alarmed.

The second circumstance arises from our discovery of new super-virulent organisms—typified by the HIV and Ebola viruses. These deadly microorganisms have proven to be very difficult to control and result in horrifying symptoms. The apocalyptic aspect of these supervirulent organisms has naturally attracted the popular press, who have to do nothing more than accurate reporting to come up with stories of hair-raising dimensions. An excellent book about this subject, *The Coming Plague* by Laurie Garrett, was published in 1994,[45] and the medical journal *Emerging Infectious Diseases*, which was launched in 1995, is devoted exclusively to this issue.[46] The World Health Organization has stated that these diseases represent a global threat that will require nothing less than a fully integrated global response if we are to cope with them.[47]

New emerging infectious diseases include AIDS, cholera (reemerging), hemorrhagic fevers, Hantavirus, Rift Valley fever, Lassa fever, Ebola, Lyme disease, Legionnaires' disease and several food-borne diseases. The reasons behind the emergence of new infectious diseases are multifold. They include sociological changes, changes in human behavior, the globalization of our food supply, environmental changes and the continuing evolution of microorganisms themselves. Localized conflicts, civil war and poverty precipitate mass emigration with the desperate refugees serving as unwitting vectors of contagious diseases. Changes in human behavior related to sexual practices and the widespread use of drugs have equally served to spread infectious diseases internationally. The sweeping destruction of fragile ecosystems has released organisms that were hitherto confined to very limited environments.

The recent globalization of our food supply also contributes to the same patterns of emerging disease proliferation. The contemporary concept of globalization is quite different from what we used to call internationalization. Internationalization normally refers to everyone looking after their own interests but cooperating internationally on particular issues to the best extent possible. Treaties about fishing limits or trading endangered species or agreements about the limitation of ozone-depleting substances are typical examples of internationalization. On the contrary, globalization removes national control of laws, policies and markets in order to bring together all people for the collective good or the common wealth. Free trade and the removal of restrictions from the movement of goods and people is symptomatic of globalization. The dismantling of national barriers results in greater efficiencies in economic growth. Because the bureaucratic mechanisms of internationalization appear so much less effective than globalization, the former is "out" and the latter is "in."

By moving together with free trade goods and services, infectious diseases also recognize no national boundaries and clearly conform to the typical globalization pattern. Every form of microorganism can cross international borders with total impunity. They journey with finished food products, raw agricultural commodities, hidden insects, visiting tourists and economic immigrants. When you walk across the border between Zambia and Zimbabwe at Victoria Falls, you remove your shoes and step through a shallow, soapy solution of murky, depleted disinfectant. This supposedly prevents the spread of cattle disease between the two countries. Imagining a more pathetic quarantine effort is hard, but at least officials are making an effort. Most other countries do not even have that. In fact, when one considers that organisms travel with the tiniest particles of dust carried in the wind and are easily swept along international waterways, one realizes that even the most rigorous quarantine procedures cannot prevent the movement of pathogens between countries.

Invisible infectious organisms inevitably accompany the free movement of goods and people. The popular demand for foreign imported products has increased our exposure to both people and goods from around the world. On the shelves of modern supermarkets one can find beef, pork and lamb from Latin America, Australia and Europe. Tropical fruits are available from Asia, Africa, Latin America and the Caribbean. You can find shrimp and exotic seafood imported from Thailand, Cambodia, Indonesia, China and Malaysia, as well as exotic delicacies from a host of other countries. These products all cross international borders with relative ease, and so do the microorganisms they can harbor.

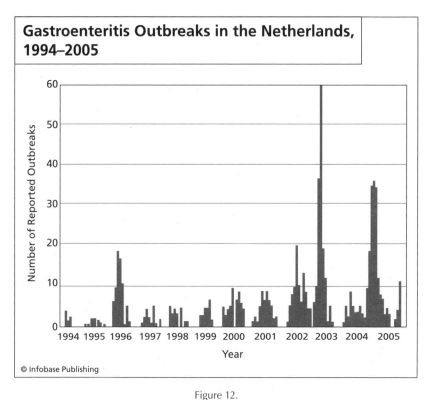

Figure 12.

Siebenga, J. J., Vennema, H., Duizer, E., Koopmans, M. P. G., "Gastroenteritis caused by norovirus GGII.4, the Netherlands, 1994–2005," Emerg. Infect. Dis. Available online. URL: http://www.cdc.gov/ncidod/EID/13/1/144.htm. Accessed January 29, 2008.

Along with the microorganisms come their particular set of virulence and antibiotic-resistance characteristics, often with devastating results. Ordinarily, pathogenic organisms come to some type of ecological balance with other forms of life in their native environment. After years of continuous exposure, people and animals will develop a form of limited immunity or adjust their behavioral practices (food, local medicine and so on) to cope with indigenous pathogens. However, when these organisms are transferred to a new environment, they will often demonstrate much greater virulence simply because natural immunity or appropriate social or medical management practices have not been established. Even though we may feel that globalization can be beneficial for international economic development, from the standpoint of public health it can be very costly.

An excellent example of this is the increase in gastroenteritis resulting from food-borne Norwalk viruses, which cause large outbreaks of gastroenteritis in environments where there is close human contact, such as hospitals, cruise ships, institutions and military bases. In recent years,

Norwalk viruses have increasingly been recognized as common causes of gastroenteritis.

From December 1993 to December 2005, a total of 1,032 gastroenteritis outbreaks were reported to the National Institute for Public Health and the Environment in the Netherlands (see figure 12).

This disturbing trend has been seen in many other countries, including the United States. From September 2 to 12, 2005, approximately 6,500 of the estimated 24,000 Hurricane Katrina evacuees visited Houston's Reliant Park medical clinic, and 18 percent reported suffering from acute gastroenteritis. A total of 44 percent of those reporting acute gastroenteritis symptoms had diarrhea alone, 29 percent reported vomiting and 27 percent said they had both diarrhea and vomiting. Medical personnel, police officers and volunteers who were in direct contact with patients also began reporting acute gastroenteritis symptoms, suggesting spread by person-to-person contact.

In the January 2005 issue of *Emerging Infectious Diseases*, CDC researchers described an investigation of Norwalk virus–caused gastroenteritis

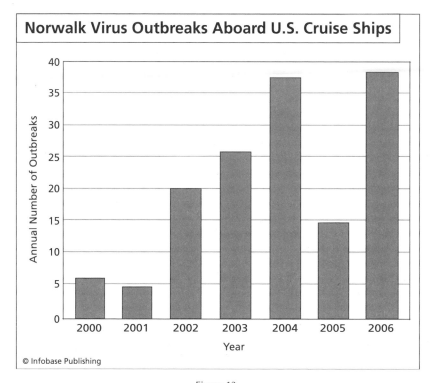

Figure 13.
Isakbaeva, E. T., Widdowson, M. A., Beard, R. S., Bulens, S. N., Mullins, J., Monroe, S. S., et al. "Norovirus transmission on cruise ship." Emerg. Infect. Dis. Available online. URL: http://www.cdc.gov/ncidod/EID/vol11no01/04-0434.htm. Accessed January 29, 2008.

outbreaks aboard a cruise ship affecting six consecutive cruises, despite intensive efforts to get rid of the virus, including a full one-week sanitization of the ship (see figure 13). A quick look at the increasing number of outbreaks is not encouraging for the future.

The bitter irony is that although these diseases spread through the unrestricted globalization process, the only means we have to deal with them is through cumbersome and slow-moving international laws and conventions. All of these depend upon the exercise of sovereign, national rights. The net result is the spread of infectious diseases by modern, efficient globalization mechanisms and a defensive reaction based on antiquated, inefficient international mechanisms. It is a one-way fight! This creates nothing less than a transnational challenge.[48]

As far as food-borne diseases are concerned, new methods of processing, changes in consumption patterns, poor practices in the food production system and globalization of the food supply have all contributed to a steady increase in serious outbreaks. From the time researchers first recognized it in 1982, the involvement of *E. coli* O157:H7 in severe food-borne disease outbreaks has increased steadily, and there are no signs of it abating. A 1996 outbreak that occurred in the technologically advanced country of Japan made over 10,000 people very sick and caused the deaths of at least ten individuals. The number of people with long-term sequelae has yet to be determined but will no doubt be very high.[49]

This mixture of increasing emergence of new, infective diseases and the rapidly deteriorating arsenal of effective weapons with which to fight them is a lethal combination. Is it time for the whole idea of modern food production to be reconsidered? If the cost of losing the most valuable tool in the fight against pathogens is factored into the price of animal feed, then we may find that the meat produced with the help of antibiotics is not cheap at all. If we are going to open up the gates to the globalization of goods and services, then we must also develop the public health mechanisms to go along with this move. Public health, too, must be globalized, as called for by the World Health Organization. The health problems of Calcutta have become the public health problems of Zurich or Philadelphia or Seattle. We have literally entered the era of the *global village*. The old precept, "No man is an island," was never more apt.

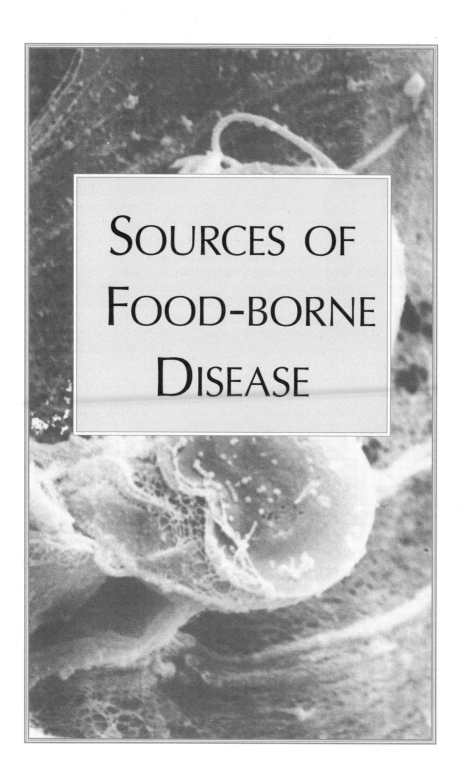

SOURCES OF
FOOD-BORNE
DISEASE

FOOD SOURCES OF DISEASE

If you're going to America, bring your own food.

Fran Lebowitz (b. 1951), *Fran Lebowitz's Travel Hints* (1981)*

The purpose of this part is to describe the various foods we normally eat and their potential to be hidden reservoirs of disease organisms. Some people may find this information shocking, while others might even find it distasteful. However, a basic understanding of our foods and the way that they are produced provides the first step in protecting ourselves against the possible hazards they pose.

Before entering into the specific details of certain types of products, we need to know some elementary characteristics common to most of the foods we consume. The first is that almost all basic food materials originate from an open or exposed environment. (The only exceptions are the fruits and vegetables cultivated in a controlled, hothouse environment. Even those are often exposed to external substances.) Grains, legumes, fruits, vegetables, meat and dairy animals, poultry, fish and seafood are all produced and harvested in a fully exposed environment or in production complexes generally open to the ambient surroundings. This, of course, means that they are exposed to all the organisms, harmful and otherwise, that exist in the environment.

The environment around us contains a multitude of organisms that have the potential, under the right conditions, to cause us harm. The soil, the water and even the air we breathe contain millions of these organisms. The old expression, "Ashes to ashes, dust to dust," provides an excellent insight into what this is all about. Understandably, dust is something that few people think about except as a nuisance that constantly has to be cleaned up. In fact, the air in a modern industrial city may contain as many as 50 million particles of dust per cubic inch. Dust itself is little more than the decomposition of mineral and organic matter in the environment, a good deal of which we produce on a routine daily basis. For example, fecal matter contains a very large number of microorganisms. When animals evacuate their feces, they produce an unsightly mess. However, within a few days, other organisms efficiently break down the feces and disperse it into the environment. Where does it go? Some of the material gets mixed into the soil, some gets washed into waterways and much of it ends up as components of windblown dust. All of it serves as a source of harmful bacteria and spores. Therefore, unless all our food is produced under sterile or near-sterile conditions, the natural environment can easily contaminate the food.

When we dump untreated sewage into the waterways, it goes away, but it does not simply disappear. It comes right back to us by infecting the fish and seafood we consume on a daily basis. The environment is therefore the starting point where food materials get their primary exposure to harmful organisms. Another major factor in the contamination of our foods is the manner in which they are produced. In the case of fruits and vegetables, irrigating crops with water containing pathogenic organisms is a common method of contamination. This occurs frequently because the water used in farming is not generally treated and its quality is not controlled as strictly as it should be. Another more recent problem results from the modern practice of organic farming. Manure is a useful fertilizer in organic farming. However, occasionally, organic farmers use material that has not been sterilized or treated to kill all the potential pathogens it contains. This results in highly contaminated fruits and vegetables, such as carrots, melons or lettuce, that are not normally considered to be reservoirs of human pathogens. People have died from consuming these products.

Mass production of foods is another important reason for the spread of disease organisms. This is not difficult to understand because the close proximity of animals to one another makes the rapid spread of contagious organisms much easier. Commonly shared water and food troughs and also the incomplete disposal of fecal matter serve to spread disease. Because many animals do not digest their food completely, fecal matter and processing by-products still contain a significant amount of nutrient materials. In order to lower the cost of feeding animals and poultry, a practice in some industries involves feeding this fecal matter and by-products to poultry and animals as a fixed proportion of the total feed ration. If these compounds are not fully sterilized or treated properly, our food animals consume the viable pathogens, and the cycle of reinfection starts all over again. Countless examples of this exist. The most dramatic has been the BSE disaster that made alarming headlines in Britain and the rest of the world.

There is also a link between climate and food-borne diseases. Support for this link comes from the changing patterns of food-borne and diarrheal illnesses during the El Niño climate warmings. In addition, weather events affect coastal water quality, which in turn can lead to subsequent seafood contamination. In particular, harmful algal blooms (HABs) are starting to come under greater scrutiny, since they have the potential to significantly affect the health of fish, mollusks, shrimp, lobsters, sea mammals and humans. A much better knowledge and understanding of the interaction between these ecosystems and our overall health are necessary. Studies have shown that the cumulative effect of multiple climatic stresses acting over time can undermine the stability of complex food webs. The statistical association with short-term temperature changes also suggests that food-borne diseases may be affected by long-term climate changes.[50]

Another source of contamination is product handling. A significant amount of food poisoning results from careless handling of products from the original producer through to the processor, retailer, restaurant and in the consumer's home as well. So many opportunities exist for contamination that it is surprising that more outbreaks do not occur. Because people consume more and more meals outside the home, handling in restaurants and food service establishments will be of particular concern in the future.

Thus, our basic foods can become exposed to harmful organisms in a great many ways. With the exception of controlled mass agricultural production in confined areas, this situation is not particularly new. Foods have always been subject to all forms of microbial contamination, and our forebears have always paid the price for eating them. The significant difference is that we now have a much better idea of what is going on and, as a result, we should be in a better position to do something about it. Unfortunately, history reveals that we do not always act upon the information we have.

The first line of defense against food contamination has traditionally been government control, and we employ an army of inspectors to ensure the safety of our food supply. Unfortunately, government scrutiny has some practical limitations. Inspectors cannot monitor every last procedure carried out in a plant, and many products simply escape their surveillance. Determining if a product contains harmful organisms takes a number of days. If a freshly harvested product has a limited shelf life before it spoils, then that analysis cannot practically prevent a contaminated product from reaching the consumer. More recently, this system has been put aside in favor of a whole new set of protocols that places the burden of control upon the food manufacturer. The system, called the hazard analysis of critical control points (HACCP) is universally regarded as a major step forward in rational food control. It is the cornerstone of future food safety initiatives and will be described in more detail later.

Another problem of food contamination is a legislative one. Because pathogenic organisms commonly occur in nature regardless of their origin, they are not typically considered to be contaminants under United States law, although they are in several other countries. This legal determination does not seem to have the consumer in mind. In all transactions between the consumer and the vendor of the food in question, the consumer naturally believes that the food is wholesome and does not pose a risk to health. If that were not the case, then all foods known to be widely contaminated with pathogens, such as poultry, should carry health warnings like those found on cigarettes.

Most of us assume that farmers and processing companies are wary of insects in vegetables and take all the proper precautionary measures to ensure that their products are free of them. Unfortunately, the products available to us reflect another reality. The FDA tolerance levels for insect infestation in produce go way beyond rigorous kosher standards. For example, the U.S. FDA Food Defect Action Levels[51] allow averages of up to 60 insects per 100 grams (3.5 oz.) in frozen broccoli and up to 50 insects per 100 grams of frozen spinach.

The following provides an idea of what these action levels are in selected produce:

FOOD DEFECT ACTION LEVELS		
PRODUCT	DEFECT	ACTION LEVEL
asparagus, canned or frozen	insects	asparagus contains an average of 40 or more thrips per 100 grams (3.5 oz.)
ground paprika	rodent filth	average of more than 11 rodent hairs per 25 grams (1 oz.)
mushrooms, canned and dried	insects	average of 20 or more maggots of any size per 100 grams of drained mushrooms and proportionate liquid or 15 grams (0.5 oz.) of dried mushrooms
raisins, golden	insects and insect eggs	10 or more whole or equivalent insects and 35 drosophila (fruit fly) eggs per 226 grams (8 oz.)
sauerkraut	insects	average of more than 50 thrips per 100 grams
thyme, ground	insect filth	average of 925 or more insect fragments per 10 grams (0.3 oz.)
tomato paste, pizza and other sauces	drosophila fly	average of 30 or more fly eggs per 100 grams
wheat flour	insect filth	average of 75 or more insect fragments per 50 grams (1.7 oz.)

In all likelihood, these levels of contaminants cause less harm than the pesticides required to eliminate them. Nevertheless, they can increase our risk of exposure to other pathogens.

The argument is made that proper handling and cooking will remove the problem by destroying the pathogens. Presumably, you could smoke cigarettes free of risk if you had a super filter or if you did not inhale, but the risk warnings would still apply. If the safety and wholesomeness of a product depend entirely upon the manner in which the consumer utilizes it, then prudence dictates that the supplier should be obliged to supply the consumer with all the relevant information on that product such as, "The surgeon general warns that this product has a strong likelihood of containing pathogenic organisms and must be handled very carefully and cooked to a minimal internal temperature of 165°F." Unfortunately, this does not currently occur. Labeling provides the consumer with little information regarding the microbial risks in foods. We can only hope that this will change.

All God's creatures have a certain degree of natural resistance to most disease organisms. If an animal or plant does not exhibit obvious outward signs of illness, assuming that it is healthy is not unreasonable. Hazards arise when organisms highly pathogenic to humans do not present the same effects on the plants or animals we consume as foods. As an example, many cattle demonstrate no obvious ill effects from *E. coli* O157:H7, an organism extremely dangerous to humans. Certain salmonella bacteria are considered commensal or normal to poultry but are hazardous pathogens to people. These microorganisms are food contaminants as far as consumers are concerned; considering them as anything else is absurd. The entire food system has the responsibility of ensuring that contaminants are eliminated from products prior to reaching the consumer. If that is not possible, then the consumer should be informed accordingly.

THE 20 MOST COMMON CAUSES OF FOOD-BORNE ILLNESS IN THE KITCHEN

Regardless of the source or type of food involved, the manner in which it is used or abused will have a critical bearing on its safety for the consumer. Thus, foods that may be perfectly safe to start with can ultimately end up being a genuine health hazard simply because of poor handling or consumption practices. Serious violations of basic sanitary disciplines or imprudent consumption habits are routine among most consumers. How many of us have consumed eggs that were not completely cooked, Caesar salad made with dressing containing raw eggs, or rare meat, rare hamburgers or raw oysters? How many consumers forget to scrub and sanitize their cutting boards after cutting raw meat or poultry on it?

In 2002, the Australian Food Safety Information Council (FSIC) released the results of a survey on hand washing.[52] Carried out by Newspoll, the survey tested peoples' knowledge of effective hand-washing techniques before preparing food. While the survey of 1,250 respondents showed that the majority knew to wash their hands using soap and water and to dry thoroughly, a significant minority thought it was safe to prepare food simply after rinsing their hands without using soap. The study observed the actual behavior of 200 men and women in the public toilets at a suburban shopping center. The results showed that only 20 percent of females and 7 percent of males were observed using the correct procedures to wash their hands. In fact, 8 percent of females and 29 percent of males failed to wash their hands at all after going to the toilet.

Another survey was carried out of consumers from more than 100 households located in 81 cities across the United States and Canada.[53, 54] The object of this survey was to determine the sort of handling practices consumers routinely employ when preparing a range of foods at home. The survey design was somewhat biased toward more educated consumers because 73 percent of the participants had a college degree and only 2 percent had not completed high school. The researchers generally felt that the selected households probably performed better than a fully random sampling would have.

Consumers were carefully observed during the preparation and serving of meals, the cleaning process and the manner with which they managed leftovers. The wide range of practices observed included personal sanitation, product storage and handling, temperature taking, routine kitchen maintenance and others. In other words, the researchers watched all the actions that one normally manages in the kitchen on a daily basis.

CRITICAL VIOLATIONS

VIOLATION	DESCRIPTION	FREQUENCY (% OF HOUSEHOLDS)
Cross contamination	The unintentional transfer of contaminants and pathogenic microorganisms from one food to another. This is chiefly due to overlooked handwashing. Other reasons are (a) storing raw materials directly over foods ready to be consumed; (b) putting utensils used for tasting back into the food being prepared; (c) using a dirty sink; (d) putting washed produce back into the original soiled container; (e) using unclean utensils to prepare foods; (f) not decontaminating cutting boards between uses; (g) using unclean scissors to open food bags; and (h) negligence in washing fresh produce.	> 75%
Neglected hand washing	Hands not washed (a) before beginning to prepare foods; (b) after touching phone, hair, body or other people; (c) after handling refuse or dirty dishes; and (d) after going to the toilet.	> 55%
Improper cooling of leftovers	Lack of rapid cooling of foods, i.e., from 140°F (60°C) to 70°F (21°C) in two hours and down to 40°F (4°C) in an additional four hours.	30%–50%
Improper labeling and storage of kitchen chemicals	Improper management of household chemicals, leading to contamination of food.	> 25%
Incomplete cooking of foods	Not cooking foods to a minimum internal temperature of 170°F (76°C).	> 20%
Improper refrigeration temperature	Refrigerator temperature too high, i.e., above 45°F (7°C).	> 20%
Improper holding of cooked foods	Not maintaining leftovers at a temperature to prevent growth of bacteria, i.e., more than 140°F (60°C) or less than 40°F (4°C).	> 10%
Neglecting appropriate use of gloves	Failure to wear gloves if the handler has open sores or bandages on hands.	> 5%
Use of severely damaged cans	Using products where the cans show obvious signs of swelling, rust, leakage and so on.	> 5%
Preparing foods while ill	Preparing foods during periods of illness, such as flu, leading to food contamination.	3%

MAJOR VIOLATIONS		
VIOLATION	DESCRIPTION	FREQUENCY (% OF HOUSEHOLDS)
Misuse of cloths/towels/sponges	Same cloths used for a variety of functions, i.e., drying dishes, drying hands, wiping counters, and so on, leading to cross contamination.	> 90%
Neglect of thermometer	Failure to measure food temperature, leading to spoilage.	> 90%
Products used past labeled "use by" date	Use of products no longer in optimal condition.	89%
Smoking, eating or chewing gum while handling food	Practices that cause hand-to-mouth contact and increase the possibility of food contamination by handler.	> 70%
Improper refrigerator temperature	Refrigerator temperature too high, i.e., above 45°F (7°C).	> 60%
Products stored uncovered	Ingredients in refrigerator or pantry exposed to contamination.	> 40%
Improper thawing practice	Frozen products not thawed (a) in a refrigerator; (b) in clean cold water within two hours; (c) as part of the overall cooking process; or (d) in a microwave (to be followed immediately by cooking).	> 30%
Evidence of infestation	Pests such as insects or rodents causing food contamination.	> 25%
Unavailability of hand towels	No towels available to prevent handler from drying hands on apron or clothes.	8%
Improper holding of cooked foods	Not maintaining leftovers at a temperature to prevent growth of bacteria, i.e., more than 140°F (60°C) or less than 40°F (4°C).	2%

The evaluations characterized the observed violations as either critical or major to the particular preparation process carried out. Critical violations were those that, by themselves, had the potential of causing food-borne illnesses or injuries. Major violations were those unlikely to cause problems independently but frequently associated as important contributing factors to food-borne disease incidents. Of course, many minor violations were observed but were not included in the report since they were very unlikely to have obvious negative consequences.

The yardstick used for comparison was the standard facility inspection program used in the food service industry. As with commercial institutions, households were permitted no critical violations at all and a maximum of four major violations in order to be considered acceptable. While these standards may at first appear to be a little too stringent, in principle, they are not. Although the consequences of a poor rating in a commercial food service facility obviously have a much greater potential for causing widespread harm than in a single household, the methodology employed and the scores arrived at were fully justified if the objective is to measure consumers' food safety practices. After all, the goal of safe food preparation is just as valid in the home.

There is one underlying cause for the incidence of food-borne diseases in the home—serious lack of food safety and handling knowledge. Despite all the media coverage about food-borne illness, people still are generally unaware of the correct techniques required to prepare and store foods safely. (Perhaps some of the more popular cooking shows should spend more time on this important issue.) People are also indifferent to the potential presence of harmful microorganisms in the kitchen environment.

In addition to a lack of knowledge about food safety and handling techniques, some of the key misconceptions consumers have regarding food-borne diseases include:

- a belief that food-borne illnesses are not serious and cause only minor gastrointestinal disorders with little or no consequences
- a belief that food-borne illnesses occur very rarely and always to other people
- an understanding that risky food is always easily detectable by appearance or smell

Obviously, this general lack of knowledge is the first issue that has to be addressed if consumers are to start eating more safely.

POULTRY

The birds that fall under the definition of poultry normally consist of chickens, turkeys, ducks and geese but may also include Cornish hens, quails, pigeons, partridge, pheasant, grouse, guinea fowl and ostriches. Poultry meat consists of muscle tissue (leg, breast and thigh), attached skin and edible organs (liver and giblets). On average, the moisture level of the edible portion of poultry varies from 55 to 70 percent, depending upon the age and type of bird. Younger birds usually have higher moisture contents, which is why they are more tender. Unfortunately, this high level of moisture makes poultry an excellent substrate for a wide range of microorganisms. Several common pathogens are associated with poultry, as listed below. For the purpose of illustration, we will focus primarily upon salmonella in commercial market poultry. Wild game birds share many of the same problems of contamination and are naturally exposed to a much broader range of contaminating organisms.

PRIMARY PATHOGENS OF POULTRY

BACTERIAL—yes	✔ *Salmonella species*
☐ *Bacillus cereus*	☐ *Shigella species*
✔ ***Campylobacter jejuni***	✔ ***Staphylococcus aureus***
☐ *Clostridium botulinum*	☐ *Streptococcus species*
✔ ***Clostridium perfringens***	☐ *Vibrio species*
☐ Enterohemorrhagic *E. coli*	✔ ***Yersinia enterocolitica***
☐ Enteroinvasive *E. coli*	FUNGAL—no
✔ Enteropathogenic ***E. coli***	PARASITIC—no
☐ Enterotoxigenic *E. coli*	TOXIC SUBSTANCES—no
☐ *Helicobacter pylori*	VIRAL—looming threat of global pandemic
✔ ***Listeria monocytogenes***	

Note:
✔ *Large bold checkmarks indicate a very common occurrence in this food.*
✓ *Regular font checkmarks indicate occurrence, but not common.*
☐ *boxes indicate no occurrence.*

BIRD FLU

A special note must be made concerning the potential for a widespread avian (bird) flu pandemic. Avian influenza is an infection caused by the various avian influenza viruses that occur naturally among wild birds. These wild birds carry the viruses in their intestines, but seldom get sick from them. The problem is that avian influenza is very contagious and can make domesticated poultry, including chickens, ducks and turkeys, very ill, often killing them.

Avian influenza can infect domestic poultry with differing levels of virulence. Low-virulence strains usually cause only mild symptoms; however, the highly pathogenic forms can spread rapidly through a flock and result in a 100 percent mortality rate within two days.

Normally, bird flu viruses refer to avian influenza viruses found exclusively in birds. We now know that infections with these viruses can also occur in humans. The risk from avian influenza is generally low for most people because the viruses do not usually infect humans. However, confirmed cases of human infection from certain types of avian influenza infection have been reported. Researchers believe the deadly H5N1 form of bird flu has divided into two distinct strains, making it that much more difficult to develop the vaccines necessary to halt the spread of the disease. Some examples of recent outbreaks are as follows:

- Hong Kong 1997. An epidemic of avian influenza caused by the H5N1 strain occurred in Hong Kong's poultry population. A total of 18 people were also stricken with severe respiratory symptoms. One-third of them died. The cause was determined to be the same strain of H5N1 as was infecting the birds. Officials determined that close contact with infected poultry was the cause of human infection. This was the first instance in which evidence was found indicating that the virus had jumped directly from birds to humans. Hong Kong health officials immediately ordered the destruction of the country's flock. In excess of 1.5 million birds were killed in three days, eliminating all cases of direct bird-to-human transmission. Some health experts say this action may have averted a pandemic.
- Vietnam 2004. Eight cases of avian influenza were found in people, six of whom died. Officials ordered the killing of millions of birds to minimize the threat to people.
- Indonesia 2005. A father and two daughters died of H5N1, although none of them worked around poultry. The WHO says it cannot rule out the possibility of human-to-human transmission of avian flu in these cases.
- October 2005. H5N1 spreads to birds in Romania, Turkey and Greece.
- In November 2005. H5N1 strain comes to Canada. Major bird slaughters are ordered to minimize the risk to humans.
- Azerbaijan 2006. Investigations revealed that contact with H5N1–infected wild dead swans was the most likely source of infection in

several cases of avian flu in children. The children were involved in removing feathers from the birds.

However, the earlier killing of millions of birds did not eliminate the threat because by March 2006 almost 100 people in Vietnam, Cambodia, Thailand, China, Indonesia, Turkey and Iraq had succumbed to the disease. By the beginning of 2007, avian influenza showed up again as Indonesia reported additional human cases, while Japan confirmed the first outbreak of H5N1 in poultry in three years. There also appeared to be evidence that the virus was spreading to flocks in Vietnam and Thailand.

Symptoms of avian influenza in humans can range from typical flu-like symptoms such as fever, cough, sore throat and muscle aches to eye infections, pneumonia and severe respiratory diseases. Studies carried out in laboratories suggest that some of the prescription medicines approved in the United States for human influenza viruses will work against avian flu. However, the viruses can easily become resistant to these drugs. Because of this, experts from around the world are watching the H5N1 situation very closely and are preparing for the possibility of a worldwide flu pandemic.

OUTBREAK INCIDENTS WITH POULTRY

Salmonella at a Medical Convention[55]

At the mouths of the Taff and Ely Rivers on Bristol Channel lies the small city of Cardiff, the capital of Wales. It is an ideal place for meetings, particularly medical conventions. And thus it happened on Friday, September 5, 1986, 266 distinguished delegates of this specialists' conference attended a buffet luncheon. Among the foods offered was breaded, baked chicken. And it was this chicken that was responsible for making 196, or 75 percent, of all the doctors attending the buffet sick with salmonella food poisoning. The specific organism in question was *Salmonella typhimurium*. The chicken used for the buffet was imported from France, but the *S. typhimurium** was found in many items produced by the kitchen, including chicken liver paté, bread crumbs and cooked beef.

The physicians attending the conference all suffered the typical symptoms of diarrhea, cramps, headaches, vomiting and fever. At the height of this outbreak, some doctors experienced as many as 15 watery stools per day. The physicians attending the conference were all experts in diabetes and more than 1,600 specialist

---

* The customary way of describing bacteria once the genus and species name is given in italics is to abbreviate the genus in italics and spell out the species in italics. Thus *Salmonella typhi* becomes *S. typhi*.

doctor-days were lost over a period of three weeks because of this particular outbreak. The disruption of services to diabetic patients was significant indicating the seriousness of a food poisoning outbreak among a concentration of specialists of any kind.

Country Club Buffet[56]

At a New Mexico country club buffet, on March 30, 1986, a large number of people came down with acute gastrointestinal symptoms, including diarrhea, nausea, painful abdominal cramps, vomiting, fever and bloody stools. The rapid onset time indicated the presence of a toxin. Sure enough, *Staphylococcus aureus* was isolated from the turkey served. But, it was also isolated from the nostrils of two of the food handlers. When the food handling procedures were reviewed, it turned out that the turkey had cooled for three hours at room temperature after cooking—plenty of time for staphylococcal toxins to develop to a poisonous level. It wasn't the first such incident for that particular country club.

These Ducks Were Not Food—At the Time[57]

For many children, the highlight of any Easter festival is the Easter egg hunt. During the Easter season of 1991, the states of Pennsylvania, Maryland and Connecticut identified 22 cases of *Salmonella hadar* in young children. Curiously, the majority of the victims had won ducklings as prizes for the Easter egg hunt. In all the winners' homes, the ducklings were kept inside and, in some cases, were even allowed to run free or swim in the same tub that the kids bathed in. The children came down with severe diarrhea, fever, abdominal cramps, bloody stools and vomiting. All of the ducklings in questions were traced back to two hatcheries in Pennsylvania. At the height of the duckling season, these hatcheries mail out over 2,000 ducklings per week. The fact that only 22 cases were registered is a good indication of the low rate of disease reporting.

PRODUCTION AND PROCESSING

The modern production of poultry starts at the farm or chicken house with eggs that could have been contaminated before being laid. These are then incubated for 21 days (28 days in the case of turkeys) at a constant temperature. Once hatched, the chicks are moved into production units where they are reared until ready for slaughter (normally six to 14 weeks), after which they are transported to a processing plant. At the processing plant, the birds are slaughtered by severing the carotid artery so that the blood can drain away. Feathers, internal organs and feet are then removed. The carcass is washed and chilled or frozen prior to shipping. Packaging can take place at the processing operation or at the retail outlet.

With little doubt, modern poultry production and processing operations have accomplished technical wonders and are responsible for bringing consumers nutritious products at an incredibly low price. On the surface, this efficient flow of products from the producer to the consumer does not appear to pose a problem. Yet, salmonella bacteria are found in 15 to 70 percent of poultry. High rates of contamination with campylobacter and *Listeria* bacteria have also been reported. If you consider all types of pathogens, the majority of chickens currently on sale are very likely contaminated with one form or another. Why does poultry have such a high rate of contamination at the retail store or supermarket level?

In order to answer this question, we must go back to the beginning. What became contaminated first, the chicken or the egg? Let us start with eggs. Eggs can become contaminated in the ovaries or oviducts by salmonella, *E. coli* or *Vibrio* bacteria. During my student days, I even found a large *Ascaris* roundworm wrapped around the yolk of an egg! In some countries, breeding flocks are carefully inspected, and if chronic bacterial problems such as salmonella are observed, the birds are quarantined or destroyed.

The rear exit of a bird is called the cloaca. It serves as the common route for both eggs and intestinal waste contents (feces). As a result, the surface of an egg can become contaminated very easily on the way to being laid. If this shell contamination is not immediately and completely removed, it can spread the contamination to the entire environment where the chicks are hatched. However, even if a producer were to start with the much more expensive salmonella-free eggs, many basic problems of contamination still remain.

Commercial poultry feeds contain a wide variety of ingredients to ensure the rapid and cost-effective growth of young birds. Some of these materials, such as rendered animal by-products (every part of the poultry or animal that cannot be sold for a better return), egg powder (which is unfit for human consumption), fish meal and recycled poultry feces are prime sources of contamination if they are not treated to kill all pathogens. Thus, the very material the birds are fed can be a source of contamination even if it contains antibiotics to prevent infection. Once they become infected, the growing birds can easily reinfect their neighbors through common eating and drinking facilities. For instance, the water troughs are an endless source of contamination until producers take specific steps to disinfect the entire system.

The young birds are not raised in a sterile laboratory environment. As the poultry litter becomes soiled, it is freely redeposited on the feathers and skin of all the birds in the vicinity. It is redistributed as dust, particularly when the birds flap their wings. Pathogens can enter through the help of insects and, in the case of free-range poultry, rodents can be agents of contamination. Wild birds, such as sparrows, pigeons, sea gulls and blackbirds, occasionally get past production barriers and add to the problem of unwanted contamination and disease organisms.

The producer is not necessarily aware of the presence of salmonella or other pathogens because the birds do not appear sick. (Only two specific varieties of salmonella are actually pathogenic to chickens, while most of the others that poultry harbor can affect humans.) As a result, these bacteria are almost impossible to eliminate. It would be the equivalent of eliminating all bacteria from the barnyard or chicken house. The only possibility of salmonella exclusion would be through the sterilization or irradiation of feed, the full sterilization of pens and litter, the complete exclusion of insects and the use of filtered air—in other words, a sterile laboratory environment. This is not a very practical possibility.

The potential for further salmonella infection can result from some of the traditional practices in getting egg-laying hens to molt their feathers faster. Currently, this is done by fasting the birds for a week or so in order to speed up the process so their egg-laying capacity can recover sooner. However, this practice makes birds extremely susceptible to infection from airborne salmonella during the process. This results in higher rates of hen infection, which translates to higher levels of egg contamination.[58] It is a never-ending story.

Disease transmission can be reduced with adequate spacing of birds, effective and continual air filtration, immediate removal of any dead birds, devices to prevent cross contamination of drinking water, frequent cleaning and sanitation and also active measures to eliminate external contaminants. Day-old chicks have even had their crops (esophagus) inoculated with the crop or intestinal material of healthy adults in an effort to reduce or prevent colonization with salmonella. With great care and attention, salmonella can be reduced significantly, but it cannot be eliminated without losing a great deal of operational cost-effectiveness.

Once raised to maturity, the load of chickens, some of which are already contaminated with salmonella, are then shipped from the producer to the processor. The proximity of the chickens to each other during transport permits a considerable amount of cross contamination to take place. Dust, feathers and litter residue all contain bacteria and are obvious sources of salmonella cross contamination.

After the birds get to the processing plant, salmonella bacteria have many opportunities to survive and spread the contamination further. Researchers have long known that salmonella bacteria have the nasty habit of securely attaching themselves to the skin of chickens.[59] Whenever the opportunity arises, this attachment happens quickly and firmly. In fact, this bond is so strong that tests have demonstrated that even after 40 consecutive carcass rinses, the level of salmonella on the poultry skin hardly decreases at all.[60]

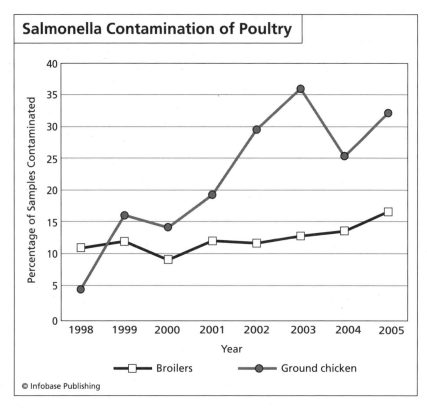

Figure 14. **Salmonella Contamination of Poultry**

The birds are slaughtered by severing the carotid artery and hung so that the blood can drain away. Considerable wing flapping during this process creates and spreads a significant amount of dust throughout all the areas that do not have dust barriers. The birds are then quickly immersed in a scalding tank in order to make the removal of feathers easier. The ideal temperature for scalding to work best is around 140°F (60 °C), but this allows salmonella and other pathogens to survive. Soil, dust and fecal matter are continually released into the scalding tanks, and the bacteria they contain are free to contaminate other carcasses.

Immediately after scalding, the chickens are transported to the defeathering machine, which is simply a device with firm rubber fingers on a revolving cylinder. Aside from removing the feathers, this machine also removes a good deal of the yellow epidermal layer of a bird's skin. This renders the remaining cuticle-free skin more susceptible to bacterial attack. Understanding why this operation serves as another prime source of cross contamination is not difficult. The revolving rubber fingers can transfer bacteria from the skin and feathers of one chicken carcass to the skin of another.

The birds are then eviscerated. Even though the vacuum equipment used is designed to minimize contamination, this operation often releases some of the intestinal contents onto the skin or meat of the bird, thereby increasing the degree of contamination. After evisceration, the carcasses are spray washed in order to clean them. However, as mentioned above, this hardly removes any of the salmonella that has attached itself to the skin or membranes. The birds are then immersed in chill tanks to lower the carcass temperature quickly and retard the spoilage process. Since salmonella easily tolerates the temperatures employed, this chilling step is a final stage where cross contamination can occur in the plant. In a number of European countries, this last step is accomplished with chilled sprays or cold-air cooling to prevent the spread of contamination. In North America, however, the chill tank is still commonly used, perhaps because the skin of the birds absorbs sufficient water to add 5–7 percent to the overall weight of the bird. One of the reasons that soaker pads are routinely found under packaged poultry is to absorb all the excess water for which consumers have payed.

If the birds are subsequently processed into parts, this spreads contamination further by exposing birds and susceptible fleshy parts to the same cutting tables. Knives, utensils and gloves that touch the poultry cross contaminate everything in the immediate environment. Even the final act of piling the parts together in consumer or bulk packages contributes to cross contamination.

In a sense, the entire modern poultry process unintentionally acts like a giant homogenizer to dilute and spread contamination among the greatest number of birds. The numbers of salmonella-positive chickens leaving a plant are invariably greater than those coming into it. As a result, up to 80 percent of the retail chickens in the United Kingdom[61] and up to 71 percent of processed carcasses in the United States[62] have been found to be salmonella positive. Salmonella-contaminated poultry rates of 15–70 percent commonly occur in most other countries.

The most recent results were announced in 2006 by the U.S. Department of Agriculture's Food Safety and Inspection Service (FSIS), the agency responsible for inspecting meat and poultry.[63] They announced their concern over an increase in salmonella contamination of broiler chickens and ground chicken. One look at the data immediately makes their concerns understandable.

Another FSIS publication that appeared at the end of 2006 reconfirmed the increase in the rate of salmonella infections in chicken. The study reported that the annual number of salmonella isolates increased more than fourfold and the proportion of establishments with *Salmonella enteritidis*–positive chickens increased nearly threefold. The number of states with *Salmonella enteritidis* in broilers increased from 14 to 24.[64] Over the years, there have been numerous claims by government and industry that the problem of poultry contamination had largely been solved. However, this latest survey shows that there is still a long way to go.

The process of mass-producing chickens in order to bring their price down to a more affordable level is not the original cause of contamination, it merely serves to spread the contamination among a greater number of birds. Salmonella commonly occurs in the environment and can therefore easily infect chickens at high levels without making them sick. In the processing plant, incoming contamination occurs on a continual basis. Even if all the equipment is thoroughly cleaned and disinfected, the arriving birds start the contamination process all over again on a daily basis. It is a chronic problem that is all too clearly demonstrated by the high rates of contamination at the retail level.

Campylobacter is a pathogenic bacterium that is even more common in poultry than salmonella. It often results in mild to severe diarrhea and fever but also has the potential to develop into a serious neurological condition known as Guillain-Barré syndrome. This pathogen is commonly found in the intestinal tracts of most farm animals and their feces are deposited on the various vehicles used to transport them to processing plants. Cross-contamination among animals is very common—a phenomenon that is replicated in the processing plant environment with the carcasses. Some of the most problematic stations on the processing line are the mechanical plucking machines.[65] This cross-contamination is not taken into account, which is why there still is a 70 percent contamination rate of *campylobacter* in poultry.

The mass processing or, for that matter, any processing of most chickens does not employ a definitive stage to exterminate bacteria. Obviously, chickens cannot be pasteurized in the traditional sense. Until a step for the destruction or significant reduction of bacteria is incorporated into the process, however, consumers cannot avoid salmonella-, campylobacter- and *Listeria*-contaminated chickens on supermarket shelves. An exception is poultry that has been irradiated, but very few retail outlets offer this product.

SECONDARY PROCESSING PRODUCTS

Once poultry is eviscerated and cooled, it can be used directly by the consumer as is. It can also be further divided into convenient pieces, such as legs or thighs, or particular cuts such as breasts. These poultry pieces can also be processed by the manufacturer or retailer into higher-value products such as breaded, battered and marinated items that are more convenient for the consumer to use at home. However, every step in handling provides the opportunity for additional contamination to take place. The resultant shelf life of these products is generally not as long as that of whole chicken carcasses.

Because of the great demand for breast meat, a surplus of dark meat often remains that must be used in a cost-effective manner. Meat can be

deboned by hand, but this is rather costly. Therefore, mechanical deboning is a very common way of removing the tiniest scraps of meat from
carcass bones, including backs and necks. This mechanically deboned
meat (MDM) has a very fine particle size and is extremely susceptible to
microbial contamination. MDM is an important component of the many
preformed and breaded poultry, cutlet and nugget products that have
become so common in supermarkets and fast-food outlets. Mechanically
deboned meat has also found an extensive use in all the poultry hot dogs,
burger and bologna products that are very popular. Because of the high
potential for microbial contamination, consumers should always observe
and adhere to the expiration dates and cook products very carefully.

Some of the most recent studies indicate that the level of contamination in poultry plants remains very high. Contamination rates for
campylobacter alone were around 40 percent and decreased very little
during the chilling process.[66] Another area of cross-contamination is the
defeathering machine.[67]

HANDLING AND PREPARATION

Because poultry usually receives high heat treatment when cooked, the
major consumer concern is cross contamination of raw poultry with
other foods that will not be cooked. From the very moment the consumer picks up the chicken at the supermarket, the cross contamination commences. Most consumers pick up moist or wet packages where
the poultry juices have leaked out to a certain extent. These juices may
contain poultry pathogens and will instantly contaminate the hands of
the shoppers. Even if your hands dry quickly, they remain contaminated
until you sanitize them. If those contaminated hands now touch fruits
or vegetables, cross contamination inescapably results. Not all vegetables
and very few fruits are cooked or sanitized before consumption. Consumers use prewashed lettuce directly in salads or as a garnish in sandwiches.
Usually, people only quickly rinse apples before eating them. Since
rinsing does little to eliminate bacteria, individuals now consume any
pathogens that find their way onto these products because the pathogens
never received any heat treatment at all. Thus, the ideal conditions for a
food-poisoning incident to occur are established.

In fact, when a consumer picks up a leaky package of poultry in the
supermarket, a process begins that has an excellent potential to expose
other consumers to pathogenic organisms. One consumer contaminated with poultry juices that contain pathogens can unintentionally
cross-contaminate many foods that will unknowingly be selected and
consumed by others. That is one of the ways that vegetarians get salmonella poisoning. What about the hardworking cashiers in supermarkets?
They handle packaged poultry and other products along with every

other product the consumer buys. Any contamination can be easily and quickly spread among all products. The conveyor belt is another source of cross-contamination. How often have we seen conveyor belts at the checkout counter that are wet because of a leaky poultry package? The most the cashier can do is give the contaminated puddle a quick wipe with a paper towel—definitely not a foolproof method of eliminating cross-contamination. Thus, cross-contamination starts well before the consumer brings the food products into the home. Grabbing a quick snack in the mall after grocery shopping without first thoroughly washing your hands is another example of what you should not do.

The consumer's kitchen is a prime location for cross-contamination. You do not need much imagination to see all the possibilities for transferring pathogens from contaminated poultry to other utensils or products in the kitchen and home. Countertops, knives, gloves, plates, hands, aprons, refrigerator trays and so forth can all be exposed to incoming contamination, and unless fully sanitized, they have the potential to cross-contaminate other foods not cooked before eating. Children who touch contaminated products at home or in the supermarket and then stick their fingers into their mouths or noses are directly exposed to food-borne pathogens without the benefit of ever eating the foods.

Needless to say, poultry can also pose a food-borne disease risk when not properly cooked. Traditional cooking procedures using frying, roasting, baking or barbecuing are well documented. Consumers are generally cautious in avoiding products not thoroughly cooked. Properly cooked meat, and particularly joint areas, should not be pink or retain a rawlike texture. If the cooking equipment is functioning properly and the recipe followed carefully, the pathogens have little chance of surviving this procedure. Conventional cooking requires that the most inaccessible part of the food reaches and maintains a particular temperature for a specified period of time because cooking is a combination of time and temperature. Since the normal movement of heat through a product takes a long time, this time-temperature relationship is simple to achieve. However, a further complication exists with microwave cooking. Because microwaves heat products to the final temperature so quickly, the time portion of the time-temperature relationship is usually not achieved. That is why many microwave recipes and instructions clearly state that once a product has reached a particular temperature, allow it to rest in the oven for a specific time without additional heating. If you prematurely remove the product before the full resting period has expired, a significant risk exists that many pathogens will survive. Controlled experiments have verified this to be the case.[68] You must observe the recommended resting period!

It is not a foregone conclusion that all poultry sold at retail outlets will contain pathogenic bacteria. Certain Scandinavian countries have a very strong program to eliminate salmonella from poultry. This program requires that chickens be raised from salmonella-free eggs and that they be fed with salmonella-free feeds. If a single chicken is found with salmonella, then the whole flock is often destroyed. This results in a very high price for chicken. It also does not provide any guarantees of freedom from other pathogens such as *Campylobacter* or *Listeria*.[69, 70] If the whole flock had to be destroyed every time a *Campylobacter*- or *Listeria*-positive chicken was found, then the price of chickens would become prohibitive. Without doubt, the rigorous sanitation practices employed in raising and processing this poultry result in higher-quality chickens, but the price is also correspondingly higher. Consumers should be made aware of differences in the average microbial quality of poultry and then be allowed to make the price/quality decision themselves. However, other options exist.

Based on all the tests and all the resulting evidence, the majority of scientists and health professionals alike feel that irradiation (also called cold pasteurization) of poultry is the most effective method of significantly reducing the public health risk of poultry-borne pathogens.[71] Results prove, beyond a doubt, the extraordinary value of irradiating poultry for the consumer and restaurant/catering trade. Researchers carried out very large-scale tests at the kitchen level to determine the effects of both irradiated poultry and irradiated spices on the overall hygienic quality of the finished foods. These tests conclusively demonstrated the potential for completely eliminating the majority of pathogens from the kitchen environment.[72] Furthermore, irradiation of chicken makes salmonella much more sensitive to the effects of heat—a critical consideration for those who like their meat and poultry on the medium-rare side.[73]

Most processors are reluctant to irradiate poultry products because they fear that consumers will resist the concept. Unfortunately, these processors have not kept up with or recognized all the latest studies, which confirm that every product market trial and commercial market introduction of irradiated foods have proven the consumers' willingness to buy such products. Despite this, most processors are still reluctant to irradiate products. The major supermarkets have also indicated that they prefer to carry poultry with the current levels of contamination exclusively rather than to offer consumers a choice of reduced-pathogen products. Until this attitude changes, the food-borne disease risk to consumers will continue. Individuals whose resistance is low at the time of exposure to contaminated products will be at a significantly increased risk—needlessly. Extending out from the North Chicago area where they were introduced by the Carrot Top Supermarket, high-quality irradiated poultry is being carried by a growing number of smaller supermarkets who appear to be more in line with the needs of today's consumers.

MEAT AND MEAT PRODUCTS

To eat steak rare . . . represents both a nature and a morality.

Roland Barthes (1915–80),
Mythologies, "Steak and Chips" (1957; tr. 1972)*

The consumption of meat has varied significantly over the years to reflect, on the one hand, the greater buying power of consumers and, on the other, their concern over the possible negative health effects of high-fat foods. The tremendous efficiency of the meat production and distribution system has resulted in products that have retained a high value-to-price ratio for decades. This has resulted in the continued high popularity for meat and meat products and the subsequent concern over their potential role in certain diseases. The very origin, nature and composition of meat make it particularly susceptible to spoilage and contamination by a wide variety of microorganisms. Thus, meat has often been implicated in the spread of several serious food-borne pathogens.

Meat is generally defined as the muscle tissue of a limited number of commercial animals including cattle, pigs, sheep, goats and, in certain specific localities, horses. Commonly, meat is presented to consumers in either raw, frozen, cooked or cured forms and can be in large cuts, sliced or ground. Meat contains about 75 percent water and is therefore an excellent substrate to support the growth of a variety of parasites and microorganisms. Furthermore, the low carbohydrate content of meat does not encourage the growth of lactic acid bacteria, an organism that can play an important role in discouraging the growth of other bacteria.

Normally, healthy animal tissue is free of microorganisms. Of course, diseased animals will harbor the organisms that are making them sick and will be more susceptible to attack from other pathogens because of their weakened condition. Even stress will decrease an animal's resistance to disease, which is the main reason why animals are treated far more carefully today than in the past. Routine veterinary inspection of animals will usually segregate diseased from healthy animals. However, the visual procedures normally employed have conspicuous limitations. Not only will the occasional sick animal escape the eye of the inspector, but no checks are made for specific human pathogens that the animals may conceal. Some diseases such as tuberculosis, anthrax, brucellosis and trichinellosis can be detected only after slaughter. It has been generally accepted that conventional inspection protocols are no longer sufficient to protect

---

* *The Columbia Dictionary of Quotations* is licensed from Columbia University Press. Copyright © 1993 by Columbia University Press. All rights reserved.

OUTBREAK INCIDENTS WITH MEAT

When Chicken Soup Just Won't Make It![74]

What do you serve at a birthday party on a frigid night in January in Alaska? Grizzly bear soup, that's what! You start off with some well-aged grizzly bear meat, cut it up into bite-sized chunks, add a few vegetables, salt, pepper, a parsnip root if you can find one and cook. There you have it—hearty, festive grizzly bear soup.

Unfortunately, most of the 16 rugged individuals who attended the birthday party came down with trichinellosis. The soup must have been great, however, because no samples of the grizzly meat were left for examination—it had all been eaten.

An Alarming New Form of Mad Cow Disease[75]

In the Spring of 1996, all of Europe quickly banned the importation of British beef following an announcement by the British health authorities that the deaths of 10 young people from Creutzfeldt-Jakob disease might be the linked to mad cow disease. Creutzfeldt-Jakob disease had always been considered an ailment of the old—the 50–70-year-old bracket—but this new form was able to strike people while they were still in their teens. Among the victims was a young student who died just before his 21st birthday. Although he was a vegetarian, he had eaten beef burgers as a youngster. Another victim was a young mother, aged 29, who had just given birth three weeks earlier. Her husband's greatest fear was that, somehow, the newborn baby might have contracted the disease and was living on borrowed time. Yet another student, aged 19, succumbed only 12 months after first experiencing depression and dizzy spells. One more youngster fell ill at the age of 16 and lapsed into a deep coma. The families of all the victims decisively linked the disease to the consumption of hamburgers.

The larger part of the European consuming public immediately began to avoid the consumption of beef. The British beef industry lost billions of pounds before the scare ran its course. The industry will never fully recover. Had there not been such an overriding focus on making cattle feed a shade cheaper by cutting corners when rendering animal by-products, perhaps these tragedies may have been avoided.

Deadly Trichinellosis[76]

The farmer from Greene County, New York, insisted that his pigs had been fed only grain. But the farmer often went hunting and fed portions of the killed game to his dogs. Maybe the pigs had a nibble as well.

After a pig was slaughtered, it was brought to New York City, where it was hung to dry for two days, before being butchered. Sausages were prepared and hung out to dry for another 10 days. This was the way of making traditional, homemade Italian pork sausages.

Within a short period, members of three related families came down with trichinellosis. All had diarrhea as well as severe muscular and abdominal pains. The most severe case, a 55-year-old woman, became feverish and had to be hospitalized. After almost three weeks in the hospital, she developed bronchopneumonia and died. An autopsy revealed several muscle samples containing Trichinella.

What a Jerky![77]

When we were young and first learned all about restaurants, one of the warnings we received was, "Never eat at a restaurant located near an alley." The implication was, of course, that they would probably serve cat meat in their dishes. But, the taboo on cat meat doesn't seem to extend to the apex feline carnivores of North America.

In early January 1995, a hardy soul from Idaho went out and shot a cougar. Once this had been accomplished, he decided to prepare jerky meat from the dead feline. He soaked the meat in brine and then lightly smoked it. Not being one to hoard the product of his labors, he distributed the meat to 14 other people. A week later, he started to experience fever, muscle aches and general fatigue.

His blood analysis indicated he had contracted trichinellosis. So did nine of the other people to whom he gave the jerky. This time the cat managed to get 10 lives not including his own.

---

consumers against more recently detected pathogens.[78, 79] A perfect example is *E. coli* O157:H7, an organism that may not show any severe negative effects in cattle but is a virulent and dangerous pathogen to humans.

The general hygienic state of animals prior to slaughter is critical to the overall quality of finished products. Plant cleanliness depends upon a number of factors, including animal-rearing location, type of transport employed and slaughterhouse conditions. Free-range animals are likely to have a significant number of soil microorganisms. Animals that receive final fattening in confined feed lots in close proximity to one another will have a greater proportion of fecal and communicable organisms. The hide or skin of meat animals is an excellent depository for filth of all kinds. Unless the animal is thoroughly washed and disinfected prior to slaughtering, it becomes a primary vector for the importation of contamination to the slaughterhouse environment.

PRIMARY PATHOGENS OF MEAT PRODUCTS

BACTERIAL—yes	FUNGAL—no
☐ *Bacillus cereus*	PARASITIC—yes
✔ *Campylobacter jejuni*	☐ *Anisakis simplex*
✔ *Clostridium botulinum*	✔ *Ascaris lumbricoides*
✔ *Clostridium perfringens*	☐ *Diphyllobothrium latum*
✔ **Enterohemorrhagic *E. coli***	☐ *Entamoeba hystolytica*
✔ **Enteroinvasive *E. coli***	✔ *Fasciola hepatica*
✔ **Enteropathogenic *E. coli***	☐ *Giardia lamblia*
✔ **Enterotoxigenic *E. coli***	✔ *Taenia saginata*
☐ *Helicobacter pylori*	✔ *Taenia solium*
✔ *Listeria monocytogenes*	✔ *Toxoplasma gondii*
✔ **Salmonella** species	✔ *Trichinella spiralis*
☐ *Shigella* species	✔ *Trichuris trichiura*
✔ *Staphylococcus aureus*	TOXIC SUBSTANCES—no
☐ *Streptococcus* species	VIRAL—possible
☐ *Vibrio* species	PRIONS—possible
✔ *Yersinia enterocolitica*	

During the actual processing, meat can become contaminated through contact with the hide, skin, feet, stomach or intestinal contents of the slaughtered animals as well as through contact with dirty floors, equipment or personnel. The degree of contamination that occurs after slaughtering reflects the standard of plant hygiene as well as the competence of the staff. Depending on the animal in question, minor differences in the slaughter procedure take place. Mechanical equipment is widely used for most operations in the dressing and processing of food animals. After the animals are stunned, they are fastened by one leg and hoisted to a continuous overhead rail system. In virtually all cases, the slaughtering is done by bleeding the animal through a sharp cut of the jugular vein. If employees do all this promptly and professionally, the blood leaves the body so quickly that death occurs almost instantaneously. However, this first step can spread contamination from one animal to another if slaughterhouse employees do not follow strict hygienic procedures to the letter. Once the animals are slaughtered, the carcasses are then transported along the rail to individual stations set up to carry out specific operations, such as skinning, disemboweling and head removal. Prior to entering the refrigeration area, employees usually cut the carcasses lengthwise down the backbone and divide them into equal halves. Sometimes they shroud the sides in muslin cloth in order to retain a white appearance of the fat.

Skin removal is the first step in the process of gaining value from the slaughtered animal. This operation must be done carefully to make sure that there is no damage inflicted to the valuable hide and that cross contamination with the carcass is kept to a minimum. In the case of hogs, the carcasses are first conveyed through scalding vats to dehairing machines. This results in a tendency toward higher bacterial loads in the carcass because the hair-removal process is not very hygienic. Sometimes, antibacterial sprays are employed to reduce the surface contamination of the carcass.

Although exposed to many of the same processing problems as poultry, meat animals are generally not as susceptible to the same high degree of contamination. In the first instance, the removal of intestinal contents is not as delicate an operation. Because of their larger size, the amount of exposed surface per unit weight of finished products is far less in meat animals than with poultry. On the other hand, the postslaughter processing and handling of meat is far more complex than poultry and makes the finished products more subject to other means of contamination.

Large meat animals undergo a significant amount of cutting and deboning in order to end up as finished products. As previously indicated, slaughterhouse employees first split the carcasses down the middle to create sides. These sides can be further processed centrally or can be shipped to retail shops where the butchers continue the process of breaking the animal down to individual consumer cuts. (Large-volume operations have the commercial advantage of making more cost-effective use of by-products and can also implement more rigorous hazard analysis of critical control points (HACCP) and quality assurance practices.) Each time someone cuts the carcass, fresh new surfaces highly susceptible to contamination are exposed. Room temperature, holding and processing times and the cleanliness of working surfaces and utensils all contribute to the overall state of finished product hygiene and quality. Immediately after slaughtering, the principal types of bacteria found on the carcass are typical animal strains. By the time the final cuts reach the retail consumer, however, characteristic human strains have taken over as the prevalent organisms, clearly demonstrating the impact of handling on finished product quality.

The consumer can fairly easily detect spoilage of meat through changes in color, odor or surface sliminess—spoiled products look, smell or feel bad. Unfortunately, the situation is not the same for products contaminated with harmful pathogenic organisms. Their presence can be determined only through microbiological tests beyond the current ability of the consumer to use. The consumer therefore totally depends upon the formal food system to guarantee the delivery of uncontaminated products. The continued incidence of serious food-borne diseases demonstrates that this food system is still woefully inadequate in fulfilling this role despite all protestations to the contrary. No better admission to this exists than the statement heard so often, "As long as consumers fully cook their meat, there is no chance of danger from food-borne disease." Finding a more crass or absurd statement would be difficult. If your meat products were dropped on a dirty floor, kissed by a tubercular handler or spat upon by a disgruntled butcher, the same statement would still apply. Such statements are testimony to the fact that the food system currently cannot supply safe, raw food products. Indeed, this concept has been institutionalized through the labeling of cooking instructions on meat.[80] It is a total abdication of responsibility. Milk and other fluid products are the exceptions since they go through a final pasteurization step to reduce the number of pathogens to an acceptable level.

In general, consumers must observe the same precautions in the handling and preparation of meat as with poultry. They should not allow juices to cross contaminate foods that they will not fully cook, such as fruits and vegetables. Given the current condition of the meat supply, people should fully cook all products to eliminate any risks of pathogens. In terms of contamination, the greater the degree of handling, the greater the potential threat. Therefore, ground or cubed meats constitute a considerably greater risk than steaks or roasts. Commercially ground meat poses a particular set of problems since pathogens from one carcass can contaminate an entire batch or spread to other batches if the equipment is not fully sanitized in between. The formulations for commercial frozen hamburger patties used by some of the major fast-food operations do not always require a country of origin that complies to particular inspection standards. They simply state, "XX% of frozen boneless beef," and so on. In other cases, the label specifies country of origin, but this is not necessarily based upon that country's reputation for hygiene. The resultant patty is multinational—the quintessential product of globalization.

The pathogens of greatest concern in fresh and frozen meat are *E. coli*, salmonella, and *Clostridium perfringens*. Cured meat concerns include salmonella, staphylococcus and the potential for *Clostridium botulinum* in sausages (after which it was named—*botulus* is Latin for sausage). Because meat is so popular both at home and in fast-food operations, these are the two areas that require the greatest attention.

FISH AND SEAFOOD

Internationally, fish and seafood come after meat and poultry as staple animal protein foods. Even though modern harvesting and postharvesting techniques have made higher quality and cheaper products more readily available, chronic problems continue to plague this industry. Higher-quality production has resulted in a greater demand. Fish stocks have dwindled dramatically, and nearly half the fish consumed worldwide are produced through farming.[81] This predicament will require far more disciplined international management of existing stocks in the future as well as the development of advanced techniques for sustainable culturing of different species.

The common consumer understanding of the term "fish" usually refers to free-swimming, finned fish of the bony or even cartilaginous (shark) type. Crustaceans include lobsters, crabs, shrimps, prawns (fresh-water shrimps) and other related species that typically have their skeletons on the outside to protect them from harm. The family of mollusks comprises clams, scallops, mussels, oysters, abalone and other shellfish types, while squid, octopus and cuttlefish belong to the cephalopod family.

The natural lifestyles of these animals usually determine the types of problems they pose regarding food-borne diseases. Fish and other creatures that inhabit waters close to the shores are particularly susceptible to contamination with the organisms contained in raw sewage, such as salmonella and vibrio. In the past, salmonella contamination of fish was believed to be something that occurred after the fish were caught, that is, the result of poor handling practices or infected workers. It was considered to be a postharvest phenomenon simply because salmonella does not tolerate salt water very well. However, scientists now recognize that salmonella contamination does indeed occur in the sea. The continual dumping of untreated, contaminated wastes into the marine environment has resulted in new salmonella mutants that are very tolerant of salt. Most fish and seafood raised by aquaculture are exposed to animal or human wastes from the local environs and can easily be contaminated by a wide variety of pathogenic organisms. Mollusks pose a particular problem because they are filter feeders and, therefore, are ideally suited to trap all bacteria and viruses, pathogenic or otherwise, that live in the waters.

Fish also host many parasites that can easily be transmitted to humans if they are not processed properly. Trematode worms such as *Clonorchis sinensis* and *Opisthorchis viverrini* and the tapeworms *Diphyllobothrium latum* (freshwater) or *Diphyllobothrium pacificum* (marine) are typical examples. Fish are also known to transmit roundworms of the genera *Anisakis* and *Phocanema* to humans.

62

OUTBREAK INCIDENTS WITH FISH AND SEAFOOD

Canary Island Blues[82]

In January 2004, two fishermen captured a huge 57-pound (26-kg) amberjack while scuba diving along the coast of the Canary Islands, Spain. When they arrived home, they dressed the fish and stored the fillets in their household freezer. Within a few days, one of the fishermen and four family members consumed some of the fish and within 30 minutes began to develop gastrointestinal and neurological symptoms. The five family members immediately sought treatment at the emergency department of Hospital de Fuerteventura and the outpatient clinic at the Infectious Diseases and Tropical Medicine Service of the Hospital Insular in Las Palmas.

The five family members exhibited a combination of diarrhea, nausea/vomiting, metallic taste, heart rhythm disturbances, fatigue, itching, dizziness and other neurologic manifestations. No hematological or biochemical abnormalities were detected in any patient. Based upon the symptomatic profiles, relationships of the patients and their common dietary histories, ciguatera intoxication was diagnosed in all. None of the patients required hospitalization. Although the neurological and gastrointestinal symptoms were resolved over several weeks, there was a continued intermittent recurrence of some symptoms for several months afterward. A small portion of the implicated fish was recovered from the fisherman's freezer at his home. After laboratory analysis, the results proved positive for ciguatoxins. Another 5.2-oz. (150-g) sample of the fish was sent to the FDA's Gulf Coast Seafood Laboratory, at Dauphin Island, Alabama, for a more sophisticated analysis. Results were positive for Caribbean ciguatoxin.

Oddly, the Canary Islands are not in the typical ciguatera-endemic zones. Now the residents of coastal West Africa have a new food-borne risk to be concerned about. Fortunately, the impact of this outbreak was minimal, but ciguatera poisoning can be a debilitating disease, and therapeutic intervention strategies are very limited.

Botulism on the Nile[83]

During May 1992, a man of Egyptian origin made three emergency visits to a New Jersey hospital because he was experiencing dizziness, weakness and respiratory failure. They were not quite sure what the problem was, but eventually had to place him on a mechanical ventilator. He stayed on mechanical ventilation in the intensive care unit until three other family members arrived with similar symptoms. It was only then that someone considered the possibility of botulism intoxication. All four were immediately given botulinal antitoxins.

The New Jersey Department of Health was able to trace the source of botulism to an ethnic fish preparation called *moloha*. The family had purchased the *moloha* at a local supermarket and consumed it without any cooking or heating. Although a family friend had also eaten some of the fish, there were no apparent symptoms, but now that everyone was convinced it was botulism, a dose of the antitoxin was given simply as a preventive measure. When the Health Department checked with the supermarket, the owner denied ever selling this type of fish. Fortunately, everyone recovered. (There is no truth to the assertion that, when asked his opinion on the whole episode, the original victim blurted out, "Moloha Sphinx!")

A Bad Bucket Off Nantucket[84]

On the sixth of June 1990, six fishermen aboard a fishing boat in the rugged waters of Georges Bank came down with severe symptoms of Paralytic Shellfish Poisoning (PSP). The men had eaten blue mussels just harvested in the deep waters. In heavy seas, over 115 miles off the coast of Nantucket Island, the men began to experience vomiting, numbness of mouth, paresthesia (burning or tingling) of arms and severe numbness of the throat. One of the fishermen even lost consciousness.

By the time they were able to return to port and check into a local hospital emergency room, most of the men were on their way to recovery, although two required a few days of hospitalization. The fishermen had fully cooked the fresh mussels prior to eating them with fish and vegetables. As it happened, an official notice had been sent out by the National Marine Fisheries Service to the effect that this particular area of Georges Bank was closed to the harvesting of all shellfish. Unfortunately, the fishermen involved claimed they had never received the notice.

Chicago, Chicago—Mahi Mahi[85]

At a private club in Chicago in February 1988 a number of patrons and employees took part in a buffet luncheon that featured mahi mahi fish. Within 90 minutes, they all began to experience nausea, headache, dizziness and diarrhea. When questioned later, three of the people seem to remember that the mahi mahi tasted like Cajun fish. All eventually recovered.

The club had purchased the frozen mahi mahi from a local distributor about a week before it was prepared. When examined later, similar lots of fish had evidence of freezer burn as well as thawing and refreezing. All samples showed evidence of high levels of histamine—scombroid poisoning—no great surprise considering the poor refrigeration history of the fish.

PRIMARY PATHOGENS OF FISH AND SEAFOOD

BACTERIAL—yes	PARASITIC—yes
☐ *Bacillus cereus*	✔ *Anisakis simplex*
☐ *Campylobacter jejuni*	☐ *Ascaris lumbricoides*
✔ **Clostridium botulinum**	✔ **Diphyllobothrium latum**
✔ **Clostridium perfringens**	☐ *Entamoeba hystolytica*
☐ Enterohemorrhagic *E. coli*	☐ *E. coli Fasciola hepatica*
☐ Enteroinvasive *E. coli*	☐ *Giardia lamblia*
✔ **Enteropathogenic** *E. coli*	✔ **Nanophyetus salmincola**
☐ Enterotoxigenic *E. coli*	✔ **Opisthorchis viverrini**
☐ *Helicobacter pylori*	☐ *Taenia saginata*
☐ *Listeria monocytogenes*	☐ *Taenia solium*
✔ **Salmonella species**	☐ *Toxoplasma gondii*
✔ **Shigella species**	☐ *Trichinella spiralis*
✔ **Staphylococcus aureus**	☐ *Trichuris trichiura*
☐ *Streptococcus species*	**Toxic Substances—yes**
☐ *Vibrio species*	✔ **Ciguatera poisoning**
☐ *Yersinia enterocolitica*	✔ **Tetrodotoxin poisoning**
FUNGAL—no	✔ **Scombroid poisoning**
VIRAL—possible	✔ **Shellfish poisoning**

Marine fish are typically harvested in the deep seas, far from processing plants. Little doubt exists that fish undergo significantly more stress prior to slaughter than meat and poultry do. Most fish are not fully processed on factory ships and must be stored frozen or chilled in ice or cold brine. Fish are usually eviscerated prior to freezing or chilling. Eviscerating the fish rids the carcass of a major source of microorganisms but also exposes freshly cut surfaces to several sources of contamination.

Fish that have not been lacerated are not very susceptible to microbial attack. However, once the surface of the skin has been penetrated, the damaged area becomes the focal point for bacterial contamination. Fish are often sold in auction houses and are openly displayed for all buyers to see. This extended exposure to an open environment containing dust, birds and rodents exacerbates the problem and adds to the contamination potential. The most fabulous fish market in the world, Tokyo's central Tsukiji market, goes to extraordinary lengths to limit spoilage and contamination. Tsukiji market sells between 20 and 25 million dollars' worth of fish per day, and you cannot detect any smells or off-odor of fish at all. Nevertheless, it still suffers many of the same problems as all other fish markets. Because of the significant handling of fish, they often carry high levels of bacteria pathogenic to humans.

The majority of fish harvested is processed into fillets, steaks and other similar products. This process naturally exposes products to workers, and hygienic practices must be constantly observed. Cross contamination in a fish-processing plant can be more critical than in a meat- or poultry-processing plant, because there is bacteria-laden slime everywhere that must be constantly washed off with chlorinated water. Initially, contamination is limited to fish surfaces. However, as more slicing or processing takes place, the contamination spreads further and deeper into the products. The level of contamination increases as you go from whole to eviscerated fish to fillets and steaks and, finally, to minced fish. The latter product is a particular problem if the equipment is not fully sanitized on a frequent basis.

Fish spoilage takes place in a rather predictable manner as the following table shows:

THE PHASES OF FISH SPOILAGE		
PHASE	CHARACTERISTICS	COMMENTS
1	Bright, clear eyes; bright gills; firm flesh; very good color; fresh odor	What consumers should look for
2	Eyes start to dull; gill color fades and appears grayish; texture softens; color fades; slightly fishy odor	Still acceptable to purchase but will not be optimal eating
3	Dull, sunken eyes; gills gray and slimy; soft flesh; dull color; unmistakable fishy odor	Do not buy this fish
4	Completely opaque and sunken eyes; slimy, bleached gills; soft flesh; dull, slimy color; strong fishy odor	Report to manager or local government inspection service

People always thought that spoilage microorganisms were able to outcompete pathogens and therefore consumers would be warned well ahead of time of any real food-poisoning problems. This has now proven to be false. Many pathogens can comfortably survive at refrigerated storage conditions and multiply before the marine products show any outward signs of spoilage at all. The pathogens of chief concern are vibrio, staphylococcus, salmonella, shigella, *E. coli* and rickettsia, a parasitic bacteria. Other concerns are scombroid poisoning in tuna due to the formation of histamine by bacteria when the fish are not cooled quickly enough.

Lobsters and crabs are generally kept alive until they are brought into port and are often sold live to consumers. Bacteria are not generally a major problem unless they are specific pathogens. Shrimps die almost as soon as they are captured and therefore must be iced immediately or they will spoil rapidly. A typical sign of spoilage in shrimp is called "black spot" and is easily distinguished by the characteristic dark discoloration of the shell tips due to enzyme degradation. Shrimp are often beheaded prior to sale in order to prevent black spot, but this does not prevent spoilage. Shrimp, prawns and crabs may also carry pathogens from sewage or agricultural runoff. *Vibrio* is a particular problem for crustaceans.

Oysters and clams are dug up or raked from the sand or sea bottom. They are usually transported live, sometimes even without the benefit of refrigeration. Since they are filter feeders, they will collect any pathogens or noxious materials contained in the waters. In fact, various shellfish have been found to be contaminated with pathogens such as vibrio so often that they are considered to be an unacceptable health risk in many parts of the United States. Never eat raw mollusks taken from questionable waters. Full cooking will destroy most pathogens of any concern but is not an iron-clad guarantee against problems such as "red tide" toxins. It is possible to purge mollusks of a significant load of pathogens through a process called depuration. This method simply allows shellfish to pump clean, uncontaminated water through their systems for an extended period of time, but this does not work well to eliminate viruses.

Freshwater fish are usually caught closer to the consumer and are more likely to be fresher. However, their very proximity to urban centers assumes that they are more apt to come from polluted waters. Quality deterioration is also a problem during summer months when even large bodies of freshwater tend to increase in temperature and become a more hospitable environment for microorganisms of all kinds. Whether from freshwater or marine sources, however, handle and treat frozen fish products in much the same way as their fresh counterparts.

Fish diseases constitute one of the most important problems and challenges confronting aquaculture. Fish in intensive culture are continually affected by environmental fluctuations and management practices such as handling, crowding, transporting, drug treatments, undernourishment and poor water quality. All of these factors can impose considerable stress on the fish, rendering them susceptible to a wide variety of pathogens. Parasites, viruses and bacteria are all causes for concern to the growing aquaculture industry. Many of these pathogens are treatable and are not pathogenic to humans. On the other hand, there are diseases that are not treatable and cause widespread mortality both in the hatchery and in wild fish. And, like *E. coli* O157:H7, there is always the possibility that a form of benign bacteria can become highly pathogenic.

Take precautions in the kitchen to avoid cross contamination with products that you will not cook. Fish products are usually laid flat before freezing. If the frozen block or fillet appears to be out of shape or grossly twisted or distorted, the product probably defrosted somewhere along the journey from the processor to the consumer. It could have occurred at the frozen storage facilities of the processor, the distributor, the retailer or even on the trip to the consumer's home. Carefully inspect such products before preparation to make sure no obvious signs of spoilage are apparent. If you have any doubt, do not consume the product.

Canned products such as salmon, tuna, sardines and mackerel all receive a full sterilization process as do other canned products. Therefore, they are free of dangerous pathogens and do not pose a problem except for the very rare occurrence of scombroid poisoning (since histamine is heat resistant). Certain products, such as mussels, cannot withstand the normal full sterilization treatment and are canned at much lower temperatures but in the presence of high concentrations of salt or vinegar. Unfortunately, this treatment does not solidly guarantee against pathogens, and problems have occurred in the past. Inspect such products carefully before purchasing, and always keep them refrigerated after opening.

Heavily smoked seafood products usually have very low moisture and do not present a great microbiological hazard. Lightly smoked products, such as finnan haddie, however, still retain a high water content and are only slightly more stable than raw, unprocessed products. Therefore, continuously store them in refrigerated conditions and fully cook them before consuming.

Barbecued or so-called hot-smoked products are among the most hazardous forms of fish available. The processing temperatures employed are only sufficient to kill growing or vegetative bacteria. Many spores survive and start to grow in the finished product. Moisture levels remain high enough to support active bacterial growth. As a result, these products have been responsible for a number of botulism outbreaks and absolutely must be fully reheated immediately before consumption.

The seriousness of fish and seafood pathogens requires that people take special care when consuming fish and seafood. Despite all the claims of freshness and sanitation associated with the consumption of sushi or sashimi, by far the majority of fish and seafood poisoning from raw fish occurs in Japan and Korea, the two countries where these foods are consumed most. Even products such as seviche (fish marinated in lime juice) can cause serious problems such as those experienced by the former president of Peru. During a period when the quality of his country's coastal waters was brought into question, he wished to demonstrate to his citizens that the press reports were exaggerated. He courageously posed for public television eating some locally prepared seviche. Very shortly thereafter, he came down with cholera. Pathogens are a biological, not a political, phenomenon. You eat raw fish at your own risk.

It is not a good idea for anyone who is making fish soup or dumplings to taste the broth in the very early stages of cooking. People often do this to make sure that the dish contains enough salt or spice. However, until the broth has boiled for some time, it can transmit hazardous pathogens. Researchers often speculated that the higher-than-normal incidences of freshwater fish tapeworms, *Diphyllobothrium*, in Jewish grandmothers resulted from their tasting the broth of gefilte fish (ground freshwater fish dumplings) too soon after it started cooking.

DAIRY AND EGG PRODUCTS

MILK PRODUCTS

Milk is generally defined as the liquid secreted by the mammary glands of female mammals. Humans consume cows' milk most widely, but other animals such as goats, sheep, buffalos, horses, camels and yaks also serve as sources. Milk is a fully integrated food containing fat, protein, minerals (calcium and phosphorus), sugar (lactose) and vitamins A and D.

PRIMARY PATHOGENS OF UNPASTEURIZED DAIRY PRODUCTS

BACTERIAL yes	
☐ *Bacillus cereus*	✔ *Listeria monocytogenes*
☐ *Brucella species*	✔ *Salmonella species*
☐ *Campylobacter jejuni*	☐ *Shigella* species
☐ *Clostridium botulinum*	✔ *Staphylococcus aureus*
✔ *Clostridium perfringens*	✔ *Streptococcus species*
☐ Enterohemorrhagic *E. coli*	☐ *Vibrio* species
☐ Enteroinvasive *E. coli*	✔ *Yersinia enterocolitica*
✔ Enteropathogenic *E. coli*	FUNGAL—no
☐ Enterotoxigenic *E. coli*	PARASITIC—no
☐ *Helicobacter pylori*	TOXIC SUBSTANCES—no
	VIRAL—possible

OUTBREAK INCIDENTS WITH MILK PRODUCTS

A Raw Deal[86]

On December 10, 2002, the Ohio Department of Health and the Clark County Combined Health District were notified of two hospitalized children infected with *Salmonella Typhimurium*. The initial investigation implicated raw, unpasteurized milk purchased at a local combination dairy-restaurant during November 27–December 13, 2002, as the cause. At the time, 27 states still allowed the sale of raw milk directly from the farm.

The dairy operation included a working dairy farm, a restaurant, a snack bar and a petting zoo with typical barnyard animals—goats, cows, calves, lambs and pigs. The entire enterprise employed 211 workers, including 16 members of the family who owned it. At the time, the dairy was the only place in Ohio that legally sold and served raw milk and milk shakes. In 2001, approximately 1,350,000 customers visited the dairy.

Further investigation indicated that a total of 62 people had the illness, including 40 customers, six household contacts, and 16 of 211 dairy workers. The other patients came from Illinois, Indiana, Ohio and Tennessee. Among the symptoms reported were regular and bloody diarrhea, cramps, fever, chills, body aches, vomiting and headache.

On December 13, 2002, following an order from local health authorities, the dairy discontinued the sale of all raw milk products. One month later, the Ohio Department of Agriculture recommended that all sales of raw milk dairy products, including bottled raw whole milk, skim milk and cream, be discontinued permanently.

On March 20, 2007, the *Boston Globe* reported that the state of Maryland was considering lifting the ban on farm-based sales of raw milk. By that time, 28 states were allowed to sell raw milk. The dairy industry in Maryland was in decline, and this measure was under consideration in order to increase incomes of dairy farmers. It remains to be seen whether selling dairy products with a greater risk of pathogens will do this, even though the taste may be improved. A much better solution would be the micro-filtered milk (available in many other countries) that never undergoes heat treatment, but eliminates pathogens through a filtration process. As of the time this book went to press, raw milk was not permitted in Maryland.

A Classic Case of Underreporting[87]

During the summer months of 1982, a large interstate outbreak of gastroenteritis occurred. Health Department tests zeroed in on milk pasteurized at a plant in Memphis, Tennessee, as the vehicle of infection and *Yersinia enterocolitica* as the responsible pathogenic organism.

Before it was over, close to 200 people with *Y. enterocolitica*-positive infections were found in the states of Arkansas, Tennessee and Mississippi. Most patients had gastrointestinal infections with diarrhea, painful abdominal cramps and fever. Many ended up with accessory infections of the throat, blood, urinary tracts and even the central nervous system. More than 40 percent of the victims were children under the age of five years. Unbelievably, most of the patients needed to be hospitalized and almost 20 of them had to undergo appendectomies!

In a post-incident inquiry to try and estimate the overall size of the outbreak, a telephone survey was made to randomly chosen households in one affected area. When all the calculations were finished, the results estimated almost 900 cases. Considering that this area only accounted for 4 percent of the milk plant's market, an estimated 20,000 people could have been affected, 100 times more than the actual number of cases reported!

Barnyard Blues[88]

On a lovely October day in 1985, a group of Northern Californian students, teachers and their family members decided to take a day off school and go on a field trip to a San Joaquin County dairy. After all, what could be closer to the country life than spending a day in the company of milk cows? Of course, part of this treat was the opportunity to drink fresh, raw milk, as close to the original source as possible. (Because of the countless outbreaks of gastrointestinal diseases that occurred among school-age children who tasted fresh, raw milk on field trips to farms and dairies, the Food and Drug Administration, in January 1985, issued an "advisory" on milk to all state school officers. It recommended that children should never be permitted to sample raw milk when making such trips. In this particular case the advice was unheeded.)

Sixty percent of those who drank the raw milk became quite ill. On the other hand, none of those who declined to drink got sick! The culprit hiding in the milk was later found to be *Campylobacter jejuni*. Among the victims was an infant who, up until then, had been exclusively breast-fed. One bottle of raw milk was all that was needed for illness to result.

The field-trippers experienced diarrhea, abdominal cramps, fever and vomiting. Many even developed bloody diarrhea. The "advisory," wasn't meant to be ignored.

Pasteurization Alone Is Not Enough[89]

On April 13, 2000, the Pennsylvania Department of Health notified the CDC of an increase in *Salmonella Typhimurium* cases. Stool samples from 93 people yielded *S. Typhimurium*. During the last two weeks of April, state and federal agencies visited the suspected dairy plant. All indications were that the pasteurization process had been adequate during the time of the outbreak. Yet a review of in-house microbial testing from January 3 to April 17 identified 13 instances where the standard plate counts were elevated and nine instances where coliforms were elevated. According to the pasteurized milk ordinance, the standard plate count should not be above 20,000/ml and the coliform count should not exceed 10/ml. Yet the highest standard plate count was 120,000/ml on April 4 and the highest coliform count was reported as more than 100/ml on April 14 and 17.

FDA inspectors found violations of sanitary standards that might have resulted in contamination of products after pasteurization. These problems included evidence of excessive condensation, which could have produced droplets that fell into open containers throughout the processing and packaging area. Several machines leaked raw milk onto the floor, and raw skim milk was held in a silo at a temperature higher than 50°F or 10°C, well above the 45°F or 7.2°C standard.

A review of records at the dairy plant identified 14 employees who were absent between March 20 and April 20. Three of them had gastrointestinal illness and all reported drinking finished products produced at the plant in the five days before the outbreak onset. The conclusion of this incident highlighted that inadequate pasteurization was an uncommon event compared to contamination after pasteurization and emphasized that additional regulatory emphasis be placed on post-pasteurization monitoring.

Chicago Style[90]

By the 16th of April, 1985, the number of confirmed cases reported to the Illinois Department of Public Health during this outbreak of milk-borne salmonellosis reached a staggering 5,770! Of the first 800 cases reported, almost 60 percent were youngsters under 10 years of age. *Salmonella typhimurium* was found in two lots of suspected milk from the same dairy plant in Illinois.

The Illinois Department of Public Health began to receive reports from three other states where the milk was routinely delivered. At the time, this was the largest number of confirmed cases ever associated with a single outbreak of salmonellosis in the United States.

Needless Tragedy[91]

The year 1985 was a tough one because, in the first half of the year, 86 cases of *Listeria monocytogenes* infection were identified in Los Angeles and Orange Counties in the state of California. Tragically, 29 fatalities occurred, including 8 neonatal deaths, 13 stillbirths and 8 deaths classified as non-neonatal. The mothers involved ranged in age from 15 to 43 years and all were of Hispanic origin. It appeared that all the cases were acquired in the local community.

Samples of Mexican-style cheeses were taken from local producers and one in particular was isolated as being a source of *Listeria*. Radio, television and newspaper ads were issued warning the public against eating the particular brand of cheese products in question. Of course, by that time, it was too late for many.

White, unpasteurized cheese from Mexico called *queso fresco* or *queso blanco* has been found to be responsible for a number of cases of listeriosis and other food-borne diseases.

Although milk from clean and healthy cows does not generally contain sufficient pathogenic microorganisms to be harmful, conditions as simple as minor udder irritation can cause the population of organisms to alter dramatically. Mastitis, which is an inflammation of the mammary tissues, often results in a massive increase in the number of infectious organisms such as *Salmonella, Staphylococcus, E. coli, Clostridium perfringens* and *Brucella.* Some cattle suffer from mastitis chronically but at subacute levels that cannot be easily detected by a normal examination. Concern for this chronic problem resulted in the application of the pasteurization technique to milk but not before interminable delays. A short history of milk pasteurization reveals how stubborn and irresponsible people can be, particularly when rational solutions are staring them straight in the face.

As described earlier, the idea of preserving foods through the reduction or destruction of the microorganisms they harbor is centuries old. In the 18th century, vigorous boiling was used to preserve vinegar (Karl Wilhelm Scheele in 1782) and various meat extracts (Lazzaro Spallanzani in 1765). In 1804, French confectioner Nicholas Appert developed canning, which ended up being one of the greatest advances in food technology. Napoleon, who always said that an army marches on its stomach, had offered up a prize-winning challenge for anyone to devise new methods for the improved preservation of foods used by the French army. Nicholas Appert found that by heating food in a glass container and then sealing it off from air, it could be kept it in an edible condition for a very long time. This was just what the army needed! Appert submitted his technology for the prize and, in 1809, won it. He was such a loyal believer in his new method that he promptly invested all his prize money in the world's first commercial food-canning plant.

Although people generally understood that these heating methods could preserve foods, the exact reasons why they worked were not understood at all. The same situation existed in the field of medicine. While controlling the symptoms of certain diseases was possible, physicians did not know the precise reasons why certain treatments worked. Microorganisms were virtually unknown, and their pathogenic effects were usually attributed to other factors.

The monumental efforts of the Frenchman Louis Pasteur changed everything. By following the trail initially set by the visionary Italians

Spallanzani and Fabroni, he began to develop the strong sense that an intimate link existed between disease and the fermentation that accompanies the spoilage of food. In his drive to determine the causes of contagious diseases conclusively, Pasteur carried out in-depth research on the various causes of spoilage in wine, beer and vinegar. These studies eventually led to the investigation of disease in silkworms and, ultimately, to his probing analysis of human diseases. Pasteur's untiring efforts eventually revolutionized the medical world and are undeniably among the most important scientific works to benefit mankind. For the first time, a sound theoretical basis for controlling microorganisms and their effects had been firmly established.

During 1860–64, Pasteur showed that wine spoilage resulted from simple microbial metabolisms. To control the problem, he suggested a low level of heat treatment, which was enough to deactivate the spoilage microorganisms (122–140°F or 50–60°C) but not enough to damage the quality or character of the finished wine. This was, and still is, the key to the pasteurization process. While he could easily have boiled the wine vigorously to kill off all the microorganisms, that would have affected the wine's taste as well—something unthinkable for a true Frenchman. He therefore set about to determine the absolute minimum temperatures required to accomplish the job without wrecking the product's traditional character. The final pasteurization technique was so effective, it was quickly applied to beer and vinegar products as well.

Pasteurization was a real boon. French consumers were no longer forced to stomach wine or beer that had spoiled. For the first time in history, a simple method was available to prevent the sort of spoilage that had always been considered a sad, but natural, fact of life. With little doubt, the commercial consequences of pasteurization were the dominant concerns for its development. However, that is not the sphere in which the technology's most extraordinary impact was ultimately realized. Wine and beer may not be absolutely essential for life but, as far as children are concerned, milk is what is most important. Thus, in the field of public health, the benefits of pasteurization were greatest. Even though Pasteur himself did not apply his technique to milk, this new method achieved its greatest success in the dairy industry. When the process was eventually applied to milk, it was christened pasteurization in due recognition of Pasteur's unequaled contribution to science, health and humanity.

Milk pasteurization did not become a commercial reality for many years after Pasteur's initial research. The pasteurization method was first commercially tested on milk in Germany in 1880. However, its main purpose was to improve the product's shelf life rather than to enhance its health benefits for consumers. Eventually, in 1886, the famous German chemist, Franz Ritter von Soxhlet, became the first respected scientist to recommend pasteurization for improving the health-related properties of milk. Before that time, people generally accepted that milk carried diseases such as diphtheria, typhoid and tuberculosis, among others. Together with an American pediatrician by the name of Abraham Jacobi, von Soxhlet insisted that only heat-treated milk was safe to feed to infants.

Shortly thereafter, a controversy developed over the relative benefits of pasteurization compared to full sterilization by lengthy boiling. European health officials generally preferred the latter method for milk destined to feed infants. Research work was also carried out on the condensation and canned sterilization of milk. However, these products differed so much from fresh milk that they could never be accepted for general consumption as an alternative to regular milk. Pasteurized milk became a reality in America once research clearly demonstrated that extended boiling was neither necessary nor desirable. Although it did not have a limitless shelf life, pasteurized milk was safe, practical and fit the everyday needs of most consumers. It had an almost identical taste and color as fresh milk and did not require any particular changes in normal consumption or cooking habits.

Yet, although these advantages were beyond doubt, establishing pasteurized milk on the market was still a struggle as can be seen from the objections shown in the following list.[92] The dairy industry together with the outspoken conservatives, who championed the incomparable qualities of natural, raw milk, delayed the adoption and commercialization of these new methods for years. However, as milk became more and more associated with the transmission of sickness and disease, public health officials and the medical community became more vocal in their condemnation of dairy products.

ORIGINAL OBJECTIONS TO PASTEURIZATION

A. SANITATION

1. Pasteurization may be used to hide low-quality milk.
2. Heat destroys great numbers of bacteria in milk and thus conceals the evidence of dirt.
3. Pasteurization is an excuse for the sale of dirty milk.

B. PHYSICAL AND BACTERIOLOGICAL QUALITY

1. Pasteurization destroys the healthy lactic acid bacteria in milk, and pasteurized milk goes putrid instead of sour.
2. Pasteurization destroys good enzymes, antibodies and hormones, and takes the "life" out of milk.

C. ECONOMICS

1. Pasteurization will increase the price of milk.
2. Pasteurization is not necessary where milk goes directly and promptly from producer to consumer.
3. Pasteurization legalizes the right to sell stale milk.

D. NUTRITION

1. Pasteurization spoils the flavor of milk.
2. Pasteurization significantly lowers the nutritive value of milk.
3. Children and invalids thrive better on raw milk.
4. Infants do not develop well on pasteurized milk.
5. Raw milk is better than no milk.

E. PUBLIC HEALTH AND SAFETY

1. Pasteurization is unnecessary, because raw milk does not give rise to tuberculosis.
2. Interfering in any way with Nature's perfect food is wrong.
3. Pasteurization will give rise to a false sense of security.
4. Pasteurization would lead to an increase in infant mortality.

As the dairy producers began to realize that the consuming public's traditional faith in raw milk was eroding in response to growing public criticism, certain dairies, in collaboration with the medical establishment, began to place their operations under a much greater degree of hygienic scrutiny and control. Farmers paid stricter attention to the cleanliness of farm animals, barns and milking utensils. The health of workers was also monitored, and all operating procedures were inspected regularly. Milk produced under these newly specified conditions received the official endorsement of the state medical milk commissions and was classified as "Certified" milk—the purest and safest form of raw milk possible to produce.

With little doubt, certified milk was a great step forward in the cleanliness and hygienic quality of milk. However, the procedures followed gave no real guarantee against the many milk-borne infections affecting consumers. The process did not contain a step actually to kill any contaminating bacteria that managed to make their way into the milk. Not surprisingly, certified milk was eventually found to be responsible for several famous outbreaks of serious milk-borne diseases. Not much time passed before it was conceded that raw milk always had the potential to be dangerous, regardless of whether or not it was certified. A way to kill any pathogenic organisms that milk might contain had to exist. This brought forth a variety of other approaches to deal with the problem of milk safety—some of which were pretty appalling. Among the chemical solutions recommended included adding hydrogen peroxide, salicylic and benzoic acids and also potassium dichromate (the crystalline compound used in explosives and in safety matches). Other substances commercially employed included borax and formaldehyde. All of this was used simply to get around the process of pasteurization.

In the United States, a New York philanthropist by the name of Nathan Straus was shocked at the mortality statistics of children fed raw milk, and he decided to wage a campaign for pasteurization. It became one of the crowning glories of his life. He established milk depots all over New York

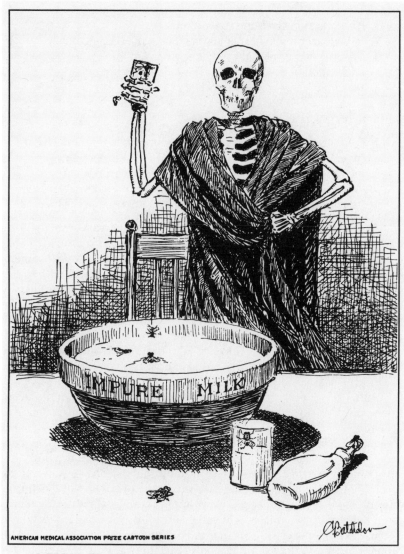

"I DRINK TO THE GENERAL DEATH OF THE WHOLE TABLE"

Figure 15. **"I Drink to the General Death of the Whole Table"**
This cartoon was awarded the first prize by the American Medical Association. (From Rosenau, M. J., The Milk Question, Houghton Mifflin Company, Boston [1913]).

City in order to make pasteurized milk available to anyone who wanted it. He even produced a gadget, called the Straus Home Pasteurizer, for those who were not able to obtain pasteurized products from the local dairy. Despite all his monumental efforts, the early history of pasteurized milk reflected a constant uphill battle. However, the practical reality of providing a reliable supply of safe milk to consumers in large urban centers was an almost impossible problem, and milk pasteurization began to be carried out in secret. The clandestine pasteurization of milk was outlawed in New York City in 1906, and an ordinance stated that all pasteurized milk had to be clearly labeled. People even demanded tests be developed to check if milk was pasteurized or not. Many eminent and influential people continued to believe that raw milk was still the best and did everything they could to persuade others. In fact, many people continue to believe it to this very day—still others pay the dear price for this belief.

The ensuing debate delayed the introduction of pasteurization for a very long time. Thousands of people, especially children, died needlessly. Yet, the overwhelming body of scientific evidence conclusively demonstrated the benefits of pasteurization for improving the shelf life of milk and preventing the diseases associated with it.[93] In the end, little doubt remains that the popular press provided the pressure and incentive for manufacturers and lawmakers finally to guarantee that pasteurized milk would be made available to the consuming public. Thus, for the first time in history, the dairy industry was able to provide consumers with milk as acceptable and nutritious as raw milk but without the risk of the diseases normally associated with it. By the 1920s, pasteurized milk was commonly available throughout the United States and Canada and was considered compulsory in most large cities. Unfortunately, in most other parts of the world, the benefits it held for consumers took much longer to be appreciated.

As an example, in 1983, Scotland was one of the last countries in Europe to institute mandatory pasteurization laws. Before that time, the rate of milk-borne salmonellosis in Scotland was one of the highest in Europe. A year after the enactment of the legislation that made pasteurization compulsory, Scotland's rate of milk-borne salmonellosis dropped to one of the lowest. A study was then carried out on the remaining incidences of milk-borne salmonellosis in the three-year period immediately following compulsory pasteurization. Of the total of 15 outbreaks reported, all occurred in rural farming communities and none in the general urban population. After analysis, the researchers explained these incidents by the fact that milk consumed in remote farming districts was exempt from the compulsory pasteurization legislation that applied to the rest of the country. All the victims were among the very few consumers who had routine access to raw, unpasteurized milk.

Even cattle kept in the most modern sanitary facilities are subject to contamination from bedding, manure and other contaminating materials that cling to the bodies of the animals. Because some of the bacterial spores occasionally found in these contaminating materials can survive the limited temperature of pasteurization, farmers must take extreme care to ensure that the animal and its udders are thoroughly sanitized.

The modern movement of milk from the cow to the consumer involves a lot of equipment. This includes milking machines, pails, milk

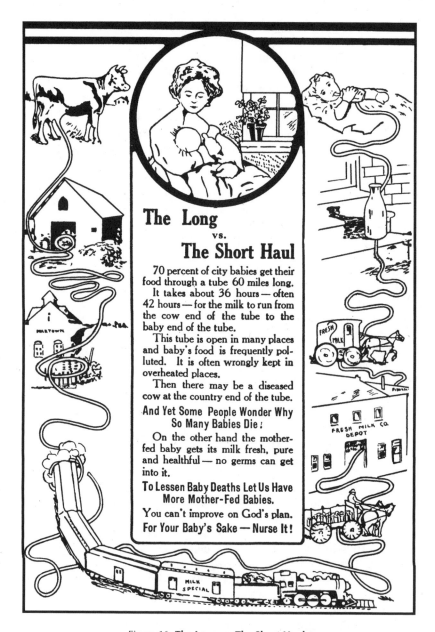

Figure 16. **The Long vs. The Short Haul**
This illustration was taken from the Weekly Bulletin *of the Chicago Health Department.*
(From Rosenau, M. J., The Milk Question, *Houghton Mifflin Company, Boston [1913]).*

cans, strainers, tubes, churns, coolers, tanks, tanker trucks and all the equipment involved in pasteurization. Milk is an excellent medium for bacterial growth. Therefore, all the surfaces, nooks and crannies of this equipment must be fully sanitized if milk and its products are to be of high quality. The sanitation and cleaning practices employed in most modern dairies achieve a very high level of effectiveness. Any neglect of continuous, strict sanitary practices can lead to residues of milkstone on the equipment. Milkstone is like tartar on teeth and can harbor large concentrations of bacteria.

The consumption of raw milk is not an acceptable heath risk. People who handle and process milk can be a significant source of pathogenic bacteria. The consumption of raw milk has caused numerous outbreaks of milk-borne typhoid fever, salmonellosis, diphtheria, scarlet fever and other intestinal diseases. Although raw milk may taste better, a century of experience with pasteurization has clearly proven the usefulness of this process in almost totally removing the risk from serious pathogens. Although not as popular in North America as in Europe, the UHT (ultra high temperature) or ultra pasteurization process allows unopened products to be safely stored for four to six months at room temperature. When these products were first introduced, they had a distinct burned milk taste. However, advances in technology have virtually eliminated this, and many expect that these products will become more popular in the future. The newer, microfiltered milk has the advantage of filtering out the bacteria while retaining a farm-fresh flavor.

Even human milk has the potential to place infants at risk. Recent studies have conclusively shown that the HIV virus can be transmitted through the breast milk of infected mothers.[94, 95] Studies published in the mid-1990s[96, 97, 98] provided estimates of the excess risk of HIV-1 transmission attributable to breast-feeding ranging from 4 percent to 22 percent. In 1997 and 1998,[99] the WHO, along with the United Nations Children's Fund (UNICEF) and the Joint United Nations Program on HIV/AIDS (UNAIDS), issued revised recommendations regarding breast-feeding and HIV-1 transmission. These recommendations called for giving women access to HIV-1 counseling and testing as well as information that would allow them to make fully informed decisions regarding infant feeding.

In addition to HIV-1 transmission, human breast milk has been implicated as a possible vehicle for the transmission of the West Nile virus.[100] Thus, the most respected nutrient in human history, delivered under the most sterile conditions, still carries a risk if infectious contamination occurs at the source of production. Fortunately, the vast majority of milk consumed is pasteurized. No better proof of the value of pasteurization can exist than the vicious spate of enterohemorrhagic *E. coli* outbreaks during the past few years. Most of these outbreaks have been associated with the consumption of beef. Milk comes from the same animals and carries the same risk. Milk could easily have been responsible for a great number of additional enterohemorrhagic *E. coli* outbreaks. Fortunately, the technology to destroy these bacteria before they reach the consumer prevents this from happening. Unfortunately, although modern technology can do the same for beef, it is not employed. Disease outbreaks inevitably result.

The same precautions employed in milk production must, of course, be followed for all other milk products such as cheeses, ice cream and dry milk products. Such items should start with pasteurized milk and be processed in a manner that will not introduce any viable pathogens into the finished products. This problem is compounded in products such as ice cream, which may have eggs or egg yolks added to the formula. If these contain pathogens such as salmonella, the entire batch of ice cream becomes contaminated. Even though ice cream is frozen and can be easily tested before consumption, this has proven to be no obstacle to food poisoning. As an example, in the summer of 1994, a contaminated batch of ice cream was shipped to more than 40 states so rapidly that thousands of people experienced ill effects before it could be recalled.

Cheeses are another category of products that have experienced occasional problems over the years. Cheeses made from pasteurized milk using sanitary hygienic practices are generally very reliable. However, certain cheeses are not made from pasteurized milk. The famous French soft cheeses made from raw milk (such as Brie and Camembert) have often been implicated in food-borne disease outbreaks.[101, 102] Even in Europe, where unpasteurized milk is not uncommon, risk exists for contracting epidemic strains of *Listeria monocytogenes,* which has been linked to outbreaks in blue-mold cheese and other hard cheeses.[103] Even when pasteurized milk is used, poor manufacturing practices or the handling of products by infected workers can contaminate products with pathogens such as *Staphylococcus aureus, Listeria,* Salmonella and *E. coli.*

PRIMARY PATHOGENS OF EGG PRODUCTS

BACTERIAL—yes	✔ *Salmonella* species
☐ *Bacillus cereus*	☐ *Shigella* species
✔ *Campylobacter jejuni*	☐ *Staphylococcus aureus*
☐ *Clostridium botulinum*	☐ *Streptococcus* species
☐ *Clostridium perfringens*	☐ *Vibrio* species
☐ Enterohemorrhagic *E. coli*	☐ *Yersinia*
☐ Enteroinvasive *E. coli*	FUNGAL—no
☐ Enteropathogenic *E. coli*	PARASITIC—no
☐ Enterotoxigenic *E. coli*	TOXIC SUBSTANCES—no
☐ *Helicobacter pylori*	VIRAL—possible
☐ *Listeria monocytogenes*	

OUTBREAK INCIDENTS WITH EGGS

This Case Is Personal!

When my daughter Heather was two years old, she accompanied her grandfather on a visit to the community medical center for his annual checkup. Once everything was completed, they decided to have lunch at the small snack bar located in the same building. The egg sandwiches looked good, so that's what they decided to have. A day later, both Heather and her grandfather came down with diarrhea. While her grandfather only suffered discomfort, which he put down to the stomach flu, my daughter quickly developed a very high fever.

We took Heather to our family pediatrician who immediately asked us to bring her to the hospital. As far as he was concerned, she was a very sick child who was exhibiting all the signs of typhoid fever. She had a temperature of 105°F that would not come down with the conventional antibiotic treatment. In order to keep her fever down, the pediatrician had her placed on a special ice-water mattress. It's impossible to forget the sight of this tiny little two-year-old lying prostrate on this freezing mattress, glistening with sweat.

She remained this way for more than a week before the fever broke and began to come down. The blood tests that the pediatrician ordered did not show *Salmonella typhosa*, but rather *Salmonella montevideo*, which was eventually traced to the eggs. As it turned out, the whole family eventually was analyzed positive for the bacteria, presumably because of close contact with one another. It took more than one month before everyone tested negative.

Thank God, Heather survived, but she has never been quite the same as far as eating is concerned. She immediately became a very fussy eater and to this day continues to have an extremely sensitive digestive system—25 years later. All this, from one lousy egg sandwich!

Salmonella Goes to College[104]

Between May 3 and May 9, 1988, almost 50 percent of the 188 students in a Fort Monmouth, New Jersey, college preparatory school contracted severe gastroenteritis. These young people experienced the full effect of a salmonella outbreak—severe diarrhea, abdominal pain and cramps, headache and fever. One-third of those that got sick had to be hospitalized. Fortunately, they all recovered. Each one of those affected tested positive for *Salmonella enteritidis*. The source of infection? Someone wanted the students to have a treat, so they brought in homemade ice cream, made with Grade A raw eggs.

EGG PRODUCTS

In the context of this book, eggs refer to chicken eggs, although eggs from ducks, turkeys, geese and quail are also available in many places. Eggs are enormously popular because of their nutritional value, convenience and easy preparation. Despite their simple appearance and preparation, eggs themselves are far more complex than they would first seem.

An eggshell is made of two layers—a thin, outer protein film called the cuticle and the thick, calcium carbonate shell itself. The liquid egg material (yolk and white) is held within a tough outer and a fine inner membrane. All in all, nature has provided the simple egg with a rather sophisticated package. Since an egg is normally sterile to start with, it does not really require refrigeration—although refrigeration does retard the natural chemical and enzymatic activities that can lower the overall flavor and functionality (such as egg white whipping ability) of eggs. Commercially, eggs are often sprayed with a very light coating of oil to protect against moisture loss.

Although eggs are normally free from microorganisms, contamination can occasionally enter through the chicken's oviduct. Over the years several large-scale incidents of egg contamination have occurred, particularly with salmonella.[105, 106] The largest of these occurred in 1988 in the United Kingdom and was ultimately responsible for the resignation of the Junior Minister of Health.

When eggs are laid, they share a common exit—the cloaca—with the intestinal contents. Consequently, the material on the eggs's surface could easily serve as a source of contamination if the complex shell did not provide excellent protective, barrier properties. The cuticle is the first line of defense. It prevents the entry of moisture and microorganisms, since the calcium carbonate shell itself is porous and would allow easy access for bacteria. The frequency and size of the pores are greatest in the blunt end of the eggs. If the cuticle is damaged, the eggs are much more susceptible to contamination.

Eggs are collected manually or, in large operations, they roll down troughs and then are sent for candling. Candling tests eggs for blood clots, fertility and growth. Once this is completed, they are then cleaned and, in some cases, oiled with a light coating of mineral oil. The cuticle is very resistant to water, but abrasion will damage it. Therefore, any washing employed to clean filth off eggs should be accompanied by only very gentle rubbing. About a week after the eggs are laid, the cuticle starts to dry out and crack, leaving the eggs susceptible to contamination.

In 2006, researchers with the U.S. Department of Agriculture (USDA) together with colleagues from Auburn University studied the frequency of salmonella, *Campylobacter, Listeria* and other pathogens in eggs that were commercially washed in cool water. Their findings were reported in the *Journal of Food Safety*.[107]

Routinely, egg processors use wash water kept at 90°F, or 20°F higher than the warmest egg entering the processing line in order to meet USDA quality standards. The eggs must also be sprayed with a sanitizing rinse that is kept at the same temperature as the wash water. The eggs are then cooled to prevent pathogen growth.

The researchers tested three different water temperature schemes. The first test used water at 120°F for both washes of the eggs. The second used water at 120°F for the first wash and 75°F for the second. The third used water at 75°F for both washes.

The results indicated that using warm water in the first wash and cooler water in the second wash could provide the greatest benefit by reducing egg temperature and microbial levels. It is likely that the temperature shock was sufficient to prevent growth of bacteria.

Eggs are generally stored with the blunt end up to prevent the yolk from drifting toward the inner membrane. At home, keep eggs dry because they are most sensitive when wet. Salmonella is the only significant pathogen of eggs, although other organisms such as streptococcus have also been implicated.[108] Although pathogens can enter the egg through the hen's ovaries, the more common route of contamination is from the outside environment. Salmonella does not affect the odor or appearance of eggs and thus gives no indication of contamination. The consumption of such eggs is hazardous unless they are cooked sufficiently to harden the yolk. This is a particular problem in commercial catering or processing operations where one egg can contaminate an entire batch of finished products such as mayonnaise.

Salmonella is the principal microbial problem in dried egg powder and has been responsible for many outbreaks through either direct consumption or cross contamination in the kitchen. Products such as cake or pancake mixes contain significant quantities of egg powder. It is a major ingredient in large commercial baking operations. Large quantities of egg powder are routinely rejected because of high microbial loads. Despite the availability of modern methods to manage this problem, contaminated products continue to find their way to the market.

FRUITS, VEGETABLES AND NUTS

Much to the surprise and consternation of everyone, fruits and vegetables are proving to be a far greater problem in the transmission of foodborne diseases than had previously been thought. A good part of the problem results from increasing produce consumption coupled with a much greater proportion of goods coming from countries where hygienic controls and agricultural practices leave much to be desired. Incidents of contamination with parasites such as *Giardia* and *Cyclospora* and bacteria such as salmonella and *E. coli* O157:H7 have been recently reported.

PRIMARY PATHOGENS OF FRUITS AND VEGETABLES

BACTERIAL—yes

✔ *Bacillus cereus*

☐ *Campylobacter jejuni*

✔ *Clostridium botulinum*

✔ *Clostridium perfringens*

✔ **Enterohemorrhagic *E. coli***

✔ **Enteroinvasive *E. coli***

✔ **Enteropathogenic *E. coli***

☐ Enterotoxigenic *E. coli*

☐ *Helicobacter pylori*

☐ *Listeria monocytogenes*

☐ *Salmonella* species

☐ *Shigella* species

✔ *Staphylococcus aureus*

☐ *Streptococcus* species

☐ *Vibrio* species

☐ *Yersinia enterocolitica*

FUNGAL—no

VIRAL—possible

PARASITIC—yes

☐ *Anisakis simplex*

☐ *Ascaris lumbricoides*

✔ *Cryptosporidium parvum*

✔ *Cyclospora cayetanensis*

✔ *Entamoeba hystolytica*

✔ *Fasciola hepatica*

✔ **Giardia lamblia**

☐ *Nanophyetus salmincola*

☐ *Opisthorchis viverrini*

☐ *Taenia saginata*

☐ *Taenia solium*

☐ *Toxoplasma gondii*

☐ *Trichinella spiralis*

☐ *Trichuris trichiura*

TOXIC SUBSTANCES—yes

✔ **Cyanogenetic glycosides**

✔ **Goitrogens**

✔ **Hemagglutinins**

✔ **Oxalates**

✔ **Pressor amines**

✔ **Solanine**

They have prompted public health officials to caution consumers to decontaminate produce before consumption.[109] Unfortunately, no simple, effective decontamination procedures exist.

OUTBREAK INCIDENTS WITH FRUITS AND VEGETABLES

Trouble in Veggie Land

Spinach has been recommended as a healthy food for hundreds of years. First cultivated in Iran (Persia) more than 2,000 years ago, spinach was introduced to China in the 600s and to Spain around 1,100 C.E. By the time of the Renaissance, the dark leafy green was well established in Europe. Spaniards brought it to America, where it eventually became the first vegetable to be frozen and sold commercially by Birds Eye Frosted Foods in 1930. Today, fresh spinach is available and distributed year round, mainly from California and Texas.

On September 13, 2006, CDC officials were alerted by epidemiologists in Wisconsin and Oregon that fresh spinach was the suspected source of small clusters of *E. coli* O157:H7 infections in those states. On the same day, New Mexico epidemiologists reported a cluster of *E. coli* O157:H7 infections in that state, also associated with fresh spinach consumption.

By September 26, a total of 183 people infected with the outbreak strain of *E. coli* O157:H7 were reported to the CDC from 26 states across the country. Among the ill, 52 percent were hospitalized, 16 percent experienced the terrible effects of hemolytic uremic syndrome (HUS) and one person died. Eighty-five percent reported the onset of their illnesses from August 19 to September 5 and 95 percent reported that they had consumed uncooked fresh spinach during the 10 days before the onset.

The health scare over bacteria-ridden spinach went nationwide, as the scale of the outbreak became apparent. The outbreak was first traced to organic bagged fresh spinach grown on a small farm in San Benito County, California. Investigators with the CDC initially speculated that the dangerous bacteria originated from irrigation water contaminated with cattle feces.

A follow-up report by the California Department of Health Services and the FDA concluded that the probable source of the *E. coli* outbreak was a 50-acre cattle ranch that had leased land to spinach grower Mission Organics.

Ultimately, more than 200 people were sickened and three died. Although the final report was unable to positively pinpoint the exact cause of the outbreak,[110] what became readily apparent was that the commercial growing of spinach—even organic spinach—was concentrated in just a few operations. One organic lettuce producer marketed products under more than 30 well-known national brand names across the country. Thus, a problem on one large farm can potentially affect the entire country in an incredibly short period of time. Strategically, this is a situation that presents a significant risk.

Considering our new understanding of the critical importance of vegetables to the diet, much greater attention will have to be paid to the food safety of this category of foods.

Just a Poona Melon[111]

June 1991—school's out, and it's time to enjoy the healthy and refreshing fruits of summer. Out of nowhere, more than 400 infections with *Salmonella poona* occur in 23 states as well as in Canada—all confirmed by laboratory analysis. Typical signs were diarrhea, nausea, vomiting, cramps and fever, in some cases lasting almost two weeks.

Extensive investigation and testing by the Public Health Laboratories of Illinois and Michigan came to the conclusion that the probable common origin was cantaloupes from the Rio Grande region of Texas. The same *S. poona* struck again in June at a New Jersey party. The 75 people attending ate a fruit salad containing the same Texas cantaloupe. No sooner had this happened then reports started trickling in from Canada. This outbreak was an excellent example of the way in which mass distribution can affect a very wide area very quickly.

Tacos—The Plumber's Nightmare[112]

The Albuquerque youth group dined at their church once a week on home-cooked food prepared by the parents. This is not the sort of function where you would expect people to come down with long-term diarrhea, but many of them did. Most of them experienced symptoms including fatigue, diarrhea, abdominal cramps and unintentional loss of weight. The required stool specimens revealed a grim story—more than 70 percent were positive for cysts of the parasite *Giardia lamblia*. With the exception of the store-bought salsa, all of the possible foods implicated had been made in the church's kitchen facilities by eight mothers of the youth group children. Five of them soon came down with diarrhea. When they were tested, three were found to be positive for *Giardia*.

As it happened, the lettuce and tomatoes used in the homemade tacos had been rinsed in the kitchen's sink, whose water came from the municipal water system. A quick study of potential cross contamination between the church's drinking water system and the sewer system revealed five possible connections. The plumbing was quickly fixed.

Fly by Night . . . and Day[113]

This unusual case is not really a normal food-borne disease incident, but it clearly illustrates the need for proper food handling. From June to August 1984, a Washington mother of a one-year-old girl frequently saw worms in her child's stool, but no other symptoms. Her doctor treated the girl for pinworm infection, but her mother continued to see worms in the bowel movement. Later that year, fly maggots were noticed in two stool specimens that the mother collected. Yet, no one else in the family had the same symptoms.

Later, more in-depth probing into the young child's dietary history showed that she had been fed over-ripe bananas that had been kept in a wire basket hanging in the warm kitchen. Flies were regularly seen swarming around that fruit basket. The exposed fruit was immediately covered and the parents made sure to wash it every time before serving. A short while later all evidence of fly maggots in the child's stool disappeared.

Intestinal myiasis arises when fly eggs that were previously deposited on foods are eaten and manage to survive the rigorous conditions of the gastrointestinal tract. It is very rare, but does occur. In fact, other forms of myiasis can occur involving the skin, eye, ear, nose, throat and urinary tract. The only way to prevent it is to control the source of the eggs—the mama fly!

Church Elders[114]

In August 1983, eight people who attended a religious conference in a remote, isolated district of Monterey County, California, came down with gastrointestinal and neurologic problems that were so acute they had to be air-lifted by helicopter to a Monterey hospital. Earlier that day, they had taken a break for some refreshments and within 15 minutes began to experience nausea and vomiting. Then came abdominal cramps, dizziness and weakness. They were in pretty bad shape when they were evacuated but, within four hours, the patients became stable and soon recovered fully.

As it turned out, the staff of the religious center had gathered wild elderberries to prepare the refreshment juice. In true natural style, the berries were crushed together with their leaves and stems in a stainless-steel juice press. The elderberry juice was blended with a bit of apple juice, chilled and then served the next day to the hard-working study group. Unfortunately, the juice must have been very good, because the degree of illness corresponded to the amount of consumed. The only individual who was hospitalized happened to have chugged down five glasses of the stuff!

While elderberries themselves are juicy and edible, their leaves, flowers, bark and roots contain a glycoside that can produce hydrocyanic acid, probably as a natural defense against insects. This breaks down in the body and means cyanide poisoning! The amount of hydrocyanic acid produced is high in the leaves. As with cassava, the roots are likely the most poisonous part of the plant and have been responsible for killing pigs and other animals that ate them.

FRUITS

A fruit is usually defined as that portion of a plant that contains the seeds. This definition includes cucumbers and tomatoes, which are more commonly thought of as vegetables. The majority of fruits are high in acidity, a characteristic that has a significant impact on the type of contamination they experience. Many of the soil-borne, dust-borne and insect-borne bacteria cannot grow well at the acidity levels common in most fruits.

Because fruit is generally fragile, it must be handled very carefully after harvesting. Once injured, even slightly, the fruit becomes very susceptible to infection and spoilage. The greatest microbial problem with fruit is mold because molds can tolerate high acidity. Not only do molds destroy the fruit quality, but they can also produce hazardous mycotoxins. Carefully check all fruits to ensure that they are free of mold prior to consumption. Do not simply remove the external evidence of mold since some of the mycotoxins produced could have entered into the flesh of the fruit.

A growing problem is also associated with fecal contamination resulting from animal or human sources. The use of untreated sewage or agriculturally contaminated runoff water for irrigation can result in highly contaminated finished products. The recent move toward organic gardening has resulted in occasional malpractice that can very adversely affect consumers of these products.

Human fecal waste—often referred to as night soil—is considered by some to be an excellent natural fertilizer. Unfortunately, along with any nutrients, it also contains all the pathogenic bacteria and parasites harbored by the producer. If the farmer applies human fecal waste directly to the field, an excellent model of a closed reinfection cycle occurs if the producer consumes his or her own products. Unfortunately, once sold commercially, the product spreads contamination to distant markets. It is therefore vital that only sterilized night soil be permitted for use. If not, problems such as salmonella in melons arise, an occurrence thought to be very unlikely under any other conditions. More recently, an increasing number of very serious outbreaks have involved fruit berries infected with *Cyclospora* parasites and hepatitis A virus.

A number of recent outbreaks with tragic consequences involving unpasteurized apple juice made with ground-tagged apples (apples that have fallen to the ground and laid there until collected) have occurred. The juice sold was unpasteurized in order to give a natural, organic appeal to consumers. Unfortunately, ground-tagged apples are exposed to high levels of dirt and manure. As a result, they are an excellent vehicle for the transmission of all types of pathogenic microorganisms, including enterohemorrhagic *E. coli* O157:H7. The results were lethal, tragic and unnecessary.

The natural acidity of fruit provides supplemental protection for canned or frozen fruit products. These items seldom pose major problems. Dried fruit, however, can support the growth of molds, such as *Aspergillus flavus*. Improperly dried products that have been infected may contain aflatoxins. Pickled products such as olives and cucumbers can spoil and get moldy, but finding any documented cases of food poisoning caused by them has been difficult. The salt and acidity of the finished products are the critical factors in controlling pathogens.

VEGETABLES

Vegetables are defined as those parts of a plant that are edible, including stalks, roots, tubers, bulbs, flowers and seeds. They are generally not as acidic as fruits and, consequently, are more susceptible to microbial contamination. Soil, dust, insects and water are the chief vectors of contaminating organisms, just as with fruit.

Like fruit, contamination can easily occur if growing areas are irrigated with water containing untreated animal or human waste. This mode of contamination can include parasites in addition to pathogenic bacteria. The use of unsterilized night soil will result in the same kind of contamination. Night soil fertilization of fruits and vegetables has been implicated in outbreaks of typhoid fever, cholera, hepatitis, and amebiasis in Asian countries.[115] Salmonella in night soil has caused outbreaks associated with celery, lettuce, cabbages and watercress. Pathogens have been found on all vegetables, including homegrown sprouts. Picking and handling of vegetables is another source of contamination, particularly if the workers employed are not accommodated in sanitary housing conditions. Vegetable products have also been recently implicated in the transmission of viruses and parasitic infections in North America.[116, 117] Even more disturbing are some of the more modern products such as bagged washed salad, which almost everyone uses without prior washing. Some of these products, which have had nationwide distribution, originated in dirty, slapdash operations. These products were completely exposed to the environment, which included cattle and their manure.

The resultant *E. coli* O157:H7-laden lettuce precipitated severe food-borne disease incidents.

Frozen vegetables have almost never been implicated in food poisoning. Once the fresh material arrives at the plant, it is thoroughly washed and generally receives a quick blanching treatment to prevent enzymatic degradation after freezing. As a result, frozen vegetables have fairly low bacterial loads. Canned vegetables do not have quite the same record of safety. Because they are lower in acid than fruits, canned vegetables must receive sufficient heat treatment to destroy all the *Clostridium botulinum* spores—the so-called botch cook.

Despite all the care taken in the commercial sterilization of products through canning, several possibilities for contamination clearly exist. In the first instance, whether it be equipment failure or operator error, products may be improperly cooked or underprocessed.[118] Despite an excellent record of quality, cans can occasionally have microscopic pin holes in them that might allow contamination to enter. Once the cooking process is completed, the cans are rapidly cooled in order to minimize heat damage to the products. The can seams themselves may not be perfectly sealed, and buckling could allow contaminated cooling water to enter. These situations occurred in the past and have lead to serious food-poisoning incidents.

Despite all this, commercial canning has an incredibly good reputation. When considering the number of cans produced annually, the insignificant ratio of spoiled products is truly extraordinary. While a few isolated cases may have made the headlines in the past, by far the majority of botulism cases result from home canning, not commercial products.

Consumers can exercise a simple precaution. Ensure that all canned vegetables and other canned foods with low acid content are cooked before consumption. Botulism toxin is very sensitive to heat, and minimum cooking easily destroys it. Even canned soups such as vichyssoise should first be cooked and then cooled prior to serving.

The most obvious sign of spoilage in canned foods is swelling. When buying canned goods, avoid products that have been damaged because the can is more susceptible to contamination. The lid of the can should always be slightly concave, not flat and definitely not bulging. If in doubt, check with the store manager. If you discover such a product at home, throw it out or bring it back to the store where you purchased it. The manufacturer will appreciate knowing that some problems exist with the company's products. The same can be said for dehydrated products. Because dried vegetables do not contain the same level of natural acids as fruits do, these products are susceptible to a wide range of microorganisms, some of which may be pathogenic. Complete cooking is the rule, even though most products have received a blanching step prior to drying.

Notwithstanding their strong smell and appearance, few, if any, well-documented cases exist of food poisoning caused by fermented vegetables such as sauerkraut or kimchi. Again, the combination of salt and acid severely limits the growth of pathogens.

PRIMARY PATHOGENS OF NUTS

BACTERIAL—no

☐ *Bacillus cereus*

☐ *Campylobacter jejuni*

☐ *Clostridium botulinum*

☐ *Clostridium perfringens*

☐ Enterohemorrhagic *E. coli*

☐ Enteroinvasive *E. coli*

☐ Enteropathogenic *E. coli*

☐ Enterotoxigenic *E. coli*

☐ *Helicobacter pylori*

☐ *Listeria monocytogenes*

☐ *Salmonella* species

☐ *Shigella* species

☐ *Staphylococcus aureus*

☐ *Streptococcus* species

☐ *Vibrio* species

☐ *Yersinia enterocolitica*

FUNGAL—yes

✔ **Mycotoxins**

PARASITIC—yes

☐ *Anisakis simplex*

☐ *Ascaris lumbricoides*

☐ *Cryptosporidium parvum*

☐ *Cyclospora cayetanensis*

☐ *Entamoeba hystolytica*

☐ *Fasciola hepatica*

☐ *Giardia lamblia*

☐ *Nanophyetus salmincola*

☐ *Opisthorchis viverrini*

☐ *Taenia saginata*

☐ *Taenia solium*

☐ *Toxoplasma gondii*

☐ *Trichinella spiralis*

☐ *Trichuris trichiura*

TOXIC SUBSTANCES—no

VIRAL—possible

✔ **Allergies**

NUTS

The nuts we generally consume include peanuts, almonds, cashews, walnuts, brazil nuts and pecans. They can be divided into tree nuts and ground nuts (peanuts). However, the susceptibility to contamination is very similar in both groups. The key problem is mold infections that produce hazardous mycotoxins. In the case of peanuts, mold contamination is almost inevitable simply because peanuts grow in the ground. The shell or seed case can prevent invasion by molds only to a limited extent. Proper harvesting and drying practices are critical in reducing mold contamination to a minimum. Even then, products must be inspected to eliminate any evidence of mold. This can be done manually or by electric-eye sorters after the seeds have been removed from their shells. Nuts must be stored under very low moisture conditions to prevent further mold growth.

Unless the shells have been physically damaged, tree nuts contain very low levels of microbes. However, they are subject to attack by birds and insects, which often break the shells. After this, contamination quickly follows. Any nuts falling directly to the ground will be tainted with whatever contaminants are present in the soil. As with ground nuts, harvesting, cleaning and drying procedures are critical in ensuring minimum damage to tree nuts. Moisture can creep into the seams of shells and split them, thus making them much more susceptible to mold contamination.

Worldwide attention was focused on *Aspergillus flavus* in 1961 when British scientists reported a rash of fatal liver disease outbreaks among animals fed commercial feeds containing Brazilian peanut meal. The condition was eventually labeled turkey X disease because of the great number of young turkeys that perished. The common occurrence of mold contamination in peanuts, combined with the severity of symptoms, alerted the entire food and medical community to the problem of aflatoxins. This ultimately led to much greater analysis and control over all mycotoxin-based contamination in the food and feed industry.

Aside from whole nuts, the consumer product with the greatest potential for mycotoxin contamination is peanut butter. Since peanut butter is generally homogenized, one or two highly contaminated nuts can ruin an entire batch. This is why peanut butter is such a highly controlled food product. Consumers who wish to make their own peanut butter or buy freshly made peanut butter at a home style supplier should make an attempt to ensure that all peanuts have been carefully inspected prior to grinding and blending. Mycotoxins are very heat resistant, and frying or roasting does not eliminate them.

GRAIN AND FLOUR PRODUCTS

Throughout the world, cereals such as wheat, rice and corn are the most abundant and most available staple foods. Food grains are all characterized by a starch content in the range of 70 to 80 percent and a protein content of 8 to 15 percent. The moisture content of these dried grains is generally between 10 and 15 percent.

Grains therefore serve as the world's chief source of food energy. To a majority of the world's population, they also provide a large portion of the daily protein requirements—usually complemented with beans or nuts. Because of their low moisture content, grains are not subject to attack by any microorganisms other than mold. They are, however, very susceptible to attack from insects, birds and rodents and also the waste materials they produce.

PRIMARY PATHOGENS OF GRAIN AND FLOUR PRODUCTS

BACTERIAL—yes	FUNGAL—yes
✔ *Bacillus cereus*	✔ **Mycotoxins**
☐ *Campylobacter jejuni*	PARASITIC—yes
✔ *Clostridium botulinum*	☐ *Anisakis simplex*
✔ *Clostridium perfringens*	☐ *Ascaris lumbricoides*
☐ Enterohemorrhagic *E. coli*	☐ *Cryptosporidium parvum*
☐ Enteroinvasive *E. coli*	☐ *Cyclospora cayetanensis*
☐ Enteropathogenic *E. coli*	☐ *Entamoeba hystolytica*
☐ Enterotoxigenic *E. coli*	☐ *Fasciola hepatica*
☐ *Helicobacter pylori*	☐ *Giardia lamblia*
☐ *Listeria monocytogenes*	☐ *Nanophyetus salmincola*
✔ *Salmonella* species	☐ *Opisthorchis viverrini*
✔ *Shigella* species	☐ *Taenia saginata*
✔ *Staphylococcus aureus*	☐ *Taenia solium*
☐ *Streptococcus* species	☐ *Toxoplasma gondii*
☐ *Vibrio* species	☐ *Trichinella spiralis*
☐ *Yersinia enterocolitica*	☐ *Trichuris trichiura*
VIRAL—possible	TOXIC SUBSTANCES—no

OUTBREAK INCIDENTS WITH FLOUR PRODUCTS

Molding History[119]

The golden age of Greece ended when Sparta began the 27-year-long Peloponnesian War by attacking Athens in 431 B.C.E. Casualties were enormous, although most were not the result of battle, but rather a devastating plague that spread throughout the city.

The plague of Athens, which played such a critical role in the outcome of the Peloponnesian War, has occupied scholars for many years. Was it bubonic plague, dengue fever, Ebola virus, influenza or measles? These possibilities are unlikely because the symptoms described by Thucydides in his comprehensive record do not match those diseases. The symptoms do, however, support a far more logical explanation that involves the consumption of contaminated food.

In *The History of the Peloponnesian War,* written in 431 B.C.E., Thucydides, who lived in Athens during the plague, gave an eyewitness account of the events. His description of the plague and its symptoms follows in this translation by Richard Crawley.[120]

> . . . people in good health were all of a sudden attacked by violent heats in the head, and redness and inflammation in the eyes, the inward parts, such as the throat or tongue. . . . When it fixed in the stomach, it upset it; and discharges of bile of every kind named by physicians ensued, accompanied by very great distress. . . . Externally the body was not very hot to the touch, nor pale in its appearance, but reddish, livid, and breaking out into small pustules and ulcers. But internally it burned so that the patient could not bear to have on him clothing or linen even of the very lightest description. . . . What they would have liked best would have been to throw themselves into cold water; as indeed was done by some of the neglected sick, who plunged into the rain-tanks in their agonies of unquenchable thirst; though it made no difference whether they drank little or much. . . . when they succumbed, as in most cases, on the seventh or eighth day to the internal inflammation, they had still some strength in them. . . . even where it did not prove mortal, it still left its mark on the extremities; the fingers and the toes, and many escaped with the loss of these, some too with that of their eyes.

This account challenges the description of most of the diseases that have been suggested, yet, more than a century ago, Rudolf Kobert[121] suggested that the plague was the result of long-term effects of ergot poisoning. This idea was originally challenged because ergot is found mainly on rye, a grain which the Athenians did not traditionally eat. However, the Athenians did eat wheat and a very similar disease resulting from moldy wheat is called alimentary toxic aleukia or ATA. Many symptoms that were described by Thucydides were also described in an epidemic of ATA that occurred in Russia during World War II. Thousands of people died a tragic death as a result.

Bagels Anyone?[122]

Bagels are not the sort of product that is normally associated with food poisoning, and niacin, one of the important B-vitamins, is not your usual type of toxin. Yet on April 27, 1983, 20 percent of the people attending a brunch came up against a harmful combination of the two. They experienced an acute rash and pruritis (itching).

Fortunately, these symptoms did not last very long. The bagels had been produced at a local bagel bakery. Investigations revealed that on three other recent occasions, individuals who had consumed bagels from the same bakery had gone to the hospital with similar symptoms.

Further investigations disclosed 60 times the normal level of niacin was added to the pumpernickel flour in order to enrich it. Based on these calculations, each individual bagel had contained two full weeks supply of niacin for the average adult!

If the Sushi Fits . . .[123]

On September 22, 1985, while still on the premises, several customers of a Maine Japanese restaurant complained of severe gastrointestinal illness. In cooperation with Health Department officials, the restaurant owner immediately closed the restaurant, pending the results of an investigation.

When contacted, the customers complained of diarrhea, nausea, vomiting, abdominal cramps and headache. This outbreak had a very rapid onset with one of the individuals experiencing symptoms within a half-hour of eating. Although most symptoms were gone within several days, some of the victims still had diarrhea more than two weeks later. Some people had to be hospitalized and placed on rehydration therapy.

Laboratory analysis of the various foods eaten was not helpful because everybody in the restaurant ate the same sort of food—stir-fried rice, chicken soup, fried zucchini, onions, bean sprouts, fried shrimp, fresh cucumber, cabbage and lettuce salad, ginger salad dressing, hibachi chicken, etc., etc. As in many similar situations, everyone had tried everyone else's dishes.

Finally, one sample of vomit and two stool specimens revealed the presence of *Bacillus cereus*. Even though fried rice is often associated with *Bacillus cereus*, no connection could be made in this case. In fact, the only *Bacillus cereus*–positive food found was the hibachi steak. This steak was seasoned with soy sauce, salt and pepper prior to being sauteed at the table, directly in front of restaurant patrons in true hibachi style. Since raw beef is an unlikely source of *Bacillus cereus*, cross-contamination with fried rice stood out as a possible factor.

As long as grain is maintained in a dry state, the contamination caused by mold is minimal. Conversely, high moisture contents can lead to significant contamination. However, pathogenic bacteria are not normally a problem because grain is produced in large operations distant from animal and human activity. The exceptions are wild rice or Asian paddy rice, which are grown in conjunction with aquaculture operations.

During dry storage of grains, mold gradually dies, and only those varieties capable of surviving at very low moisture contents remain. As indicated, certain types of rice that contain heavy loads of microorganisms pose a particular problem. Once dried, however, the number of organisms in the rice is significantly reduced. Cooking usually brings this down to an insignificant level. Currently, these products are treated with a methyl bromide fumigant. However, this practice will be eliminated shortly due to the ozone-depleting and potential carcinogenic effects of this chemical.

Contamination with mycotoxins is the most important microbiologically based health concern of cereals. Although relatively rare, ergotism, alimentary toxic aleukia and aflatoxicosis outbreaks have occurred in the recent past. Symptoms of the various mycotoxin-related diseases will be described later. Although the moisture levels of most grains are too low to support the active growth of bacteria, they can carry very large numbers of viable spores. Once these grains or the flours derived from them are used in formulated foods, the introduction of moisture allows the spores to germinate and recover their destructive potential.

When grain products are processed into flour, baked goods, pasta, breakfast foods and convenience foods, their economic value increases dramatically. As a result, they are subject to more careful control and inspection to ensure that this added value is not lost. Microbial loads in heat-processed products are naturally lower. The problems presented by pathogens are diminished unless introduced through other ingredients, such as the eggs in egg noodles.

Heating flour to 130°C (265°F) for four minutes will markedly reduce the level of bacteria, but this is not done commercially. At home, heating a one-inch layer of flour in an oven at 100°C (212°F) for 15 minutes has much the same effect. Only mold spores are able to survive baking temperatures above 100°C (212°F) at the center of the loaf. All subsequent mold problems in baked goods result from spores in the environment, on slicers and on cooling and wrapping equipment.

Because no cooking step occurs in the manufacturing of pasta, microbes have a tendency to increase rapidly during mixing and extrusion. As a result, microbial counts can be very high in pasta. The boiling required to cook pasta fully kills most of the microorganisms. Since people usually consume pasta shortly after it is cooked, this presents no hazards. Pasta salads are a special case and do pose potential problems, particularly if the dressings used do not have sufficient vinegar or acid to limit microbial growth. Salmonella can survive in dried pasta for several months. Do not mix pasta with moist foods unless first cooking it. No one should make a habit of chewing dried pasta.

Fresh pasta poses another type of problem. It is usually made by small operators, many of whom are not fully trained in hygiene and sanitation. Since by definition fresh pasta is not dried, it remains an excellent medium for bacterial growth. Aside from salmonella, *Staphylococcus aureus* can easily survive and multiply in this environment. If the *Staphylococcus aureus* produces a toxin, it will not be destroyed nor will it be fully leached out into the water during the cooking process. Therefore, the potential exists for staphylococcal poisoning. You must have confidence in the pasta maker and his or her cleanliness.

Cream- or custard-filled pastries are well-established agents of foodborne disease. These fillings are excellent substrates for the growth of all types of microorganisms. Staphylococcal food poisoning is a frequent problem here because of the poor handling practices and sanitation often found in small operations. (Half of the general population tests positive for the presence of *Staphylococcus aureus* on their skins.) Recently, several other pathogens have been implicated with the consumption of these types of products. You must keep such products refrigerated until ready to eat, although bacteria such as *Listeria* can survive and grow at reduced temperatures.

OTHER FOODS

SPICES AND HERBS

With very few exceptions, commercial spices and herbs are all grown and dried in the open air. Even when they are covered with screens, insects, birds and rodents manage to deposit their excreta directly onto these exposed products. Herbs and spices can also be contaminated by fine, windblown dust particles that contain essentially the same contaminants. This happens in even the most hygienic operations. Once the bacteria or molds take hold on the fresh herbs or spices, they cling tightly and are not easily removed. Although they often harbor a very high load of spores, herbs and spices are not good substrates for the active growth of microbes once they have been dried. However, whenever these ingredients are incorporated into high-moisture foods, such as sauces or prepared meats, the spores quickly germinate and severely contaminate the final products.

PRIMARY PATHOGENS OF SPICES, COCOA AND TEA

BACTERIAL—yes

✔ *Bacillus cereus*

☐ *Campylobacter jejuni*

☐ *Clostridium botulinum*

✔ *Clostridium perfringens*

☐ Enterohemorrhagic *E. coli*

☐ Enteroinvasive *E. coli*

✔ **Enteropathogenic *E. coli***

☐ Enterotoxigenic *E. coli*

☐ *Helicobacter pylori*

☐ *Listeria monocytogenes*

✔ ***Salmonella* species**

☐ *Shigella* species

☐ *Staphylococcus aureus*

☐ *Streptococcus* species

☐ *Vibrio* species

☐ *Yersinia enterocolitica*

FUNGAL—yes

✔ Mycotoxins

PARASITIC—yes

☐ *Anisakis simplex*

☐ *Ascaris lumbricoides*

☐ *Cryptosporidium parvum*

☐ *Cyclospora cayetanensis*

☐ *Entamoeba hystolytica*

☐ *Fasciola hepatica*

☐ *Giardia lamblia*

☐ *Nanophyetus salmincola*

☐ *Opisthorchis viverrini*

☐ *Taenia saginata*

☐ *Taenia solium*

☐ *Toxoplasma gondii*

☐ *Trichinella spiralis*

☐ *Trichuris trichiura*

TOXIC SUBSTANCES—no

VIRAL—no

From 1980 to 2000, the annual per capita consumption of spices in the United States increased from 2.2 to 3.5 pounds per person per year. Despite the fact that spices harbor various molds, fungi and bacteria, relatively few reports have documented this group of food ingredients as a cause of illness. More recently, however, the FDA observed an increased number of recalls of dried spices due to bacterial contamination. From 1970 to 2003, the FDA monitored 21 recalls involving 12 different spices contaminated with bacterial pathogens; in all but one case the recalled spices contained *Salmonella*, and paprika was the spice most often implicated in the recalls.

OUTBREAK INCIDENTS WITH SPICE PRODUCTS

Hot Pink Paprika?[124, 125]

Who would think that you can get sick from eating potato chips? Yet, if the conditions are right, you certainly can—and you would be in the company of many others. Between April and September of 1993, there was a national outbreak of salmonellosis in Germany that was traced to potato chips made by an internationally known company. Not surprisingly, most of the estimated 1,000 cases were in children below the age of 14 years.

In fact, the salmonella was traced to the paprika powder (called Hot Pink Paprika) that the chips were coated with. Spices are often the source of pathogenic microorganisms, but rarely in cases of dry finished products, such as potato chips, do they cause disease outbreaks. The high percentage of victims in the one- to four-year-old age bracket gave some cause for serious reflection. It was concluded that the generally lower gastric acid level of these children made them much more vulnerable than older people. It also dispelled the notion that salmonella activity is exclusively associated with active bacterial growth in the product consumed.

More than 3,000 tons of snack products seasoned with the contaminated paprika were recalled by the manufacture at a cost of approximately $25 million.

The level of spoilage and pathogenic microorganisms carried by herbs and spices is generally so high they must be decontaminated in some way prior to use. The actual components that give the distinctive flavors to herbs and spices are called essential oils. Most consumers are familiar with garlic, pepper or clove oils. Heat or steam treatment in various forms has been recommended as a means of destroying bacteria on herbs and spices. However, the flavorful essential oils are generally heat sensitive. Therefore, the most practical way to treat these materials is by a cold process. In the past, toxic gases such as ethylene oxide were used to kill the microorganisms on herbs and spices. Ethylene oxide, in particular, had critical operational problems. Aside from being a toxic gas, ethylene oxide can form a flammable and explosive mixture with air and thus poses a genuine hazard to workers. Nevertheless, it was the most popular treatment for the elimination of bacteria in spices for many years. Most consumers were not aware of this, because food labels never indicated this treatment even though residues could remain on the products. As a result of the foregoing problems, many countries either ban or severely restrict the use of chemical fumigants. Since the dilemma of pathogens in herbs and spices still remains, scientists generally consider food irradiation to be the most effective and safest method for their control.[126]

PRIMARY PATHOGENS OF MAYONNAISE, SALAD DRESSINGS AND OIL-BASED PRODUCTS

BACTERIAL—yes	✔ *Staphylococcus aureus*
☐ *Bacillus cereus*	☐ *Streptococcus* species
☐ *Clostridium botulinum*	☐ *Yersinia enterocolitica*
☐ *Clostridium perfringens*	PARASITIC—no
☐ Enteropathogenic *E. coli*	TOXIC SUBSTANCES—no
☐ *Helicobacter pylori*	VIRAL—possible
☐ *Listeria monocytogenes*	FUNGAL—yes
✔ *Salmonella* species	☐ Mycotoxins
☐ *Shigella* species	

OUTBREAK INCIDENTS WITH MAYONNAISE AND SALAD DRESSINGS

Et tu, Brute![127]

In October 1991, 15 persons who ate at a restaurant over a nine-day period developed severe gastroenteritis. With the exception of one individual, everyone had eaten Caesar salad. During the same outbreak, one-third of the restaurant's 78 workers also came down with diarrhea, cramps, nausea and fever.

The restaurant's Caesar salad dressing was prepared with three dozen egg yolks, olive oil, anchovies and garlic. Surprisingly, lemon juice or vinegar was not included. The dressing was then kept refrigerated approximately 8–12 hours until the restaurant closed. When the investigation was eventually concluded, the culprit was found to be *Salmonella enteritidis* in the eggs.

MAYONNAISE AND SALAD DRESSINGS

These products, which often contain potentially contaminated ingredients such as eggs and spices, are not normally a major problem because of their high acid content from vinegar or lemon juice. Nevertheless, improperly formulated mayonnaise has caused countless cases of food poisoning.[128] Unless the product has sufficient acid levels, the potential for microbial growth and consequent food poisoning is real.

Fresh, homemade mayonnaise poses a particular problem. Controlling the acid level is extremely difficult, and the final product is very often consumed before the acid has sufficient time to kill the pathogens. As a rule, the consumer should use 5 to 10 percent more acid than called for in the recipes and hold the product for at least two days before using it.

MARGARINE AND BUTTER

Margarine is not an item of concern except for certain diet products that have a high level of water and can therefore support the growth of bacteria. Even then, if the products are kept refrigerated, few problems arise. The situation is similar for butter except for those instances where unpasteurized milk is used or where the plant sanitation is poorly maintained.

OUTBREAK INCIDENTS WITH COCOA PRODUCTS

This Money Should Have Been Laundered![129]

In autumn of 1985, there was an international outbreak of salmonellosis traced back to Belgian chocolate. The products were the familiar gold foil-wrapped coins that parents so often give to kids as rewards or treats. The number of confirmed cases reported in Canada and the United States was limited to less than 40. However, the symptoms were fairly mild, so that it is likely that there was a higher degree of under-reporting then usual. Again, the majority of victims were very young children, underscoring their susceptibility to salmonellosis in low-moisture products that do not have active salmonella growth.

COCOA

One does not normally think of cocoa as a source of pathogens, but it is. Cocoa is derived from cocoa beans by a rather complicated process. Throughout this process, opportunities arise for cocoa to become contaminated. If the strictest of sanitation practices are not followed, the finished product can pose a potential hazard.

Cocoa pods are about the size of large avocados. Each pod contains about 30–40 beans together with the surrounding pulp. If the pod is undamaged, the beans and pulp are virtually sterile. Problems begin once the beans and pulp are removed for the fermentation process. The very act of removing the pod contents exposes these contents to the microorganisms commonly found in the soil and the environment. Just as with grapes, the organisms that initially dominate the fermentation process are yeasts. As the fermentation proceeds, however, the mass of pulp and beans becomes less acidic and also warmed by naturally generated heat. This permits other microorganisms to flourish, including various pathogens such as bacillus.

Tropical countries produce cocoa beans, and the conditions employed in the fermentation process can vary tremendously. In technically advanced operations, the beans are brought to a central facility and fermented under highly controlled and sanitary conditions. In other cases, the beans and pulp are simply laid out on the ground underneath the same trees from which they were harvested. Here, they are exposed to all the dust, birds, insects and animals, together with the attendant microorganisms, that occur in the local environment. Predictably, the hygienic quality of the final products reflects the conditions employed in the fermentation process.

After fermentation, the beans are dried, occasionally after washing off residual pulp. Again, the conditions employed can vary tremendously. In some tropical countries, I have witnessed beans drying on or beside an asphalt road fully exposed to all the elements. While the combination of sunlight and black asphalt provides an excellent source of heat, it also subjects the beans to dust, animal droppings and the ubiquitous oil and diesel fuels so common on these roads. The sun-drying process can require up to three to four weeks in areas of high humidity. Imagining the degree to which beans can be exposed to contamination during that time is not difficult. Artificial drying requires only two to three days. Unless the beans are fully dried, they will be subject to mold growth and the consequent production of mycotoxins.

The next step of bean roasting can be done in two ways—with or without the skin or shell. They are usually roasted whole, and the nib or meat of the bean (cotyledon) is then separated from the shell. Since roasting does not kill all the contaminating organisms (between 1 percent and 10 percent survive), from the hygienic point of view removing the shell before roasting is better.

The next operation is milling of the nibs, a process that yields a final chocolate product with over 50 percent fat and very low moisture (2 percent). This is a time-consuming process. Any microorganisms that survive it have had the opportunity to adjust to the low moisture levels.

This allows these organisms to survive for surprisingly long periods of time. Milk chocolate is made by the slow mixing of chocolate with milk powder, a process called conching.

The pathogen of greatest concern in cocoa and chocolate is salmonella. This organism has often been isolated from chocolate and has been known to survive in it for years. One recorded incident involved several hundred people and had a surprisingly high hospitalization rate of close to 40 percent. Postincident calculations estimated that several hundred thousand people may have been at risk from that one incident.[130]

Chocolate was one of the first products that provided strong evidence that large numbers of salmonella were not necessarily a prerequisite for human infection. Furthermore, it demonstrated that some food ingredients had the ability to protect salmonella against the harsh acidic conditions of the stomach. Even small numbers of salmonella present in the product could pass through the stomach with few losses and colonize the lower gastrointestinal tract to produce clinical symptoms. One of the more recent well-documented outbreaks of salmonella food poisoning associated with chocolate confirmed that international trade has the potential to introduce new or different food safety risks into the food supply of a great many importing countries at the same time.[131] From mid-October 2001 to February 2002, German health authorities received almost 400 reports of *Salmonella oranienburg* infections. More than 150 of the reported cases were of children younger than 10 years.

Chocolate from a particular supermarket chain was found to be the responsible agent. In addition to Germany, the chocolate was soon found to be responsible for similar outbreaks in Denmark, Sweden, Netherlands, Canada, Austria, Belgium, Australia, Finland and Croatia.

A growing problem with cocoa is that the countries of origin carry out more and more of the processing operations. Shifting the processing closer to production can theoretically result in a better product. However, unless these operations scrupulously adhere to the hygienic and sanitary standards required, an increased potential for contamination exists. Unfortunately, a consumer can do almost nothing about such a product because it exhibits absolutely no signs of potential contamination. This makes a high level of microbiological quality control essential for this industry.

TEA AND OTHER INFUSIONS

The pharmacological properties of tea and other infusions have been known to humankind for thousands of years. Certain infusions such as tea are stimulating, while others such as chamomile are relaxing. Some infusions prevent diarrhea, and others relieve constipation. Acetylsalicylic acid, the active, pain-killing ingredient of aspirin, originally came to us centuries ago as an infusion of the bark of willow trees. Excellent marketing, combined with our desire to have warm, soothing beverages to linger over, has spurred a tremendous growth in the consumption of various exotic infusions.

Infusions cover the entire range of hot or cold beverages prepared by steeping plant materials in water. The many varieties of tea currently available barely reflect the multiplicity of infusions commonly consumed around the world. These infusions are seldom considered as sources of pathogenic organisms. However, when considering their origin and method of home preparation, why they are becomes abundantly clear. The materials used for infusions can be the leaves, berries, petals, bark, stalks, twigs or even roots of various plants. These plants all grow wild or are cultivated in the open, exposed to all the dust, birds, animals and insects the environment has to offer. Furthermore, infusions are seldom washed or cleaned in any way (other than sifting) prior to drying. Certain infusions, such as tea, are dry fermented in the open air. Many are sun dried in the field or by a roadside. As a result, unless they are fumigated with ethylene oxide or treated by irradiation, the consumer receives plant materials that contain a very high load of microorganisms, many of which are pathogenic.

Most infusions are not boiled, they are simply steeped. Therefore, a large proportion of the original organisms survive prior to consumption. Fortunately, since many infusions contain components such as tannic acid that retard microbial development and most are consumed immediately after steeping, conditions for growth are limited. Nevertheless, infusions can be a source of particularly hazardous pathogens. Since detecting any potential problems or high levels of contamination is very difficult, choose a reputable supplier.

RESTAURANTS AND FOOD SERVICE

One of the most important tasks of any restaurant or food service establishment is the procurement of raw materials and ingredients of satisfactory hygienic quality. Once this has been done the ultimate quality and safety of the foods served will depend upon the hygienic practices employed throughout the entire handling process. As can be seen, this does not always measure up to par.

OUTBREAK INCIDENTS IN RESTAURANTS AND FOOD SERVICE

Let's Check Out the Drive-In?[132]

In 1983, in the tiny town of Marietta in Love County, Oklahoma (county population 7,800), there was a drive-in restaurant where everybody just loved to go. In fact, when more than 200 people became ill with hepatitis A, they found that 92 percent of them had eaten there before they got sick. Many of the people in town who work as food handlers in other restaurants had eaten there. So did some people who worked at a local bakery that distributed cookies nationwide.

The situation got so bad that the Oklahoma State Health Department recommended that immunoglobulin shots be given, and they were. A total of 5,500 doses were given in the little town of Marietta! The drive-in closed for a month.

Simon Says?[133]

In July 1989, more than 60 children attending a day-care summer program in Florida suddenly experienced gastrointestinal illness. The symptoms occurred within minutes after the lunch was concluded and involved cramps, nausea, headaches and dizziness. Most of the kids had even vomited. Fortunately, the symptoms didn't last too long but, just to be on the safe side, all those children who had obvious symptoms were quickly sent to emergency departments at the local hospitals. Fortunately, within a few hours, everyone started to feel better. The children went back to the center and no further problems were reported.

What they all ate was a prepackaged lunch made up of a ham and cheese sandwich, some diced pears, chocolate milk and apple juice. The first child to get ill was a 12-year-old girl, who said that her food tasted bad. Within a short period, she developed nausea and threw up. Immediately thereafter, more of the children got nauseous and vomited and some of the staff members hinted to the other kids that the food may have been contaminated.

When the kids were later interviewed in person they could not precisely correlate any one food with the symptoms. When the FDA was called in to test some meal samples, they could not detect pesticides, staphylococcal toxin or evidence of *Bacillus cereus*. Sophisticated atomic absorption analysis for heavy metals, copper or zinc also proved negative. A careful review of the day-care center's food handling and preparation system also revealed nothing. The extremely costly and thorough investigation could not identify anything usual about that day at all. What could it be?

Have you ever seen what happens when one kid sees another kid throw up? That's right—the second kid throws up! They even have a name for it. It's called line-of-sight vomiting! The Florida Department of Health and Rehabilitative Services came to the final conclusion that this outbreak was the result of mass sociogenic illness (MSI).

Heidel-Burger Medium Rare[134]

On June 22, 2004, the local public health department of Edmonton, Alberta, received multiple reports of gastrointestinal illness from individuals who had consumed a meal, some hours before the onset of symptoms, at an Edmonton buffet-style restaurant specializing in South Asian cuisine. The initial reports of illness linked to the restaurant were received through separate telephone calls to a local health service. Transcripts of the calls were then sent to the local public health department and initiated the outbreak investigation.

Officials visited the restaurant to conduct inspections and interview the management regarding their food handling practices. Employee stool specimens were collected for salmonella screening and submitted for analysis. Additional reports of illness linked to the restaurant kept coming in to the health service. A total of 32 cases of *Salmonella Heidelberg* were identified during the outbreak period, one of whom was an employee of the implicated restaurant.

No improper food-handling practices were noted at the restaurant during the investigation. However, it was confirmed that the employee infected with salmonella was involved in food-handling activities as part of his normal duties. Salmonella-infected food handlers are frequently cited as reservoirs in food-borne salmonella outbreaks. It has long been known that salmonella bacteria survive on the fingertips for several hours and that food can be contaminated through contact with fingertips. The Edmonton incident highlighted the fact that even slight breaches in hand hygiene, resulting in microscopic fecal contamination of fingertips, could result in such an outbreak.

RESTAURANT FOODS

Most consumers have no idea of the size of the restaurant industry in the United States. In order to gain some perspective about the volume of business it incorporates, consider the following statistics prepared by the National Restaurant Association:

- In 2007, yearly restaurant sales were estimated at close to $540 billion.
- The restaurant industry employs almost 13 million people and is the largest employer after the government.
- In 2007, restaurant industry sales equaled 4 percent of the U.S. gross domestic product.
- The average annual expenditure for food away from home was $2,634 per person in 2005.

Obviously, this is an immense business. When combined, meals consumed in restaurants and in school and work cafeterias total close to 50 billion meals annually! The vast reach of this industry imparts an exceptional degree of responsibility upon it, particularly in the area of food safety and hygiene.

Most of the routine problems of food hygiene encountered in the home are also experienced in the restaurant and catering trade (collectively known as the food service industry). These problems are compounded by the fact that each establishment can be responsible for preparing foods not simply for a few family individuals but for hundreds or even thousands of people. The sheer volume of meals prepared also contributes to the difficulties encountered. Far more fish, meat, poultry, fruits, vegetables, spices and other products and ingredients are lying about in contact with one another. This becomes a particular problem of cross contamination when defrosting takes place and the fish, poultry or meat juices drip unnoticed onto surfaces used to prepare other products. The constant frying that takes place in the food service industry sends an extraordinary amount of oil vapor into the air to clog filters and condense as grease in cracks, corners and hard-to-clean areas. This entraps dust and dirt distributed by the human traffic of cooks, dishwashers, busboys, waiters and delivery people. It also attracts mites and other insects. The net result is a significant amount of contamination that is difficult to control properly.

The high volume of food and the high cost of ingredients can also make a cook, pastry chef or manager reluctant to discard prepared products such as mayonnaise, salad dressing or pastry creme that have been standing out for too long and are far past peak condition. Their guess is that no one will be able to tell the difference once the product is blended in with a fresh batch. This is probably correct. The same goes for fish or meats that may end up being chopped or ground up and served under a highly flavored sauce. Understandably, the higher the value of the ingredient, the greater the reluctance to discard it. The judgments made are highly subjective and based on smell and overall appearance. Unfortunately, the potential that these less-than-prime ingredients hold for harboring high levels of food-borne disease organisms or toxins is seldom a conscious part of these decisions.

Another major problem in the food service industry is training. More than 40 percent of individuals employed in the U.S. food service industry did not complete high school. Moreover, the turnover rate in the food service industry is much higher than anywhere else.[135] Although some rudimentary guidelines are usually given regarding personal and product hygiene, very few organizations provide the training commensurate with the responsibilities of feeding a great many people. Even then, consumers have no guarantee that this will reduce poor practices.[136, 137] A major proportion of food service industry staff consists of the lowest wage earners in the country. Most employees are either at the minimum wage or just above it. Little doubt exists that the many illegal immigrants who work in this industry are being exploited, receiving even less than the minimum wage. While some individuals work diligently regardless of the level of remuneration they receive, low wages have a direct bearing on the sense of responsibility, self-esteem and loyalty workers exhibit toward their jobs. More significantly, low wages directly bear upon the view held by employers of the value and responsibilities of the job and the need for a fully trained individual. Anyone investing so little in staff wages will probably not turn around and spend money on hygienic training programs.

Unfortunately, in our food system, a very large proportion of restaurant service income is derived from tips and gratuities. Our understanding of service is completely superficial. It reflects our own egos far more than an understanding or appreciation of the food we eat. When we go to a restaurant, the activities we classify as service are really only the tip of the iceberg of integrated activities required to get food to your table and to remove the refuse. The maître d', servers and support staff appear to spend far more effort massaging a client's vanity than ensuring the quality of his or her food. All the other services—not the least of which involves ensuring that food is treated in as hygienic a manner as possible—go completely unnoticed and largely unappreciated. It is unfortunate that all jobs in the food service industry are not properly salaried. In Europe, the service and gratuity are generally included in the price of the meal simply because the entire staff is considered equally. A disagreeable waiter, busboy or maître d' makes everyone look bad and usually does not last long. The slow speed of activity commonly found in European restaurants reflects normal meal-time etiquette more than poor service. The client pays for the food and all the requisite services together. A small gratuity, such as 5 to 10 percent of the bill or simply small, leftover change is really for outstanding services. Food service workers seldom anticipate tips, and the local clients who make up the bulk of the business almost never offer them.

When eating at a restaurant or dealing with a caterer, take particular note of the appearance and smell of the establishment and the cleanliness of its staff. Unfortunately, most of us have become so accustomed to the smell of rancid frying oil, we hardly notice it anymore. If a restaurant does not smell fresh and clean, the chances are it is not. Any restauranteur who has no interest in changing the oil before it goes rancid is unlikely to be willing to spend the money required to keep the place clean and hygienic. The system of grading restaurants on the basis of food safety standards that began in Los Angeles in 1998 started to tackle this problem.[138]

The Department of Environmental Health carries out inspections focusing on the critical concerns of proper food handling practices, such as raw material and ingredient storage, preparation and cooking procedures, holding and serving practices, as well as insect and pest infestation and the condition of restroom facilities. An alphabetical card grading system indicating an "A," "B," or "C" rating is given. These cards must be posted where clients can see them.

- A is a score of 90–100 percent
- B is a score of 80–89 percent
- C is a score of 70–79 percent

Any establishment that receives a score of less than 70 percent does not qualify for a letter grade card, but does get a scorecard that shows the actual scoring. This remains posted until the next routine inspection, when the inspector issues a grade card if the establishment deserves it. Any establishment that scores below 60 percent more than twice within a 12-month period, may be closed and taken to court. This program has served as an effective incentive to maintain a consistently high level of hygiene in Los Angeles restaurants.

Anyone who wants to see the actual ranking of Los Angeles area restaurants can do so on the Internet at http://ph.lacounty.gov/rating.

A follow-up to this program was recently carried out to determine its long-term effectiveness.[139] After trend adjustments were made, the analysis indicated that the restaurant hygiene grading program was associated with a 13.1 percent decrease in the number of food-borne disease hospitalizations in Los Angeles County in the year following implementation of the program (1998)—a decrease that continued to be sustained over the next years. The results suggested that the system of restaurant hygiene grading with public posting of results was an effective way of reducing restaurant-related food-borne disease outbreaks.

Restaurant reviewers should start earning their living with a little less pretense and a lot more professionalism. Many of us get ideas and suggestions about eating out from these journalists. They should have more than a passing knowledge of what constitutes good food and its preparation. Providing consumers with useful guidelines about eating out is a task of increasing importance, because we are eating more and more of our meals away from the home.

Much of the information we currently get about restaurants is cosmetic. Some reviewers have fine, discriminating palates and do take the trouble to explain the refinements of the food served. Many others are impressed with decor, service and, particularly, the size of the portions, considering this to be a measure of the good value that one can find when eating out. Of course, all this information is subjective and largely a matter of taste. However, hygiene is not a matter of taste. It is a matter of health and safety and is something that most consumers would be too shy to look into on their own. Someone would have to undergo only one good bout of salmonellosis or staphylococcal poisoning to learn that hygiene is far more important than decor, service or portion size. Yet, it is almost never a subject of newspaper reviews and is seldom, if ever, referred to in the published restaurant guides.

Journalists who review restaurants should be given appropriate courses or briefings about food service standards and hygiene. It would be very useful if a proper scoring system, easily understandable by consumers, could be developed and agreed upon to rate the state of restaurant cleanliness. This would require an examination of the kitchen, storage and refrigeration areas; the appearance of the staff and evidence of hygienic consciousness as evidenced by hand-washing signs in the kitchen and washrooms; and so forth. A simple 10-point scale should provide consumers with an idea of the overall state of the restaurant's hygiene. Any restaurant that refuses to allow a journalist to see the kitchen should be so noted in the review. Such reviews will put the issue of food service hygiene into proper perspective. Good restaurants have clean kitchens and employ people who are conscious of the need for hygienic practices when preparing food. Poor restaurants really do not care. Consumers should be aware of the importance a restaurant gives to this matter. The food service industry is a major contributor to food-borne diseases.

Although there is little doubt that consumers are keenly interested in a restaurant's service and decor, their main interest revolves around food quality. However, quality is not limited to taste and presentation, it also includes food safety and hygiene. In order to provide consumers with a useful perspective on a food establishment's dedication to safety and hygiene, journalists should give some thought to using the following form to prepare such evaluations. The outcome is fairly straightforward—the higher the score the cleaner the establishment and the safer the food.

FOOD SERVICE/RESTAURANT HYGIENE SCORE					
AREA/PROCESS	NOT ACCEPTABLE	POOR	ADEQUATE	GOOD	EXCELLENT
SCORE	1 2	3 4	5 6	7 8	9 10
Raw Food/ Ingredients' Storage					
Raw Food/ Ingredients' Quality					
Staff Washroom Facilities					
Food Handler Hygiene					
Food Preparation Facilities (counters, and so forth)					
Food Handling Practices					
Delivery of Food to Customer					
Waiter/Busboy Hygiene					
Sanitation of Dishes/Utensils					
Customer Washroom Facilities					
Overall Score					

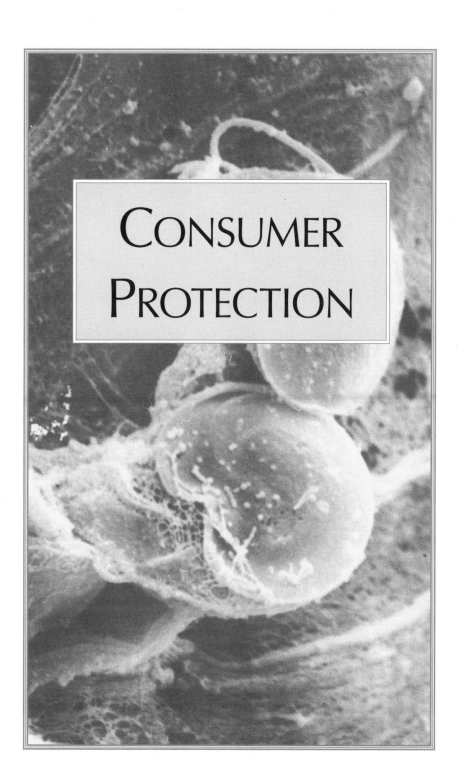

CONSUMER
PROTECTION

INCIDENCE AND COSTS OF
FOOD-BORNE DISEASES

In mid-December 2006, the *Wall Street Journal* published the results of their new Wall Street Journal Online/Harris Interactive health-care poll,[140] which focused on food-borne diseases. From December 12–14, 2006, Harris Interactive carried out this online analysis in the United States using a nationwide sample of more than 2,000 adults.

About 13 percent, or one in eight adults, said someone in their household had suffered a food-related illness during the past year. However, in only one-third of the cases did anyone report the incident to a doctor, the place where the food was purchased or local health officials.

Surprisingly, 95 percent of respondents said that they closely follow food safety warnings, such as when products are recalled or when warnings are issued that certain products are suspected of making people ill. The poll asked which agency or institutions should bear primary responsibility for establishing the regulations for food handling, production and packaging to ensure the safety of these consumer products. Here, the response was curious, with less than 60 percent stating that the FDA should bear primary responsibility. The remainder felt that either local health agencies or the food and restaurant industry should bear the brunt of the responsibility.

Following this survey, Thomas Hargrove described an investigation carried out by Scripps Howard News Service.[141] Close to 6,400 food-related disease outbreaks were reported from January 1, 2000, to December 31, 2004—almost two-thirds of which were declared to be of unknown causes. Doctors and medical examiners have been increasingly likely to list food-borne and intestinal diseases as the primary cause of death in recent years, suggesting a growing sensitivity to the threats posed by food- and water-related diseases.

According to federal records based on death certificates, only 1,370 Americans died of infectious intestinal diseases in the year 2000. However, food- and water-borne deaths rose to 1,586 in 2001, to 2,496 in 2002 and to 3,142 in 2003, the last year analyzed. The more than doubling of deaths in just four years is quite shocking. Further analysis indicated that almost 84 percent of the 2003 deaths were people over 70 years of age—testimony to the fact that the food safety system in place does not adequately protect the elderly.

While the number of individuals over 70 was about 9 percent of the population in 2005, this is expected to increase dramatically in the near future. For example, by 2025, the U.S. Census Bureau projects there will be 44 million people, or more than 12.5 percent of the population, over

70. Unless a significant improvement is made in dealing with the impact of food-borne disease on senior citizens, a great increase in the number of deaths will occur.

THE COSTS OF FOOD-BORNE DISEASES

Most now concede that food-borne diseases occur far more commonly and have far more significant effects than most people previously believed. As unpleasant as the subject is, all must be aware of it because the money

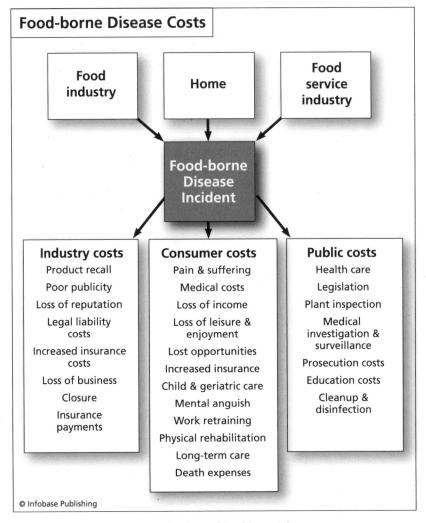

Food-borne Disease Costs

| Food industry | Home | Food service industry |

Food-borne Disease Incident

Industry costs	Consumer costs	Public costs
Product recall	Pain & suffering	Health care
Poor publicity	Medical costs	Legislation
Loss of reputation	Loss of income	Plant inspection
Legal liability costs	Loss of leisure & enjoyment	Medical investigation & surveillance
Increased insurance costs	Lost opportunities	Prosecution costs
Loss of business	Increased insurance	Education costs
Closure	Child & geriatric care	Cleanup & disinfection
Insurance payments	Mental anguish	
	Work retraining	
	Physical rehabilitation	
	Long-term care	
	Death expenses	

© Infobase Publishing

Figure 17. **The Costs of Food-borne Disease**

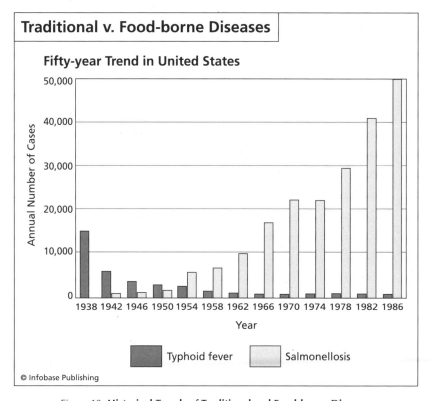

Figure 18. **Historical Trends of Traditional and Food-borne Diseases**

required to pay for their consequences comes straight out of our pockets. Preliminary appraisals of the cost of food-borne diseases indicate that they have considerable economic impact.[142–144] When taking into account factors such as lost labor or income, medical and hospitalization expenses, legal fees and other associated costs, the estimates run into billions of dollars (see figure 17). The most recent figures for the United States, based on 1996 estimates, place the total costs resulting from intestinal infectious diseases from six major pathogens at $6.7 billion annually.[145] This includes medical costs as well as the cost of lost productivity.

Even though these figures might seem like an enormous sum, it is probably only the tip of the iceberg. The value of lost opportunities, ruined reputations and grief due to sickness and death are virtually impossible to calculate with any true meaning, particularly for the victims. Any consumer-based issue worth $6.7 billion or more should warrant everyone's attention.

What is particularly disturbing is the historical tendency associated with food-borne diseases. While modern science and medicine have been extremely successful in bringing many of the conventional infectious diseases under control, the incidence of food-borne diseases continues to rise. This pattern becomes evident when certain food-borne diseases are compared with a historically important disease such as typhoid fever. Figure 18 gives the data for a 50-year period.[146] The trend points out that modern medicine and hygiene have been very effective in thwarting certain diseases, but have been unable to stem the consistent rise in food-borne diseases.

This distressing trend has a direct impact on the steadily rising costs of medical care. In any proposed government campaign to reduce the cost of medical care, policies directed at minimizing food-borne diseases are essential elements. Because the vehicle for the transmission of these diseases is food, a product manufactured and controlled under close supervision, the degree of risk can be controlled. A perfect example is milk, where the method of pasteurization was employed to eliminate virtually all disease risks associated with its consumption. The same has occurred with other products like fruit juices. Relatively few cases of food-borne disease occur with beverage products that have received proper processing. The same can be said for canned products. The trend in food-borne disease incidents

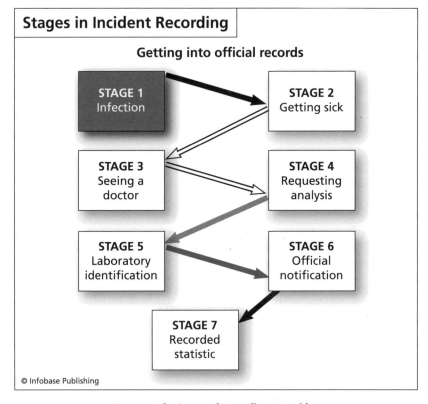

Figure 19. **The Stages of Recording an Incident**

exhibited in the previous figure highlights the neglect in taking similar positive actions for untreated solid foods such as meat, poultry and eggs.

For the majority of people, the unpleasant experience of food-borne disease probably lasts only·a few days. However, a significant number of cases can be very serious and cause long-term chronic gastric problems and other related difficulties. The very young, as well as older people, are particularly at risk from food-borne diseases. Some rather spectacular and well-publicized outbreaks of food-related poisonings or infections have occurred. Unfortunately, though, most incidents of food-borne illness go almost totally unreported.

When considering all the stages that have to be passed through before an incident officially gets into the records (see figure 19), one can see why food-borne diseases are grossly underestimated. The whole process starts with someone becoming infected—stage 1. Stage 2 is the process of getting ill. Depending upon the severity of the illness, the victim may or may not seek medical attention. Very often, people simply endure the sickness, take a few days off work and never see doctors at all.

The act of seeing a physician is stage 3. Depending on the patient's symptoms, the physician may or may not obtain a stool sample or other form of specimen for typing. Obtaining a specimen and sending it in for analysis is stage 4 in the process. One does not need much imagination to realize that very few stomachaches, cases of cramps, diarrhea or bouts of nausea ever get to this stage. If they do, stage 5 is the laboratory identification of the organism, followed by stage 6—making an official report to the local health department. Depending upon the local, state or national infrastructures, many incidents may not be reported further. If they are reported, stage 7 involves the process of moving this information to the national epidemiological statistics agency, which places it into the official records. Of course, the official bureaucratic process and flow of paper may be quite different, but the above pattern describes the basic activities involved.

Health professionals have variously estimated that anywhere from one in 25 to as few as one in 5,800 of the true number of cases are actually reported.[147] A number of reasons explain this. In many cases, people simply do not think that the symptoms are serious enough to warrant the time and expense of consulting a physician and furnishing samples for analysis. The symptoms, which are typically diarrhea and stomachache, are not uncommon. Most people feel that they will inevitably improve without resorting to a doctor. Even if they do see a doctor, unless blood or stool samples are taken and analyzed, no one can know the exact cause of the episode. Consequently, the incident goes totally unreported. It does not take much to recall the number of times this has happened to each of us. ("Gee, I just had a bout of diarrhea. The next time we buy that terrific pasta salad, let's make sure it was made the same day." End of story.) Of course, not all cases of diarrhea are due to food-borne diseases, but the majority of such incidents are. The fact that the episode was not more damaging was little more than a chance at the roulette wheel of pathogens we repeatedly face. The odds against us are mounting, not getting better. When a reasonable estimate is made of the health and economic effects of food-borne diseases, we can readily see why food and health experts consider them to be the greatest of all the food-related risks we face.

MAJOR FOOD POISONING OUTBREAKS SINCE 2000

Since the year 2000, there have been a number of large-scale food poisoning outbreaks reported to the Centers for Disease Control. Many of these outbreaks are not well known because state departments of health seldom report them publicly.

Despite all the efforts that have taken place, food-borne disease outbreaks continue to plague us. As a telling example, the following table illustrates that the recalls related to *E. coli* were greater in 2007 than they were in 2002.

E. COLI RECALLS IN U.S. 2002–2007		
YEAR	NUMBER OF RECALLS	POUND OF PRODUCT RECALLED
2002	21	23,984,590
2003	11	1,872,746
2004	6	1,198,600
2005	5	1,248,450
2006	8	181,900
2007	21	33,358,521

Brasher, P. "Scientists study possible link between ethanol byproduct and E. coli" *The Des Moines Register* January 27, 2008. Available online. URL: http://www.desmoinesregister.com/apps/pbcs. dll/article?AID=/20080127/NEWS/801270330.

The following are some examples that occurred over the years:

2007

In September 2007 the Topps Meat Company of Elizabeth, N. J., recalled 21.7 million pounds of frozen hamburger patties because of *E. coli* O157: H7 contamination, making it the second-largest ground beef recall in U.S. history. At least 21 people reported illnesses associated with the recall of hamburgers, which had been shipped mainly to states in the Northeast.[148]

Salmonella bacteria were recovered from national brands of peanut butter in 44 states. By March 7, 2007, the outbreak had grown to 425 cases.

The CDC said it is believed to be the first salmonella outbreak associated with peanut butter in U.S. history.[149]

2006

(a) *E. coli* O157:H7 from a fast-food chain in New Jersey and New York. Thirty-nine victims were sickened, with a number of them suffering from hemolytic uremic syndrome. At first it was believed the *E. coli* came from green onions. However, it was later suspected that lettuce was the cause of the outbreak.

(b) *E. coli* O157:H7 in bagged spinach packaged by a national producer resulted in three dead and 198 people sickened across 25 U.S. states and one Canadian province.

2005

In December 2005, following an outbreak in the state of Washington, the FDA warned the public against drinking raw milk because it may contain *E. coli* O157:H7. Eight illnesses were reported in Washington, several of which were in children. Health authorities identified locally sold raw milk as a source of the outbreak and ordered the unlicensed dairy to shut down.[150]

2004

A food-borne disease outbreak affecting more than 700 people was reported in January 2004 in Texas, according to CDC files. However, Texas health officials said they could find no records of this outbreak. No other information was available.

2003

(a) Hepatitis A associated with green onions in a Pennsylvania restaurant resulted in approximately 555 people coming down with the disease. At least 13 restaurant workers and 75 residents of six other states who dined at the suspect restaurant became ill with the disease and three people died.

(b) An outbreak of *Clostridium perfringens* at a Louisiana prison sickened 880 inmates in November. State health officials said the disease was spread by food maintained at improper temperature.

(c) An outbreak of *Shigella sonnei* bacteria infected 964 people in seven West Texas counties during a four-month period in 2003. More than 70 percent of the victims were children under 12. The outbreak began as a food-borne illness, but also spread through person-to-person contact.

(d) A cafeteria at the St. Louis Children's Hospital was the source of an outbreak of *Salmonella javiana* that sickened 641 people in 2003, according to CDC files. Investigators diagnosed the disease, but were

unable to confirm how it spread, although they suspected a food handler who worked the salad bar on the two days of the outbreak.
(e) More than 500 customers of a Pennsylvania restaurant were sickened by Hepatitis A from infected raw green onions used to make salsa. Three people died. Investigators failed to identify the exact cause of the infection in the fields where the onions were grown.

2002

(a) Roast beef with mashed potatoes and gravy was responsible for making close to 1,000 inmates of the Illinois River Correctional Center sick. Investigators determined the gravy was contaminated with the *Clostridium perfringens* bacteria.
(b) Following a conference at a Dallas hotel in March 2002, Texas health officials began receiving reports from all over the nation. More than 700 people fell sick from the *Salmonella enteritidis* bacteria. The outbreak lasted more than five weeks. Investigators eventually identified an infected hotel employee who had prepared the food.

2001

(a) *Shigella flexneri* bacteria were responsible for an outbreak that began at a restaurant in New York, and quickly spread to four other restaurants. Almost 900 people were affected. Investigators concluded that an infected worker at a produce distribution plant had contaminated a shipment of bruised tomatoes.
(b) A large *norovirus* outbreak in Nashville, Tennessee, in January 2001 sickened 811 people. Despite an extensive investigation, health officials were not able to determine the cause.

2000

Watermelon contaminated with beef juices served at a children's buffet at a Milwaukee restaurant was found to be responsible for spreading *E. coli* to 736 people in July 2000. One child died of hemolytic uremic syndrome.

LONG-TERM SEQUELAE

In medical jargon, any pathological condition that results from a disease is called a "sequela," from the Latin word *sequi*—to follow. The plural form is "sequelae" and refers to all those disorders and conditions that develop as a consequence of a disease incident. Sometimes, they are also referred to as the "long-term complications" arising from a disease, and that is how most people understand them. They are not the immediate symptoms of the disease but rather the extended aftereffects. For example, the major cause of death for people with high blood pressure is not high blood pressure itself but rather the complications that result from it, such as stroke or kidney failure. In the case of food-borne diseases, some of the sequelae are far more critical than the immediate effects of the original incident.

Although long-term chronic sequelae are characteristic of many food-borne diseases, they have not received the same degree of attention that the primary, acute symptoms have. Most victims and their physicians are happy to get over the short-term effects and seldom worry about future consequences. Because of the difficulty in calculating the impact of long-term sequelae upon the health care system, they are seldom considered when determining the full impact of food-borne diseases. Long-term chronic effects are also overlooked simply because the data about them is not systematically collected. As a result, directly linking them to an originating cause is difficult. In fact, the significance of long-term sequelae is only now starting to be considered more comprehensively. The conclusions indicate that they can be very serious. Food-borne diseases have been implicated in reactive arthritis, Guillain-Barré syndrome, hemolytic uremic syndrome, Reiter's syndrome, ankylosing spondylitis, meningoencephalitis, meningitis and other neurological syndromes.[151, 152] Long-term sequelae often destroy an individual's morale and general enjoyment of life. Not surprisingly, extended chronic effects are often accompanied by measurable changes in personality.

Arthritis

Several food-borne bacteria have been implicated with the development of arthritic conditions, including *Campylobacter jejuni*,[153] *Salmonella* sp.,[154] *Shigella* sp.,[155] *Yersinia enterocolitica*,[156] *Brucella melitensis*[157] and *Streptococcus* sp.[158] The most frequent type of long-term arthritic sequelae is "reactive arthritis"—an inflammatory arthritic condition that occurs in the joints in response to the presence of bacterial antigens even though the bacteria themselves are not present. Preliminary estimates indicate that more than 2 percent of people who get food poisoning will develop arthritis.[159] This means that a large outbreak involving 250,000 people will result in more than 5,000 individuals experiencing long-term arthritis. Another related disease that has been shown to be a sequela of food-borne infection is Reiter's syndrome, the most common form of arthritis in young men (normally transmitted sexually). Its symptoms include urethritis, conjunctivitis and psoriasis in addition to joint pain and swelling. Yet another form of joint disease is ankylosing spondylitis, which literally means rigid spine in Greek. It is characterized by pain and soreness in the spine and joints of the trunk region. After some time, the vertebrae grow together, and the typical bent-over posture of the condition develops.

Guillain-Barré Syndrome

Guillain-Barré syndrome is a serious disease that can result in paralysis, breathing difficulty and death. The condition is the aftermath of the inflammation and destruction of the myelin sheath of the nerve fibers. It is generally associated with bouts of infection, and food-borne pathogens have been implicated in many cases. The symptoms usually begin with numbness and tingling in fingers and toes. They continue to evolve into widespread muscle fatigue and difficulty in breathing. Treatment usually consists of supportive hospital care but in some cases, may require respiratory assistance. The mortality rate is about 4 percent. About 10 percent of the remaining cases are left with some form of permanent impairment. The food-borne organism most commonly associated with this condition is *Campylobacter jejuni.*

Meningitis and Meningoencephalitis

The brain and spinal column are protected by spinal fluid and tough membranes called meninges. If these become infected, the condition is called meningitis, and it can be extremely serious. The causative microorganisms can enter the bloodstream via several routes, including contaminated food. Symptoms can include fever, headache, fatigue and even seizures. It can be a highly dangerous condition that requires immediate medical attention. If not treated properly, it can result in brain damage, hearing loss and mental retardation. It is particularly a concern for infants. Meningoencephalitis is an infection and inflammation limited to the brain. The primary food-borne organism implicated is *Listeria,* although *Campylobacter,*[160] *E. coli,*[161] *Streptococcus*[162] and *Brucella* sp.[163] have also been involved.

Hemolytic Uremic Syndrome

The recent rash of food-borne ECO157 disease outbreaks around the world has focused much attention on hemolytic uremic syndrome (HUS), one of the severe sequelae of this infection. HUS occurs far more readily in infants and young children than in older children and adults. It usually starts with diarrhea and abruptly progresses to hemolytic anemia—a condition where mature red blood cells are broken down faster than the bone marrow can produce new ones. Aside from the symptoms of anemia, the urine may also appear brown, because the hemoglobin from the ruptured blood cells is liberated into the blood, where it can put an impossible load on the kidneys. This is followed by a rapid loss of kidney function and ensuing neurological conditions. HUS very often requires kidney dialysis and blood transfusions. If not caught in time, it results in permanent kidney damage, loss of other organ functions and death. Because of the rapid and virulent nature of this disease, it is one of the few sequelae generally accounted for in tallying up the impact of food-borne disease outbreaks. Because it seems to favor infants and young children, it is also one of the most heartbreaking of the sequelae.

Inflammatory Bowel Disease

Inflammatory bowel disease covers both Crohn's disease and ulcerative colitis. While both are chronic inflammatory diseases, the primary pathologic effects are gastrointestinal. The acute clinical characteristics are diarrhea, abdominal pain, fever and weight loss. Abdominal abscesses are a common and difficult complication of Crohn's disease, while in ulcerative colitis, abdominal perforations may lead to peritonitis. Crohn's disease involves the ileum or colon while ulcerative colitis appears limited to the colon.

Although the cause of inflammatory bowel disease is unknown, research has recently focused on food-borne pathogens. Organisms such as pseudomonas, *Mycobacterium, Enterococcus fecalis* and *E. coli* have been isolated from affected tissues. Occasionally, infected cows shed *M. paratuberculosis,* and the organism has been found in pasteurized milk. The proposed mechanism suggests that a susceptible infant first ingests the organism in commercial dairy products. This causes a low-grade chronic inflammation. The immune response to this inflammation increases in severity over the years, ultimately producing the symptoms of Crohn's disease. Recent research has demonstrated a connection between *Listeria monocytogenes, E. coli* and *Streptococcus* and Crohn's disease as well.

DETERMINING THE COSTS OF FOOD-BORNE DISEASES

Making a reasonable estimation of the costs of food-borne diseases is not an easy task. It requires that all the possible costs resulting from an incident be accounted. Many such estimates have been made by professionals. The general approach is to break costs down into direct and indirect costs. Going through such an exercise is instructive and serves to provide an excellent perspective about what is actually involved.

DIRECT AND INDIRECT COSTS

The direct and indirect costs associated with food-borne diseases are manifold. They are related to the medical and health care establishment, the public service and industry. While some costs are easily determined, others such as a loss of reputation are almost incalculable.

Medical Costs

The medical costs of food-borne diseases include the

- costs of visits to physicians (transportation, doctors' fees, laboratory tests, medication and so on)
- costs of hospital visits (ambulances and their crews, hospitalization fees, charges for physicians and other professional staff, laboratory and specialized equipment costs, medication, intravenous feeding and so forth)
- convalescence costs (medication, special equipment for dialysis, private nurse, special diet and so on)
- costs in case of death (autopsy, morgue charges, death certificates, burial costs and so forth)

Public Service Costs

The public service costs of food-borne diseases involve the

- costs of local and national medical professionals to investigate incidents and maintain statistics about outbreaks (laboratories, examinations, epidemiological analysis and so on)
- costs of food and drug, public health and agriculture professionals to investigate incidents and recommend remedial measures and policies (laboratories, statistics and so forth)
- costs of local and national ongoing food inspection services (laboratories, statistics and so on)
- costs of public information about food-borne diseases and their prevention (brochures, television, advertisements and so forth)

General Industrial Losses

The general industrial losses of food-borne diseases include the

- loss of production due to labor interruptions and reduced productivity
- costs of bureaucracy and paperwork associated with labor absence, replacement and insurance
- medical and insurance costs
- costs of ensuring the problem will not be experienced by other employees
- costs of replacement labor

Food or Food-Service Industry Costs

The food or food service industries also experience costs associated with food-borne disease. These include the

- loss of product
- costs of product recall
- loss of reputation

- legal and liability costs
- costs associated with correcting the original problem

When all the above factors are totaled, it is not difficult to see how statisticians arrived at a figure of 25 billion dollars. Once this figure is added to the sorrow, anguish and distress that these incidents cause, the monumental impact food-borne diseases have upon our society begins to take focus. Since we are only beginning to consider the long-term sequelae, many more factors must still be accounted for.

METHODS TO REDUCE
FOOD-BORNE DISEASES

FOOD PRESERVATION

Throughout history, our food supply has been secured from the extensive variety of species present in the plant and animal kingdoms. Because they are all products of the natural environment, the supply of food commodities is not always constant. Its availability very often follows normal cycles of boom and bust. With very few exceptions, foods are perishable and quickly lose their quality following harvest or slaughter. Since obtaining food was always such a struggle, once food of some type was secured, our ancestors had a natural tendency to consume it completely before going out and getting more. If the food on hand happened to be a whale or a mammoth, this posed certain practical problems of food safety and acceptability.

We cannot really know our early ancestors' reaction to spoiled food. In the animal kingdom, large carnivores do not appear to exhibit any particular aversion to spoiled meat. Lions and tigers, for instance, will continue to return to a carcass for days until fully consuming it (assuming it has not been scavenged). As time progressed, our predecessors must have noticed a relationship between the consumption of spoiled food and an increased level of community mortality. The need to better preserve the food they managed to obtain soon became evident. The first forms of raw meat preservation employed by our hunter-gatherer antecedents are largely a subject of speculation. Likely, air drying on the ground or using tree branches or simple racks probably ranks high in the short list of possibilities. Although the bacterial loads of these dried products were undoubtedly elevated, air drying was a long-sought improvement. The technology took hold and has been continually in use until today.

The factual, scientific basis of disease and food spoilage was not known until the late 19th century, although the theoretical foundation of this knowledge had slowly built over the preceding centuries. In the last few years of the 18th century, Nicholas Appert's research uncovered a practical method for preserving foods. He sealed the foods in glass containers, immersed them in boiling water for various lengths of time and then simply cooled them. Appert himself was not quite certain why this process worked. However, he speculated that heat was the chief factor responsible for the preservation phenomenon. One of France's most renowned scientists, Joseph-Louis Gay-Lussac, disagreed and attributed the preservation effects to the complete lack of oxygen in the bottled products. Since Nicholas Appert was only a humble confectioner, he could not compete with the reputation of Gay-Lussac. Attention drew away from heat as the fundamental factor in this type of preservation. Very little else was published on the subject until Pasteur reexamined the issue. He rather diplomatically pronounced Appert correct and Gay-Lussac excellent at analyzing oxygen but considerably off the mark regarding his theories of food preservation.

The success of Appert's technology had enormous impact upon the supply of food. For the first time in our history, we could take advantage of the great volumes of food available during seasons of plenty and preserve them for those times when they were ordinarily not available. Previously, this was only possible for certain grains or foods that had been dried. As a result, fruits, vegetables and an enormous variety of formulated foods such as soups, stews and prepared meats were manufactured. Appert's discovery ushered in the era of commercial food processing.

Canning

Surprisingly, Appert's process has not undergone very many changes during the last two centuries. Of course, a great many refinements were made, but the basic principles remain the same, that is, high heat treatment in a sealed container. Close upon Appert's initial breakthrough followed modifications of his procedure to allow the use of a wide range of containers, including those made of metal, called "canisters" or simply "cans." Around 1840, another step forward was made by adding the salt calcium chloride to the cooking water bath. This increased the cooking temperature from 212°F to 240°F, which allowed a decrease in cooking times from six hours to 30 minutes.[164, 165]

The next major advance in canning occurred around 1875. Large, steam pressure cookers called vertical retorts were introduced to replace the traditional calcium brine baths. Since the cans did not move during the cooking process, these new cookers were called static retorts. These did not differ very much from the pressure cookers found in many homes, except that they were much larger and were heated by injected steam rather than from an electric or gas burner. This allowed greater control and temperature consistency. Shortly thereafter, the theory of canning began to be studied systematically. The time-temperature requirements for processing various products placed the industry on a sound practical basis.

The ultimate goal of canning is to produce a product free of critical pathogens—a commercially sterile preparation. Safe production dictates that the temperature required to kill bacterial spores must be attained at the hardest place to reach—the geometric center of the can. Because the heat takes longer to reach the center of the can, the rest of the product is generally heated to a much higher temperature than necessary. This is why so many canned products are overcooked. More recently, retorts have

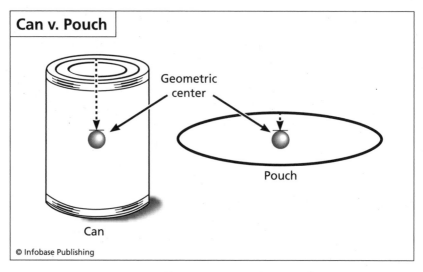

Figure 20. **Can v. Pouch**

been modified to allow cans to rotate horizontally throughout the heating process. This agitation distributes the heat evenly throughout the can and effectively reduces the need to achieve a particular temperature at the geometric center. The resulting products are cooked much more rapidly and have much higher quality and acceptability for the consumer. Another means of reducing the degree of overcooking is through the use of a thin pouch rather than a can (see figure 20). This occurs because the uniform transfer of heat happens much faster throughout a thin pouch than in a round can.

Canning has achieved an incredible record of commercial success during this century. When considering the billions and billions of canned products that have been processed, the number of food-borne disease outbreaks has been negligible. By far the majority of botulism cases that occur are due to homemade preparations, not commercially canned foods. When considering the abuse that cans routinely undergo during distribution, it is surprising that more spoilage has not occurred. People use canned products without a second thought, and consumers rarely see a swollen or spoiled can. Despite the fact that high-temperature thermal processes such as canning destroy certain nutrients and seldom produce gourmet products, very few technologies in the food industry can boast the same record of safety and success as canning.

Because of the nutritional and quality changes that result from high-temperature processing, a tremendous amount of research has been carried out to develop new methods of treating foods. Some of them are already commercial, while others still require fine tuning to make them competitive with technologies currently being used. Although the destruction or inhibition of unwanted disease and spoilage organisms is the common goal of these technologies, the resultant end products can be divided into two types. The first category includes heat processed foods, which do not resemble natural, raw products in any way. The major advance is in the manner with which the thermal treatment occurs. The second type of process seeks to destroy or eliminate unwanted microorganisms without significantly changing the basic character of the food. This would allow the consumer to utilize the food as a fresh product but without encountering the risks of food-borne disease.

Ohmic Heating

In order to improve the uniform transfer of heat to food products, researchers made attempts to carry out the thermal treatment in heated mixers called scraped-surface heat exchangers followed by packaging in aluminum cans under sterile or aseptic conditions. This worked well for uniform fluid products such as smooth puddings but failed when larger particulate materials, such as fruit pieces, were incorporated. Problems occurred simply because the particles heated more slowly than the surrounding fluid.[166] As a result, the entire process had to be slowed to ensure that the particles were properly treated. It seemed like an impossible problem to solve—then along came ohmic heating.

Ohmic heating itself is not a new concept. What was new was its application to the thermal processing of food. Many readers will remember the cheap home humidifiers that worked by passing a current of electricity through a solution of water containing a small amount of salt. The same principle was used in those little portable steamers that people carried with them in the hope of removing all the wrinkles from their clothes during travels. These devices work on the principle of electric resistance heating. This principle has now been turned into a commercial reality to process foods that contain high levels of particulate matter, such as very thick sauces or even soups containing small chunks of solid particles. With this process, an electric current passes through the food, and the solid materials heat up as fast as or even faster than the surrounding fluid. The electric current heats all the particles more quickly and efficiently so that the final temperatures required to kill or inhibit bacteria are reached with far less total cooking. This is supposed to result in products with improved quality. Unfortunately though, products treated by ohmic heating are not specifically labeled, so consumers cannot determine if better quality actually results.

High Electric Field Pulse (HEFP) Treatment

This process seeks to destroy unwanted bacterial cells without the application of heat in order to have a product remain in its raw natural state but without viable contaminating organisms. The method employs a series of high-voltage shocks to weaken bacterial cell membranes to a point where holes or pores form. When the voltage applied is high enough and when a sufficient number of shocks or pulses are delivered, the bacteria become irreversibly injured. The fact that low levels of treatment may result in reversible minor injury begs the question of whether microbial cells will be able to develop resistance to increasing levels of treatment before irreversible damage is achieved.

Since the utilization of this technology for the treatment of food is still in the experimental stages, many unsolved problems still remain. One hang-up is that the process is not particularly selective, and it also damages intact cells of the food. This may lead to changes in the texture of those foods, such as a loss of crispness in carrots or increased mushiness in meat. Another concern is that most bacterial spores are very resistant to this treatment.[167] Since spores are a particular problem in natural plant products, the applicability of this technology to fruits and vegetables will be severely limited if this hurdle cannot be overcome through the employment of other combination treatments. At the present time, this process in not in commercial use, but it may one day become a reality.

High-Pressure Processing

High-pressure processing is a method designed to maintain foods in their raw, natural state and destroy only the contaminating organisms. This technique is not new and was first applied to milk almost a century ago.[168] When organisms are placed under conditions of very high pressure, their proteins will be denatured with a resultant loss of enzymatic and biological activity. The organisms lose their viability and perish. This is much more easily accomplished with vegetative, or growing, bacteria than with spores, which require much higher pressures.

This method is currently being applied to fruit products such as jams and juices, particularly in Japan. Raw materials are placed in chambers under very high pressure for 10–60 minutes prior to opening the release valve. Both the equipment and the process are costly. As a result, the major commercial limitation to this method is economic rather than technical. As a commercial process, high-pressure treatment can significantly increase the cost of foods. This has limited the wider adoption of this process and will probably continue to do so for some time to come.

Manothermosonication

This method of food preservation sounds like everything but the kitchen sink. It involves using elevated pressure, elevated temperature and sound waves similar to those sonic cleaners that jewelers use. The trick is that all three treatments are used at lower levels than they would be if used individually. The goal is to kill microorganisms without damaging the original raw material. This method is currently not used commercially. Most likely, a considerable amount of time will pass before this will happen because of the difficulty in penetrating solid foods with ultrasonic energy.

Food Irradiation (Cold Pasteurization)

Food irradiation is a process where foods are exposed to a highly penetrating form of energy—gamma rays or high-energy electrons. Radioactive isotopes such as cobalt 60 (the same material used in cobalt medical treatments) are used to produce energy in the form of gamma rays. Gamma rays have high energy and can penetrate fairly deeply into solid materials such as foods. No other form of energy, other than accelerated electrons, can penetrate as evenly throughout a solid food.

Because these forms of energy can evenly penetrate solid foods, gamma rays and high-energy electrons can uniformly inactivate the DNA of unwanted microorganisms without changing the basic nature of the treated food. For this reason, food irradiation is also referred to as cold pasteurization. Fresh, irradiated foods with exceptional hygienic and eating qualities are virtually indistinguishable from fresh, untreated foods, except for the label and, in many cases, an improved appearance. The gamma rays and electrons used in the process are simply energy, just as heat, light or microwaves are—they are not particles and therefore do not leave any residues. Food irradiation does not make foods radioactive.

Food irradiation factories are virtually identical to the many irradiation facilities currently in use to process a wide range of materials such as medical supplies, blood, pharmaceuticals, plastic packaging films and wine corks. In the case of cobalt 60 facilities, irradiation takes place in a heavily walled concrete chamber to ensure that no gamma rays can escape. When the cobalt 60 source of gamma rays is not in use, it is simply lowered into a pool of water that converts the energy to heat. The water is routinely cooled and, of course, does not become radioactive. In the case of high-energy electron factories, irradiation usually takes place on a shielded conveyor belt since electrons can penetrate a product thickness of only about four inches. Electron irradiation facilities are simply turned on and off with an electric switch, just like a lightbulb.

Food irradiation is a safe process approved by international and national health authorities and medical associations. Public health officials all over the world highly recommended it. It can be used on most fruits, vegetables, meat, poultry, fish, shellfish, seafoods, spices, potatoes, grains and a host of other commodities. Currently, it is used on spices, certain fruits and vegetables and poultry in the United States. It is also approved for beef and shellfish. Depending upon the food product and treatment in question, the cost of food irradiation varies between one and five cents per pound. When considering the improvements it provides to the practical and hygienic qualities of foods, this is a fairly small price to pay for the corresponding health benefits it brings to consumers.

If food irradiation holds such benefits for the consumer, why is it not used more commonly? The answer lies in our generic fear of the unknown. Ever since the first atomic bomb was dropped, we have a great fear of the word radiation. Radiation-related incidents at Three-Mile

Island and Chernobyl have only heightened these fears. Therefore, semantics has played a major role in the confusion surrounding the subject of food irradiation. To confound the issue further, antinuclear lobbyists have publicly done their best to build frightening images of the technology. While this disinformation may have had some influence with the public in the past, the endorsement of food irradiation by all medical and public health authorities has had an even greater impact. A review of the studies carried out by universities and national polling organizations during the last 10 years indicates that current consumer fears of food-borne diseases far exceed any lingering fears of food irradiation. Consumers will purchase irradiated foods, particularly when they are made aware of the improved hygienic quality of the food. Since food irradiation is the only physical process that requires clear labeling, these products will be readily apparent in the marketplace. (All the other processes, including fumigation, electrocution and so on do not require such labeling.)

Access to safer products is therefore not a problem of consumer resistance—it is a problem of industry resistance. The food industry, the supermarket industry and the food service industry are as busy as possible pumping out as much food production as they can. They get very nervous and upset when the subject of food-borne diseases comes up and do not wish to incorporate improvements into their system unless absolutely necessary. Their major fear is that the public might decrease buying their products at the rate they currently do. The biggest culprit here is the supermarket industry, which consistently says that consumers will not accept irradiated foods. They say this despite the fact that all the studies, including those commissioned by the Food Marketing Institute, an association fully supported by the same supermarket business, indicate otherwise. Supermarket executives, out of touch with reality and their own commissioned studies, fear antinuclear protestors more than they do consumers who might start boycotting the contaminated products that are on sale. Like heat pasteurization before it, food irradiation will take some time before it gets a very wide application. It continues to be the most practical and effective way to provide solid foods with the same degree of protection from food-borne diseases as pasteurization does for liquids.

Minimally Processed Foods

While modern food preservation methods were developed to kill the microorganisms present in food, many other methods, some of them thousands of years old, are employed simply to control their excessive growth. Since the minimum infective dose of pathogens is fairly high for many food-borne diseases, these methods have played a very important role in maintaining food safety over the centuries. Common examples of these methods are acidification (such as in pickled vegetables), fermentation (as illustrated in certain European sausages or yogurt), the use of high concentrations of salt or sugar, freezing or cooling and drying. These methods continue to be very popular in the manufacture of traditional food products. In fact, this approach has been broadened into a new class of foods described as "minimally processed." In order to increase the eating quality of contemporary ready-to-eat processed foods, a battery of gentle techniques has been combined into a fully integrated treatment. The philosophy behind this approach is based upon the notion that each technique alone might not destroy microorganisms. However, when employed together, they are very effective. The concept of minimal processing theoretically involves the care of foods from the farm gate all the way to the consumer. This minimal-processing approach is also called hurdle technology simply because a series of hurdles is placed in the way of the microorganisms' growth and survival. The process includes combinations of weak acid treatments with modified atmosphere packaging, or mild heating with reduced moisture activity, or alternate doses of mild heating and chilling and so on.[169]

The marketing concept for minimally processed foods is based upon the perceived consumer desire for more natural, less-processed, high-quality homemade-style food preparations. Chilled ready-to-eat or ready-to-heat foods are a very rapidly growing segment of the market. Some of the best examples of this are the so-called *sous-vide* or vacuum-packed products. These products are prepared under very rigorous hygienic conditions, packed under a vacuum and cooked at fairly low temperatures. The cooking profile is not predicated on the need to destroy bacteria but rather upon the culinary requirements of the product. This latter factor has meant that the shelf life of *sous-vide* products is normally limited to one to three weeks.

Other technologies applied to minimally processed foods include the addition of antimicrobial agents such as enzymes and other natural compounds that suppress the growth of bacteria. Again, they constitute one step in an integrated hurdle approach that must usher the product from the farm to the consumer.[170] This technology is gaining particular ground in Europe and will likely follow suit in North America. Unfortunately, this desire to employ a combination of less-severe treatments in the hope that, together, they will ultimately accomplish the task of inhibiting undesirable organisms may lead to other problems.

While the hurdle approach has demonstrated its effectiveness in reducing the rapid growth of bacteria in foods, recent evidence has revealed that those bacteria that have survived the treatments may develop increased virulence.[171] From what we have seen thus far of the incredible adaptability of microorganisms, this may not seem all that surprising. In his book, *On the Origin of Species*,[172] Darwin asserted that the evolutionary mutation of species always arose from totally random variations that the environment happened to favor. Yet, we are now seeing something completely different. The mutations we see do not appear to be random at all but rather specifically designed to meet new hurdles in the surroundings. These deliberate adaptations arise in direct response to challenging environmental factors rather than spontaneous mutations—a far more sobering consideration.

When conditions for growth are excellent, microorganisms seem to direct all their energies toward that purpose alone. However, as soon as challenges are introduced into the environment, these same organisms apparently slow their growth and immediately begin creating and testing adaptations that will allow them to survive under the new conditions. These adaptations can be in the form of altered metabolic systems that make more efficient use of available nutrients or enzymatic systems that can neutralize toxic materials introduced into the surroundings. In the case of pathogens, the virulence or heightened ability to infect and multiply within the host would be such an adaptive response to environmental challenges and stresses.

All processes that do not achieve the death of microorganisms leave the door open for adaptive mutations to occur. In the past, we have seen that subtherapeutic doses of antibiotics in feeds or improper use of antibiotics in hospitals have resulted in wide-scale antibiotic resistance in bacteria. No particular reason exists for us to believe that the same type of subacute hurdles seen in minimal-processing technologies will not result in the same adaptive responses that will ultimately arise in resistance to that hurdle or in organisms with increased lethality. When we consider the extreme virulence and low-infective doses of the newly emerging food-borne pathogens, this is a frightening prospect. Although the reasons for employing new minimal-processing techniques are understandable, unless they comply with long-term public health needs, their adoption must be considered very carefully.

HAZARD ANALYSIS CRITICAL CONTROL POINT SYSTEMS (HACCP)

In order to improve food safety and to reduce the levels of rejected products, during the early 1970s, the food industry began considering the same sort of "total quality management" and "zero-defects" concepts employed in the aerospace industry. The application of this approach to the food industry eventually resulted in a system of control (particularly microbiological) called Hazard Analysis Critical Control Point or HACCP (pronounced "hassep").[173] This system emphasized the fully integrated analysis of the entire production process for each product. This included ingredients, the individual process steps and even the potential for consumer abuse. The goal was to determine when and where things could possibly go wrong with the microbiological safety of the finished product. The basic thrust of the HACCP concept shifted the emphasis of control from the testing of end products (when it was too late to do anything about contamination) to preventative control of all critical operations of the process. From the very early stages of development, the government inspection services showed a great interest in this concept.[174]

Although this idea was slowly accepted during the 1970s and 1980s, the concept seemed to gain terrific momentum in the 1990s. The majority of food companies and many established food service operations have now adopted it. The HACCP system not only pays off in dividends of product safety, but it also results in far fewer rejects. Fewer rejects mean fewer losses, and food manufacturers are always ready to look at any system that will result in savings. In fact, HACCP will soon become a mandatory part of the overall food inspection scheme once the government obliges all processors to institute such plans.[175] Then, the government will simply be able to check the company HACCP records to confirm that it has carried out all the correct procedures.

Many people, particularly those from industry, feel that the use of the HACCP system will significantly reduce the need for traditional government inspection.[176] A major weak link in the whole system of HACCP, as it is presently constituted, is related to the presence of microorganisms in foods. Everyone readily acknowledges that all natural raw materials such as poultry, meat, fish, fruit and vegetables carry pathogenic microorganisms. Since the first critical control point is the receiving door of the plant, how can contaminated raw materials be allowed in? Yet, they are.

Once these contaminated raw materials have been allowed to come into a plant, an incredible amount of remedial work has to be carried out in order to ensure that these microorganisms are killed during processing and that cross contamination does not take place. Since many products so exposed to cross contamination do not have some definitive step to kill bacteria in their processing, the end result could well be contaminated products. Although it is a significant improvement in overall control, HACCP is definitely not a panacea for problems of microbial contamination in foods. All recommendations for the relaxation of zero-tolerance policies for food-borne pathogens should be treated with great caution.[177]

Finally, bear in mind that the HACCP process must extend all the way to the consumption of the foods. Foods must be handled properly when distributed from the processor to the retailer. They must be stored at the proper temperature and must be maintained under the most rigorous hygienic conditions. Once in the store or supermarket, HACCP still applies. In fact, a form of HACCP has to follow through to the home kitchen and up until the time the food is served. The same goes for foods served in restaurants or fast-food outlets. If not, all the effort put into bringing safe products to the consumer may be wasted.

IN THE CONSUMER'S INTEREST

If we were to believe everything that has been written and said about the food we eat, then the American consumer is without any doubt, the luckiest person in the world. Just about everyone associated with the food industry is hard at work toiling in the sole interest of the consumer. Intrepid consumer advocates, conscientious government agencies, earnest industry executives and the strident media all seem to be totally devoted to ensuring that the American consumer has the safest, best, cheapest and most abundant food supply in the world. Their efforts seem to have been sidetracked somewhere along the way, because America now boasts the most obese population in the developed world—a population that is informed that certain antacids are a calcium-laden food supplement and that the unlimited consumption of synthetic chemicals, such as artificial sweeteners and fat replacements, are better than a reduced intake of the real thing. It is a population that appears to have lost a good deal of its common sense perspective and self-control regarding diet. All those working in the "sole interest of the consumer" do bear a significant share of the responsibility for this fiasco.

Consumer advocacy groups regularly hold press conferences to announce that products such as the enormous sticky buns people routinely eat for breakfast contain 800 calories and 32 grams of fat. They beat the drum about the relationship between hamburgers and cardiac arrest. They warn the public against the dangers of ethnic eating because of the MSG in Chinese food, or the alkalized corn flour in Mexican tacos and the hot spices in East Indian and Caribbean foods. Consumer advocates do their best to make what should be obvious sound like new and startling revelations just to stress a point. They are also effective with the press because they always come up with something striking to write about—even if it is something we all knew about before.

Consumer advocates have routinely pointed the finger at the establishment, usually big industries or institutions such as the government. It would likely be important for the sake of credibility to look less at the magnitude of the establishment involved and focus more upon the specific issues. For example, while it may not appear to be in vogue to go examine some of the negative characteristics of certain natural foods, such as organic vegetables fertilized with unsterilized manure, these products do pose a hazard to the public. The same can be said for any food products that do not benefit from the scrutiny of close inspection and sanitary regulations. It may be bad form to go after the poor smallholder farmers in Central America who scrape out a living selling waxed cassava roots to American supermarkets. However, until regulations and labeling provide

140

the consumer with information on any possible cyanogenic compounds that may be present in the roots, there can be exposure to undue risk.

There are two distinctly different advocacy groups that represent the consumer.[178] The first is the traditional consumers' advocacy group that has the consumer as its singular focus and priority. The second, more prominent type of group is somewhat different because, although it too works solely in the interests of consumers, its actions, and agenda are somewhat different. This latter group is commonly referred to as consumer activists. They are feisty; they are literate; and they are effective in attracting the press and arousing the emotions of their membership. They are an extremely persuasive force in the food system. Indeed, they have made both the government and industry sit up and take notice.

Traditional consumer representatives are deeply interested in defending the cause of consumers, and they go about it two slightly different ways. The first is to represent the actual views of the consumer, while the second is to represent the legitimate interests of consumers. Representing the views of consumers can be a difficult matter because, if their fears or concerns are not rational or well-founded, the consumer can end up being the ultimate loser. Obviously, a large part of this function must be directed at ensuring that consumers have the most authoritative information available to them. In this way, at least they are representing the views of properly informed consumers.

In representing the interests of the consumer, the consumer advocates must be certain that they, themselves, are fully and objectively informed on the issues. Responsible consumer representatives usually approach the most qualified and recognized authorities they can for this information. Once this is secured, they pass this information to their members in language that is factual, objective and comprehensible. When all aspects of a particular issue have been analyzed and evaluated, a position representing the overall interests of the consumer is taken.

Consumer advocates have been very successful in ensuring that consumers are well informed about the pros and cons of the foods they eat and have made the food industry much more responsive to consumer concerns in general. Most traditional consumer groups try to avoid being single-issue advocacy groups, simply because this seldom leads to a balanced perspective for their membership.

The tactics of the more aggressive consumer activist groups seldom resemble those of traditional consumer advocates. They often characterize many issues as moral imperatives, rather than technical, economic or health problems that have to be dealt with pragmatically. Despite the fact that their arguments are occasionally distorted, the vigorous pursuit of issues and their compelling manner have made government and industry much more conscious of the need to compete for the attention of consumers. Together with traditional consumer advocates, their pressure tactics have benefited consumers in countless ways, including access to better labeling legislation and more consumer-oriented products.

The impact of the highly focused, single-issue advocacy has not been quite as positive. Although most of the causes they champion, such as protection of the environment, are important, they often do consumers a disservice by concentrating almost exclusively on emotional controversies rather than hard facts. However, they are invariably excellent debaters and very effective in a town-hall setting, where statements don't necessarily have to be corroborated. A favorite tactic is to shake the public's confidence in modern science and technology—this has often proved to be very successful. A fear of the unknown is almost universal, and most consumers view scientists with suspicion. The positions of these activists are often amplified by the media, because the controversy they generate sells news. Even well-known traditional consumer advocacy and activist groups have been seduced or hijacked by some of these single-issue activists and the attention they command in the press.[179]

In most advanced economies, the production and marketing of food is almost exclusively in the hands of the commercial private sector. It is the role of the government to develop policies and implement legislation and, in this way, they have an effect on the quality, price and availability of the foods consumers eat. Trade regulations and barriers determine the price and availability of most imported goods. The government also establishes the many food quality and safety standards that are required to ensure a wholesome food supply. The responsibility for the provision of nutritional advice and safety information to consumers also falls under government agencies.

National and international policies involved in establishing food pricing and availability often reveal the intricate relationship between the producers, the government and consumers. However, notwithstanding the expanding impact of advocacy groups, consumers continue to have very little effect upon government policy in these two areas. With the exception of programs designed to subsidize food for specific groups at risk (for example, food stamps), the development of policies about food pricing and availability remains an issue exclusively between producers and the government.

Consumers and their representatives have had a rather limited impact, thus far, on policies governing food quality. Food quality policies generally involve product standards and safety considerations. Standards can be as basic as fruit grading or as complex as the specifications for products such as chicken frankfurters or enriched breads. In the latter case, specifications are also set out for the flour used (vitamin and mineral supplements, maturing or bleaching agents and so on) as well as preservatives, emulsifiers, fats, milk, dough plasticizers and various other ingredients.

Food safety standards normally take shape through mediation between producers, processors and the concerned government agency. The major criteria employed to arrive at these standards are scientific data about food safety or toxicity together with the practical problems of food production. Consumers have always been subjected to all types of toxins, whether they come from the general environment or from the food and water supply. Biological mechanisms concentrated in the liver have evolved over history to neutralize most of the toxins we are faced with effectively. The problems arise when the levels of these toxins exceed our ability to deactivate them. Therefore, when food safety limits are set, the average tolerances to toxins are determined, and a very considerable margin of safety is added.

When decisions are made about food safety standards, it is in everyone's interest that they should be arrived at objectively and with the minimum of outside interference. This is not always that easy, because certain decisions can have significant political and commercial consequences. For example, standards prohibiting the presence of certain pathogenic bacteria in poultry could be very costly to the broiler industry. These costs would have to be passed on to consumers, who might react by reducing their levels of poultry consumption. This would, in turn, elicit a strong response from politicians whose constituents are poultry producers. Often, decisions that should be made based on biological or physiological criteria alone are compromised by other considerations.

When microbiologists examine the risks related to certain food products, they have to consider several matters in order to arrive at a meaningful conclusion. These might include the presence of certain sensitive ingredients, such as raw eggs, that might render the finished product more susceptible to pathogenic bacteria. They must determine whether the process used to prepare the food incorporates a decisive step to kill all unwanted microorganisms. They must also give further thought to any possible problems that might be involved in the way products are stored in warehouses or the manner in which they are distributed to supermarkets. The analysts must even be aware of problems that routinely occur in supermarkets, such as defrosting and refreezing of frozen foods or keeping foods past their expiration date. Finally, any assessment of the overall risks must reflect the manner in which consumers normally handle their foods in the home.

Setting food safety standards can be a very complicated process. Of course, anyone can come up with hypothetical standards that might sound good but will have no relation to the practical realities of production for the marketplace. For example, many have suggested that we follow the Swedish method for producing commercial poultry. Indeed, in some countries such as Sweden, the standards set for poultry are very high, but so is the cost of the poultry sold. Would consumers in America buy poultry if it cost two to three times its current price? In fact, whether the American poultry industry would have economic viability with such prices is questionable. So, decisions are made that reflect a compromise between what is ideal and what the realities of commercial food production dictate. This compromise differs somewhat from country to country. The only thing that is common is that safety standards seldom satisfy everyone.

When consumers disagree with these standards, they buy alternative products. The phenomenal growth in the organic food market is a good example. Even though the current levels of additives allowed in foods are considered to be safe, many consumers prefer products that do not contain them. Without certain additives, many products end up with a shorter shelf life or a substandard appearance. However, a growing number of consumers prefer these more natural products over the ones containing additives. The growth in sales of organic and natural foods over the last two decades has clearly demonstrated this. That is what freedom of choice is all about. However, these organic products must adhere to the same safety standards as commercial products. If someone can objectively demonstrate that these products provide an even greater degree of safety, then so much the better for the consumer.

Once government policy decisions have been made, the food production, processing and retailing sectors determine the price, quality and appearance of foods available on the market. Most companies continue to feel that price is a key criteria for consumers. As a result, they give priority to providing food to consumers at the lowest price. Upscale marketers, on the other hand, are confident that they can sell more expensive products by featuring exotic ingredients, elaborate packages and, most important, an exclusive image. In recent years, this form of product marketing has proven to be incredibly successful.

Supermarket retailers have always been extremely influential, and they continue to make most of the decisions regarding which foods will be offered to the public. Retailers make the important decisions regarding the priority given to products in terms of shelf space. Shelf space has become so important in the sales potential of products that supermarkets actually sell their space, in one way or another, to food manufacturers. Many small operators with the tastiest or most creative products have been completely excluded from selling in large supermarket chains because they could not raise the up-front money to pay for the shelf space (which sometimes runs into the six-figure bracket). Profitability, rather than acceptability, nutrition or safety, is the key consideration. Many retailers have for a long time known about the poor microbiological quality of products currently on the market. However, most supermarkets have done little to encourage processors to employ technologies that would eliminate pathogens from the mainstream food supply. On the contrary, even when such products are available, most retailers do not carry them. For example, very few supermarkets offer consumers a choice between regular and cold-pasteurized (irradiated) poultry.

Although the media does not like to assume the responsibility, it has always had an important role in educating the public. Today, more than 99 percent of American homes have at least one color television. In addition to the more than 11,000 newspapers, Americans can listen to in excess of 500 million radios. For many consumers, the media has effectively displaced government and academia as their formal source of knowledge. Unfortunately, the prime motivation of the media is profitability. This has had a major impact on determining the way in which information is presented, which has, in turn, had a profound impact on the perspectives developed by consumers.

News has become a form of public entertainment. While most journalists make a genuine effort to provide the facts, presenting a balanced perspective can be boring, time consuming and unprofitable. The more sensational or controversial issues will always get top billing. Outspoken, single-issue consumer activists will normally get more coverage than scientific or government authorities. Sadly, intense and fiery consumer advocates are usually more animated and interesting to interview than dull scientists.

More recently, the Internet has become a global information network for the public. Home computers can access text, images, e-mail, files, programs, sound, video and interactive discussions. The sheer quantity of information available is mind-boggling.

Publishing on the Internet is free from conventional constraints, so there is considerable variation in the quality of information. As a result, it is important that the reader distinguish what information is accurate. This is a particular problem for matters related to food-borne diseases because it is difficult to determine if the source of information is reliable, such as a government agency or a university, or the ranting of a commercially or lifestyle-oriented advocate. As an example, it is interesting to look at the results of a "benefits of raw milk" search on Google. It is not surprising when the public ends up with a somewhat distorted understanding of food and food safety.

Food safety and nutrition have never been considered a really interesting topic for the public. Very few television or radio shows address this issue per se, and few of the shows devoted to cooking or eating spend any time in this area. Indeed, I have seen a number of programs extolling the virtues of the great gourmet chefs of the world while, at the same time, demonstrating some of the worst hygienic practices imaginable. Surely, someone can assume a limited degree of responsibility to ensure that consumers are provided with decent examples of how to prepare foods safely.

Food safety education must start at the elementary school level and follow through to college. Children who have been taught about the dangers of tobacco and smoking come home and lecture their parents about it. The same can be done regarding children's knowledge of food and its preparation. The countless educational television shows we see are ideally suited for short spots about the promotion of safe food preparation and good hygiene habits. With little doubt, the media has a great role to play in bringing food safety to the consumer. Whether they will do it is another matter.

SELF-HELP

WHY IS SELF-HELP NECESSARY?

Our biosphere literally teems with life of every imaginable form. Microorganisms appear to occupy every nook, niche, cranny and crevice on the planet. They frequently contaminate the food and water we consume and, if not removed or destroyed, place us at continual risk. Many different pathogenic microorganisms are resistant to routine handling and preservation techniques, thus constituting a hazard in foods if they are consumed without further treatment. Certain foods, which pose no problems at all to most consumers, can be extremely dangerous to others who, for whatever medical reasons, are permanently or temporarily at an increased risk. Despite government legislation and control measures, and notwithstanding the rigorous quality assurance schemes of manufacturers and retailers, pathogen-containing foods continue to find their way into the homes of consumers. In all these instances, once pathogens make it through the front door of the home, the consumer must assume the role of ultimate manager of food safety. It is a demanding role and, judging from the evidence, one that people do not carry out as effectively as they should.

Although the precise incidence of food-borne illness is not known, the authoritative and widely read Council for Agricultural Science and Technology (CAST) report of 1994[180] estimated that the annual number of cases of food-borne illness in the United States was somewhere between 6.5 and 33 million. Other estimates go as high as 81 million cases,[181] and even this figure has been considered conservative.[182] These startling and disturbing numbers represent the net efforts of all actors and actions in the food system, which were unable to safeguard the consumer from food-borne diseases. While little doubt remains that everyone involved in bringing food to the consumer bears a large part of the responsibility for this deplorable situation, a good part of the responsibility also rests with consumers themselves.

Unfortunately, the old expression, "If you want something done, you have to do it yourself," applies far too often. Protecting yourself from the dangers of food-borne diseases is a case in point. Despite all the good intentions and progress made in improving the food supply, you still have to exercise a good deal of prudence and common sense to avoid the ill effects of food-borne diseases.

During a 1995 national telephone inquiry,[183] more than 1,600 randomly selected U.S. residents who were at least 18 years old and resided in households with kitchen facilities were quizzed about their knowledge of food-borne pathogens, of foods that pose a particular risk for transmitting diseases and of safe food-handling practices. One-third of the respondents recounted poor and unsafe food preparation practices. They did not wash their hands frequently nor were they aware of the precautions required to prevent cross contamination in the kitchen. Men reported unsafe practices more than women did. Oddly, adults in the 18- to 29-year-old bracket indicated worse habits than persons older than 30 years. These results confirm the need for consumer education and self-help.

In a comprehensive survey of food-borne disease outbreaks from 1973 to 1987, researchers determined that in approximately 20 percent of the cases, the implicated foods had been prepared in the home.[184] The same survey revealed that 92 percent of the botulism outbreaks were due to home-prepared foods, particularly canned foods. Likely, the number of cases of food-borne diseases that originate in the home is considerably higher than that reported since very few of these cases are actually reported. An analysis of the home-based cases revealed that a great many consumers lacked knowledge of the most basic principles of hygienic food preparation and preservation. The following table lists the most significant factors in the mishandling or the mistreatment of foods by consumers in the home. A review of the factors leaves us wondering how these easily preventable situations continue to occur on such a wide scale—yet they do. It is a clear example of where a little self-help can prevent an enormous amount of needless suffering and unwarranted expense.

MAJOR IN-HOME CONTRIBUTING FACTORS TO FOOD-BORNE DISEASES	
RANK	FACTOR
1	Improper storage and holding temperature
2	Use of contaminated foods or ingredients
3	Inadequate cooking or heat processing
4	Food obtained from unreliable source (e.g., polluted waters)
5	Improper cooling of food
6	Long delays (12 hours or more) between preparation and eating
7	Infected person handling and preparing food
8	Poor personal hygiene of food handler
9	Cross contamination in the kitchen

The modern food system extends from the farm to the consumer's plate. If the consumer is to have some measure of freedom from food-borne diseases, then a systematic approach to food safety must be maintained throughout the system. There is a limited value to the food industry adopting elaborate HACCP programs (see page 138) if foods will then be abused in the home. For example, research has shown that although foods may be fully cooked, allowing them to stand unrefrigerated for long periods before consumption can result in high risks for consumers.[185] Therefore, self-help is a critical component of any fully integrated program designed to ensure food safety for all the family. The good news is that the most important element of any self-help effort is plain, common sense coupled with a basic understanding of how food goes bad.

INFORMATION SOURCES OF FOOD-BORNE DISEASES AND THEIR PREVENTION

The amount of information available about food-borne diseases and how to avoid them is surprising. Newspaper articles, television programs, books, brochures and pamphlets are available from municipal, state and national government health departments, food companies, consumer groups and innumerable advocates promoting one lifestyle or another. For those that have computers equipped with modems, the motherload of all information is available—the Internet. A supplement containing several major Web sites has been appended to this book. All you have to search for is "food-borne disease," and a wide range of information sources will turn up. At times, however, this mind-boggling array of information can be more of a risk than a benefit, because a good deal of it comes from dubious sources that promote their own interests rather than those of the consumer.

The Internet swooped down upon us like no other phenomenon in history. In the period of a few short years, we have embraced an information technology that permits any individual with access to a computer to communicate with the entire world. The Internet also allows individuals to portray themselves in any way they wish—from forthright images to elaborate fantasies, from gurus to presidents of multinational corporations to benevolent leaders of international charities. All one has to do is design a home page representing the particular image in question and then place it onto the World Wide Web. No controls, no rules and no internationally accepted conventions exist. With very little effort, the proverbial snake oil salesman can come off looking like a professor of pharmacology who just won a Nobel prize in medicine and take advantage of people online desperate for advice—any advice. The Internet is a source of information, but it does not guarantee the quality of the information it contains.

People without computers may be able to access the Internet with the help of their local libraries. Government departments, universities, private companies, hospitals, research institutions, various societies and associations as well as individuals are all on the Internet, and they all have free information to offer. It is utter chaos—which is both the Internet's strength and weakness. The lack of controls over the quality of the material on the Internet permits the widest range of information and opinion to be available. However, this also requires that the user discriminate between the reliable and the ridiculous.

Food-borne diseases are serious, and anyone seeking advice should make sure the information is authoritative. As a rule of thumb, it is always best to go to those sources who have the primary responsibility of protecting the public—your local department of public health. You may not get the most animated or glitzy information, but it will generally be rational and balanced. The information it has to offer is usually available in paper form, such as brochures and information leaflets, for those who do not have access to the Internet. The well-designed home pages from various health departments usually have links to many other related sites from around the world. These same departments often have toll-free telephone or fax numbers for consumers to call to get answers to specific questions they may have. These sources are the first ones to try in the search for authoritative information. If the service they provide is not up to expectations, then you can usually complain to a higher authority.

Many universities, particularly those with active departments of food science or schools of public health, provide highly qualified information about food-borne diseases. If they do not print their own materials, then they will generally be able to direct you to an authoritative source of information. Most universities have excellent home pages with interesting links to related information, including nutrition and diet. A certain amount of discretion and common sense is required here, because universities do not always validate the information put out by their staff. Although remote, the possibility always exists that an individual or a group promoting themselves or a particular philosophy may hijack the reputation of the university for their own parochial purposes.

Other interesting sources of information are international health organizations and food technology associations. They often have excellent documentation, written in simple language, that deals with the subject of food-borne diseases in general as well as with specific problems or issues of current interest such as large food-poisoning outbreaks. These organizations all have home pages with useful links to other sources of related information. Agencies such as the World Health Organization (WHO) or the Pan American Health Organization (PAHO) are prime examples of such institutions. The Institute of Food Technologists represents a good model of a food technology association dedicated to providing up-to-date, authoritative information about all aspects of food. It publishes a monthly journal and has printed materials in simple language about specific food-related topics. It also has an excellent home page.

Many consumer organizations provide information about food issues in both printed and electronic form. Of all sources of information available about food-borne diseases, this source should be one of the most useful but, sadly, this does not always occur. In fact, some of the best-known consumer organizations provide almost no information at all about the subject. It is a great pity and a lost opportunity, because many consumers believe implicitly in their advocacy organizations and do not treat them with the same critical eye as they would, say, the government. In these cases, influence over the consumer is squandered by approaching all issues as political confrontations and treating them with moral indignation rather than simply providing high-quality, practical information that can be of some use to their members. While no doubt exists that certain circumstances in the food system can evoke bitterness or dissatisfaction, resorting to highly charged rhetoric does not make the consumer more accurately and usefully informed.

When dealing with food-borne diseases, avoid information from fringe groups with very specific agendas and instant answers to all the questions. Authoritative advice about any issue requires an in-depth knowledge of what is going on—a level of specific professional expertise seldom available from these fringe groups. Consumers should not be impressed by a Ph.D. after anyone's name, unless it accurately reflects the experience and expertise that it strives to portray. I have known Ph.D.s in psychology or sociology pass themselves off as nuclear experts. Although they may have been more animating to listen to than nuclear physicists, they did not provide the facts needed to make rational judgments about the issues.

CONSUMER EDUCATION

Just as professional food handlers must learn the basic principles of hygiene and all the procedures required to minimize the chances of causing food-borne diseases, so must anyone who prepares food in the home. Consumers who understand the rudimentary principles of safe food handling are well equipped to make the routine risk-benefit decisions needed in the kitchen on a daily basis. Should the leftovers be kept another day, or should they be thrown out? Is it safe to make Caesar salad with raw eggs, or should you coddle them first? If the meat is slightly discolored, does that mean it is spoiled? Should the hollandaise sauce, accidentally left out overnight, be used the next morning for eggs Benedict? These are all risk-benefit questions that require some knowledge to minimize risk and maximize benefit. Above all, everyone must appreciate that very few, if any, activities in life are without some risk, even if it is minuscule. The same goes for food safety—no foods can be made entirely free of risk—all you can do is minimize risk. Without understanding this simple premise, consumers may abdicate their own obligations. They will end up taking advice from carpetbaggers peddling magic bullets and instant solutions to serious food safety issues.

Basic hygiene and food safety should be introduced to children at an early age. It is an ideal subject for children's educational T.V. programs. Animated cartoons can introduce the world of microbes, and basic hygienic principles can be easily demonstrated by actions and imitation. The fundamental concepts of food handling and storage can also be made into a demonstrative activity. It is a practical knowledge that will be reinforced every day throughout life, and it may one day save lives. Seeing the numbers of adults leaving washrooms with combed hair but unwashed hands is astonishing. The same can be said of children and teenagers. Hygiene must be made more interesting, and the educational process must continue throughout life. Schools, in particular, must have visible reinforcing signs in kitchens and washrooms to ensure that students and employees always observe basic hygiene.

Adult consumers could also benefit from hygiene education. However, getting an older person to have the patience to sit through lectures about the subject is generally difficult. It might be useful if cooking shows would make a special effort, without being ponderous, to incorporate good handling practices and tips during the course of the show. People at an exceptionally high risk from food-borne diseases must be made especially sensitive to the importance of proper hygiene and food-handling practices. When considering the large and growing number of people in this group, having a cooking program that specializes in the preparation of foods that provide the greatest degree of freedom from food-borne diseases would be very useful. The same can be said for those cookbooks, cooking magazines and newspaper sections devoted to the home preparation of food. Consumers should not be put off by such a prospect, because the most delicious and appealing foods can also be the most hygienic.

REDUCING FOOD-BORNE DISEASES IN THE HOME

Most practices involved in preventing food-borne diseases in the home are little more than common sense and may appear to be trivial. They do, however, constitute the difference between good and poor home practice. The following lists were designed for you to check off, so that you can have an idea of how you rate. Before starting out, it may be worthwhile to take a look at a list of the materials and gadgets you will need to comply with good handling and good sanitation practices.

Tools of the Trade

Check off each tool of the trade that you have access to when cooking:

- ☐ oven, refrigerator and meat thermometers
- ☐ tempered glass or easy-to-wash plastic cutting board
- ☐ dishwasher or draining rack for cutlery and dishes
- ☐ holders or hooks for separate hand and dish towels
- ☐ rubber gloves, in good condition
- ☐ sink disposal system and/or convenient waste receptacle with a disposable and sealable liner

□ assortment of clean sponges, wipes or cloths
□ easily accessible paper towels (preferably white and not recycled)
□ hand soap (regular and antibacterial) and moisturizing hand cream
□ disinfectant counter spray or hypochlorite bleach for dilution
□ self-stick labels to make sure you know what everything is
□ easily washable cotton aprons

Acquiring Foods

Check off each method that applies when you acquire foods:

□ make sure the supermarket is a spotless establishment, particularly
the meat and fish areas as well as the fresh salad section—see that
the ice in the fish and seafood display is fresh and clean—supermarket hygiene is costly and, despite head office policies, store managers
occasionally cut corners.
□ ensure that grocery shopping is the last item on the agenda before
returning home—delays in refrigerating foods often result in multiplication of microorganisms
□ when purchasing foods, examine them carefully, check expiration
dates and buy all refrigerated foods last so you can get them home
quickly (well-managed stores always place their freshest goods at
the rear of the displays in order to sell the oldest goods first)
□ choose foods that have been processed to ensure a greater degree
of safety, such as pasteurized or microfiltered rather than raw
milk, and select poultry treated with ionizing irradiation if it is
available (World Health Organization *Golden Rules for Safe Food
Preparation*)
□ packaged poultry, meat and fish may leak juices containing pathogens—handle them with the plastic gloves or the plastic bags freely
available in the produce department—if not, juices from these products can be easily transferred to hands and then to fruit or vegetables that you are going to eat raw and unpeeled—simple cold-water
rinsing would not eliminate the contaminating organisms—keep
them in a free plastic produce bag until you get home
□ check canned and bottled goods carefully to ensure that the top lid is
slightly concave, indicating a partial vacuum—products with lids that
are level or bulging should be checked out with the store manager
□ fish and shellfish from polluted waters are tainted and are a hazard—
consuming these products is an unacceptable risk—the same goes for
wild game hung for tenderness until it is "ripe"

Proper Storage of Foods

Place a check mark next to each method of properly storing foods that
you employ:

☐ make a point of checking the temperature of your refrigerator/freezer regularly or leave a thermometer in it permanently—the refrigerator should be held between 40°F and 42°F, and the freezer should be kept at 0°F—refrigerators lose their coolant gas with age and should be recharged if not cooling properly

☐ refrigerate all perishable items as soon as you arrive home—certain fruits such as bananas are very sensitive to cold and should be kept outside in a cool place protected from flies—it is generally not necessary to store potatoes in the refrigerator, so long as you keep them in a cool, dark place if you are going to consume them within a week

☐ keep meat or poultry that is to be consumed within 48 hours or less in the refrigerator—the rest goes into the freezer

☐ refrigerated meat, poultry and fish should be packaged so that they do not leak juices over other products—loose plastic wrap or new plastic bags are well-suited for this purpose

☐ keep eggs refrigerated, as they will last longer and contaminating salmonella, if present, will be more susceptible to cooking[186]

☐ wrap frozen foods carefully and tightly with a minimum of air—do not jam the freezer because it will not properly circulate the cooling air

☐ check the refrigerator daily, and throw out anything perishable that is moldy or has been around for more than four to five days—try to plan the consumption of foods *before* you have to throw them out

☐ refrigerate all dressings and sauces such as mayonnaise, ketchup, salad dressings and so on after opening them

☐ do not keep sensitive products in the door panel of the refrigerator since this is the warmest location of the unit

☐ defrost and thoroughly clean the refrigerator and freezer according to the manufacturer's instructions—stick a label on the inside door panel with a reminder of the next defrost date

☐ in all storage situations, follow the same rules as supermarkets do— rotate the goods so that the freshest are at the back and the oldest come forward to be used first—this way, you will avoid being faced one day with four-year-old tomato sauce in a rusty can that looks like it was salvaged from the Titanic

☐ keep cupboards uncluttered and scrupulously clean—at the first sign of insect infestation, remove everything and throw out all open boxes, bags (including ones with bag ties), and containers with loose tops—try to find the source of infestation (flour, bread crumbs, dried fruit and so forth) and throw it out—clean up everything and for the next two weeks, check daily for signs of insect reemergence

☐ clean up all cupboard spills immediately, and occasionally check the bottom of all containers to make sure no leakage or residue is occurring from capillary action (which is common with oil bottles or dispensers)

☐ clean under all rotating cupboard racks

□ if your home is not air-conditioned, be aware that all storage problems are aggravated during the hot summer months, which is also the period of the greatest frequency of food-borne diseases

FOOD STORAGE TIMES		
FOOD PRODUCT (properly wrapped)	RECOMMENDED STORAGE PERIOD	
	Refrigerator (40°F) (days)	Freezer (0°F) months
Chicken—whole or parts	1–3	6–9
Chicken—in long-life package	4–6	9–12
Pork—roast and chops	3–5	4–6
Pork—ground	1–2	1–3
Beef—roasts and steaks	3–6	6–9
Beef—ground	1–3	1–3
Fish—whole and slices, lean	1–2	3–6
Fish—whole and slices, fatty	1–2	2–4
Fish—smoked	2–5	2–6
Cured meats	2–4	1–3
Cooked stew	2–4	2–4
Cooked soup	1–3	2–4
Cooked vegetables	1–3	2–4
Eggs in their shells	15–20	—
Cooked rice—pudding and pilaf	2–4	1–3

Personal Hygiene

Place a check mark next to the personal hygiene methods you use:

□ while ridding hands of the normal population of bacteria (including those hiding in hair follicles and microscopic cracks and creases in the skin) is virtually impossible, thorough washing and proper hygiene will significantly reduce the number of pathogenic bacteria picked up from unfavorable sources (nasal passages, fecal contamination and raw animal products)

□ washing means thoroughly scrubbing with soap and warm water for 20 to 30 seconds and drying with a clean towel (preferably a disposable paper towel)—safe hand disinfectant solutions are available but of limited use since most depend upon the action of a residue film and are very slow to work

□ have a good-quality nylon nail brush handy, because microbes love to hide under nails and cuticles—change the brush before it begins to look like a scouring pad—few sights are less appetizing than seeing someone preparing foods looking like they just finished greasing a lawn mower

□ after handling raw fish, meat or poultry, never touch foods intended to be eaten raw without first thoroughly washing your hands

□ the three most critical sites of contamination for the hands are the toilet, the nose and raw animal foods (including soft unpasteurized cheeses)—you must presume that even minor contact results in significant contamination, and personal hygienic actions must follow accordingly—very thorough washing (30 seconds minimum) followed by drying with a clean, dry towel—wait at least five minutes before handling foods that will not receive heat treatment (raw fruits and vegetables, cream fillings, precooked seafood like shrimp)—keep the handling of these products down to a minimum

□ do not prepare foods if you are ill with diarrhea or viral diseases because they are easily transferred to foods—if you absolutely must, exercise due caution—if at all possible, stay out of the kitchen entirely, and do not share your hand towel with anyone else

□ your clothes and appearance should be neat, clean and consistent with the responsible task of preparing safe and healthy food

Food Preparation and Consumption

Check off each method you use when preparing and consuming food:

□ raw eggs in their shells are a high-risk food and should not be consumed without fully cooking them—soft-boiled, sunny-side up and any cooked form of eggs where liquid yolk remains may still contain *Salmonella*[187, 188]—mayonnaise, Caesar salad dressing, homemade ice cream and any food containing raw eggs should not be consumed by anyone who is even slightly immunocompromised—pasteurized liquid egg or egg replacement products can be used for these purposes—a letter in the *British Medical Journal* recommends that recipes and magazine articles about cooking should never recommend the consumption of foods containing raw eggs[189]

□ defrost foods overnight in the refrigerator or in the microwave according to instructions—foods should not be left out for long periods in the kitchen to defrost because that will promote the growth of microorganisms

□ plan the sequence and strategy of your cooking—you will be better organized, you will make better use of space and utensils and it will prevent cross contamination of foods and needless exposure to incorrect temperatures

□ avoid all contact between raw and cooked foods

□ make sure foods are thoroughly defrosted before cooking, and make sure they are cooked throughout—a minimum internal temperature of 155°F should be reached for beef and lamb, 160°F for pork and 175°F for poultry

☐ although those cute little pop-up timers that come with some turkeys are quite accurate as far as temperature is concerned, they penetrate only to a limited depth so that they do not actually reflect the same amount of doneness for different-sized turkeys—they work well for birds up to 10 pounds—above that, use a good-quality meat thermometer inserted into the deepest part of the meat[190]

☐ use clean, sharp knives and a cutting board that is easy to clean (plastic or tempered glass is best)—discard the cutting board when it is so used that normal cleaning will not remove all the residues— never allow residues on the cutting board from one food to contaminate another food—this is a very common way for cross contamination to occur

☐ do not allow anyone to taste foods before they are fully cooked—no tasting of cake or cookie batters that contain raw eggs—no tasting of raw or partially cooked gefilte fish or fish soup (taste and season them after they are cooked)—do not be tempted to eat while cooking or barbecuing

☐ sashimi, sushi, steak tartare, oysters, seviche, lightly smoked products and all other uncooked animal-based products pose a great risk— adventuresome consumers should be prepared to pay the piper

☐ wash all raw fruits and vegetables thoroughly

☐ wash hands frequently while preparing foods and particularly well after a visit to the washroom

☐ never prepare foods if you have open cuts or wounds of any type— wear gloves if you must—never smoke at the same time as you are preparing food—pin back long hair—all this is done in an army field kitchen, it is the least you can do at home

☐ make sure the lids of cans are clean before opening them because dust and dirt can easily enter during the opening process—keep the cutting blades of the can opener clean to prevent contamination

☐ when you barbecue foods, remember that everything that is not cooked is contaminated—if you use a plate to bring raw foods to the barbecue, do not use the same plate to bring the cooked products back unless you have thoroughly washed and dried it—keep the turning spatula near the coals for a short period before you remove products from the grill to ensure that you do not recontaminate a cooked product

☐ if any product smells bad, cooking will not improve it—throw it out

☐ eat foods as soon as possible after they are cooked—do not let them stand around—if they are not to be consumed immediately, keep hot foods hot (140°F or above) and cold foods cold (45°F or less)

☐ do not cut corners when microwaving foods—follow manufacturer's directions carefully, and observe all resting or standing periods

☐ when foods are required to be reheated, bring them to a minimum temperature of 160°F to 165°F—you can use a thermometer to be sure

- [ ] refrigerate foods destined to be leftovers immediately after eating—not after washing the dishes, but immediately—place them into shallow containers to ensure rapid cooling—do not stack one container over the other as this will slow cooling considerably—refrigerator manufacturers should make racks capable of holding warm plates—refrigerated foods should be consumed within three to four days (unless they are frozen)
- [ ] when preparing spicy or aromatic foods that may end up as stored leftovers (such as basmati rice pilaf), make sure the spices and herbs receive high-heat treatment (prefrying in oil) prior to adding rice— natural spices or herbs can contain high loads of microbial spores that can be very resistant to simple cooking or simmering and pose a risk if they start growing in great numbers
- [ ] avoid foods susceptible to *Listeria* (for example, unpasteurized soft cheeses), and remember that this bacteria can multiply at refrigeration temperatures
- [ ] if anybody insists that a little bit of dirt is good for you, take them out to the garden, and have them swallow a thimbleful of the stuff

Kitchen Hygiene

Place a check next to each phrase that applies to your kitchen:

- [ ] keep the entire kitchen spotless and clean up as quickly as possible— do not wait until residues dry, because removing them will be move difficult
- [ ] keep counters clean with soap and warm water, and regularly wipe them with a disinfectant solution, which could be chlorine based (mild solution of bleach such as two teaspoons per quart of water) or any commercial consumer product—a new waterless sanitation system for bacteria removal using a handy sanitizer wipe was recently tested by the U.S. Army and proved to be very effective in eliminating several food-poisoning microbes[191]
- [ ] use a dishwasher with hot-air drying, if available—if not, wash with soap and warm water and allow to drain and air dry
- [ ] change hand and dish towels frequently and do not use them when they are damp because, in that state, they are more of a microbial liability than an asset
- [ ] do not soak soiled dishes in warm water without soap or detergent— it is an ideal breeding ground for microbes
- [ ] at least twice a month, pour a mild solution of bleach (three teaspoons per quart of water) down your kitchen sink drain and allow to stand for at least 10 minutes
- [ ] clean utensils, food processors, meat grinders and graters thoroughly with warm water and soap

□ never store any kitchen utensils or containers unless they have completely dried
□ when you are finally sure that you can eat off the floor, make sure you do not

A WORD ABOUT MICROWAVE OVENS

Microwave ovens have become one of the most popular appliances in the modern kitchen. They work in a manner totally different from a conventional oven, and few people are aware of the idiosyncrasies they possess. As an example, microwave heating has a tendency to produce cold spots in the oven, which result in uneven heating and a risk of undercooking.[192] As a consequence, some concerns exist regarding their ability to deliver properly cooked foods to the consumer consistently.[193] Questions also exist regarding the proper use of packaging and utensils for microwave cooking.[194]

MICROWAVABLE PACKAGING AND COOKWARE

Follow these guidelines when using microwavable packaging and cooking:

□ all products specifically designed for microwave use are clearly labeled to that effect—they are very stable to high heat and will not leach out chemicals into the food
□ never use container types expressly excluded by the microwave manufacturer
□ never use recycled paper or bags since you cannot know what they may contain
□ cold-storage plastic containers (e.g., plastic yogurt or margarine tubs) were made for the cold and not the microwave—they might even melt
□ remove the store packaging prior to defrosting in order to avoid chemical migration from white foam trays and plastic wrap into the food—these materials were designed for low temperatures
□ when using a microwave to defrost foods, carry on with the final cooking immediately—defrosting sometimes sets up warm spots in the food that make a good area for the multiplication of bacteria
□ avoid salting foods before they go into the microwave—salt saps microwave energy, and the foods will not get the level of heat treatment you expect[195, 196]—if food has been salted, compensate with a longer microwave time or check the food with a thermometer
□ microwave heating can be very uneven, especially with tall, thin containers such as baby bottles[197]—take these out, mix them two to

three times during the heating process and thoroughly shake and temperature-test them before feeding to infants in order to prevent scalding

☐ remove large bones, if possible, before cooking since they will interfere with even heat distribution

☐ if, after microwave cooking, a dish has to be finished by browning in a conventional oven, do it right away—do not allow partially cooked foods to stand around and spoil

☐ if you have the option, cook meat at lower power for longer periods in order to achieve greater uniformity of heat distribution

☐ always follow the manufacturer's instructions regarding a waiting period after microwave cooking—even though the food may have reached the proper temperature, it may not have been at that temperature for a sufficient time to kill all pathogens[198]—this is also true for reheating cold foods[199]

☐ when reheating leftovers, they should be brought to a minimum temperature of 160°F to 165°F

☐ particular concerns regarding microwavable foods are targeted at children and teens[200] because the risk of severe burns due to uneven heating is real[201]

☐ at times, microwaving of certain products, such as bacon, is actually considered safer than conventional methods[202] because the fat can be easily drained off and fewer nitrosamines form

AVOIDING PROBLEMS IN RESTAURANTS AND TAKEOUTS

With people consuming more and more of meals away from home, food safety in restaurants and take-out establishments is becoming a major issue of concern. Consumer confidence in restaurant food is questionable. A 1995 University of Georgia study demonstrated this: 84 percent of the participants said they would like all chicken served in restaurants or fast-food places to be irradiated.[203] In fact, the restaurant industry has started to carry more insurance specifically for food-poisoning incidents.[204] Although the restaurant trade commonly receives some form of government inspection, it continues to be one of the most unregulated industries in the food system. Foods do not have to be labeled, employees do not require proof of hygienic training or strict health certification and consumers depend entirely upon the good faith of the restauranteur to assure their food safety. Years ago, when people ate relatively few meals away from home, this issue was not that critical. However, now, away-from-home eating accounts for more than 50 percent of all food consumed in the United States.[205]

Restaurants, both gourmet and fast-food varieties, have been responsible for food-borne disease outbreaks due to poor hygiene, poor cooking practices, the purchase of contaminated raw materials and general negligence. Problems have ranged from anisakid parasites in sushi[206] to *E. coli* O157:H7 in hamburgers to the sale of ciguatera-prone fish.[207] Consumers are well-advised to approach restaurant eating with the same or even greater caution than eating at home. Just as high-quality food is available from the most modest local operations to nationally known gourmet extravaganzas, such is the case with poor-quality food. Do not be impressed with fancy decor and pretentious waiters named François—unless he and his establishment are scrupulously clean. The quality of the food ultimately causes food-borne disease—not the decor or the waiter. This is not a condemnation of all restaurants but simply a note of caution for consumers to include hygiene and food safety in their overall understanding of what food quality really is. The following checklist offers some guidelines to lessen the risk of eating out:

- check out the cleanliness of the entire place—the tables, floors, table tops or tablecloths, china, glassware, cutlery and any equipment you can see—some consumers do not hesitate to inspect the kitchen, and no one can prevent them from this prerogative
- check out the appearance of any food on display, such as antipastos, fish displays or desserts—the more out in the open the food, the more trust must be placed in a restaurant
- check the appearance of the staff, their appearance should indicate that they respect themselves
- if all else appears in order, do not neglect to trust your senses—simply do not consume food that looks or smells bad—have it taken back and leave the restaurant, preferably without paying, because restaurants know exactly what they serve you
- if you are not familiar with the restaurant, use caution when ordering all products particularly susceptible to storage and temperature abuse—custards, creme fillings, zabaglione and so on
- ask if the Caesar salad dressings are made with pasteurized eggs—it is not as impressive as a waiter cracking an egg and making the dressing in front of you, but the risks are considerably lower—if you insist on the show, the waiter should use a coddled egg
- eat raw foods at your own risk—never eat steak tartare from wild game, take up skydiving instead—it is probably safer

Remember, you are the client—trust yourself, and trust your instincts. If worse comes to worst, a minor embarrassment is much easier to handle than a life-threatening disease. The food that goes into your mouth can nourish or sicken your body—you are in control. Do not cede that control to others without some prudence.

AVOIDING PROBLEMS WHILE ABROAD

The variety of food available around the world is really quite incredible. It is difficult to think of Thailand without its Tom Yum (lemongrass) soup or China without its sautéed sea cucumbers and 100-year-old eggs. One of the tastiest fish meals I ever had was barbecued bluefin tuna jaw at a tiny, second-story hole-in-the-wall restaurant in Manila. Eating local food is an integral part of the travel adventure and experience. Unfortunately, all too often, tourists come down with food-borne diseases, some very critical. Because of the serious nature of this problem and because of the difficulties in keeping up with traveling tourists, staff from the Walter Reed Army Research Institute carried out a study on expatriate residents living in Kathmandu, Nepal.[208] The results linked food-borne-related diarrhea with younger ages, the duration of the stay, eating in restaurants and warm weather—not a very surprising conclusion.

People generally adapt to their particular environment. Long-term residents (including expatriates) develop an immunity to certain endemic disease organisms. This is, of course, not the case with temporary visitors or newcomers. Therefore, take all precautions, and even that may not be a guarantee. Years ago, I was traveling through the heart of Nigeria with a colleague and, every morning at the same time, we both took exactly the same protective pills against malaria. We were never out of each other's sight. A month after our return, he came down with a near-fatal case of cerebral malaria, and I never experienced any symptoms whatsoever.

The standards of cleanliness and hygiene that we routinely take for granted do not apply in many other parts of the world. Economically developed countries usually have similar or even better standards of hygiene—therefore they require the same amount of prudence as one would use back home. Developing countries represent a wider range of hygienic conditions—and even within one country, broad variations exist. Well-known restaurants and modern hotel chains cater to international business people as well as tourists and generally provide food that is very low risk. Small restaurants and street vendors can be a problem, particularly if they have not received any training in hygienic food preparation.

The popularity of travel and the wide range of problems encountered warrant particular attention. A separate chapter has been devoted to it.

SIMPLE PRECAUTIONS

Below are a few simple hints considered the most basic preventives:

- see your doctor or public health department, and get advice about traveling to your destination country (this may range from simple precautionary advice to shots for yellow fever and hepatitis as well as prophylactic pills for known microorganisms)

- carry antidiarrheal medicine such as Imodium and a gentle bulking fiber such as Metamucil to slow water loss—carry a few packets of rehydration salts
- while it is great fun to eat with the people, it does involve certain risks—consider it carefully
- most street foods are acceptable if they are freshly cooked and piping hot, but that is not always the case—when not properly handled, they can be a major source of contamination[209]
- if not adequately trained, street food vendors will allow unconsumed foods to stand for long periods until they are sold (sometimes unrefrigerated overnight[210])—eat only from vendors who appear clean and busy, and eat at the height of mealtime to increase the chances of getting the freshest food
- buy only bottled water, and check that the cap is tightly sealed—it is no guarantee, but it is the best you can do
- in certain countries, eating with fingers from communal bowls is a habit and you are charged for only what you consume—avoid these opportunities because they present an exceedingly high risk of contracting food-borne infection
- cruise ships experience occasional problems, particularly with undercooked seafood such as scallops[211]—exercise caution when on shore excursions
- camping or picnicking can also pose problems if foods are kept at ambient temperature for long periods—make sure to use a coolerbox[212]
- getting sick can ruin any vacation, so exercise caution regarding what you eat, where you eat and how much you eat

WHAT TO DO IF YOU GET SICK

If, after all the precautions you have taken, you do manage to get ill, you can do a number of things to minimize the negative impact and put yourself on the road to recovery. Considering what has happened it is most important.

What Are Your Symptoms?

- nausea, vomiting, retching
- abdominal pain, diarrhea
- dizziness, weakness
- chills, fever, sore throat
- rash, swelling, tightening of throat
- cramps, bloody stools

What and Where Did You Eat During the Last Day or So?

- home-cooked meals
- restaurant, fast food
- cafeteria
- meat, fish, poultry
- eggs, dairy products
- salads, side dishes
- baked goods
- any suspect foods

How Long Since Your Last Meal or the Suspect Meal?

- less than one hour
- one to two hours
- two to four hours
- six to 16 hours
- 12 to 24 hours
- more than 24 hours

Record your symptoms, and seek medical attention immediately. Many food-borne disease incidents are self-limiting and disappear by themselves. However, you have no way of knowing what the outcome of your own episode will be. Do not treat symptoms lightly. Seeing a doctor and relating exactly what your symptoms are is best. You can also indicate what you feel may have brought on your condition. If you have abdominal pain or cramps, diarrhea, bloody stools or decreased urine output, make sure a stool culture is taken. Hemolytic uremic syndrome is characterized by diarrhea followed by hemolytic anemia (rapid loss of blood platelets, brown urine) and loss of kidney function—it is very serious. Follow the physician's instructions carefully. Seek a second opinion if you lack confidence in the first diagnosis and course of treatment.

If you experience rapid-onset symptoms, call your physician and ask whether you should go directly to a treatment center—this will be critical in cases of toxic poisoning. Physicians seldom have the sort of equipment or antitoxins required to deal with poisoning incidents. Powerful toxins do not leave much time for treatment. It is best if your physician can arrange to have you admitted to the treatment center and follow-up with you afterward. If you are experiencing much water loss with diarrhea, drink water with salts, and occasionally take a gentle fiber-bulking agent. If no packets of rehydration salts are conveniently available, have some form of sports beverage handy for this purpose. They normally contain a moderate level of replacement electrolytes (salts) and sugar for energy. Fresh coconut water is also an excellent alternative in tropical countries.

Depending on how you feel and the severity of your symptoms, inquire with your physician if you could eat yogurt. Yogurt with live lactobacillus cultures may help improve digestion, particularly after you have had antibiotic treatment. The live lactobacillus in certain brands of yogurt may also compete with and help to displace some of the pathogens you harbor.[213]

In order to provide some guidance as to the onset times and types of symptoms associated with the more common food-borne diseases, a table based upon these elements follows. Remember that the table represents averages and is only a guideline. Variations can result from the dose of pathogen or toxin ingested, the general health or immunocompromised status of the individual and even the time of the month. As unique individuals, our own particular constitutions will play a significant role in determining the variations from the average figures.

ONSET TIMES, DURATION, SYMPTOMS AND LIKELY CAUSE OF FOOD-BORNE ILLNESSES		
SYMPTOM ONSET TIME AFTER EATING	MAIN SYMPTOM	LIKELY CAUSE
Less than one hour	headache, nausea, dizziness, facial flush, itchiness, vomiting	Scombroid poison
	tingling, numbness, pallor, drowsiness, slurred speech, breathing difficulty, loss of reflexes, staring	Paralytic or neurotoxic shellfish poison tetrodotoxin
	perspiration, excess salivation, asthma, irregular pulse, gastroenteritis	*Muscaria* mushroom poisoning
one to four hours	nausea, retching, vomiting, perspiration, abdominal pain, diarrhea	*Staphylococcus aureus* enterotoxin
	tingling, numbness, pallor, gastroenteritis, drowsiness, slurred speech, breathing difficulty, loss of reflexes	Ciguatera toxin
six to 24+ hours	nausea, retching, vomiting, thirst, diarrhea, pupil dilation, collapse	*Amanita* mushroom poisoning
	sore throat, fever, nausea, vomiting	*Streptococcus pyogenes*
	dizziness, blurred vision, loss of reflex to light, difficulty swallowing and breathing, weakness, slurred speech, respiratory paralysis	*Clostridium botulinum* toxin (can occur from 12 to 36 hours)

SYMPTOM ONSET TIME AFTER EATING	MAIN SYMPTOM	LIKELY CAUSE
six to 24+ hours	nausea, vomiting, perspiration, abdominal pain, cramps, diarrhea	*Clostridium perfringens, Bacillus cereus, Streptococcus faecalis*
	vomiting, abdominal pain, cramps, diarrhea, headache, occasional high fever, chills, prostration	*Salmonella* species *E. coli* species *Campylobacter* species *Shigella* species Other enterics
	with bloody/mucoid (fatty) diarrhea	*Vibrio* species
	bloody diarrhea/hemolytic uremic syndrome	*E. coli* O157:H7
	with flulike symptoms	*Yersinia enterocolitica*
12 to 48 hours	nausea, vomiting, diarrhea, stomach cramping, low-grade fever, chills, headache, muscle aches, and a general sense of tiredness. Children experience more vomiting than adults.	*Norovirus*
24 to 72 hours	vomiting, abdominal pain, cramps, diarrhea, headache, fever	Enteric viruses
More than four days	gastroenteritis, fever, muscle pain, perspiration, chills, breathing difficulty, puffiness about the eyes	*Trichinella spiralis*
	fever, headache, nausea, retching, vomiting, abdominal pain, constipation, red spots, bloody stools	*Salmonella typhi*
	fever, headache, muscle tenderness, rash	*Toxoplasma gondii*
	abdominal pain, mucus-like diarrhea, loss of weight	*Giardia lamblia*
	abdominal pain, diarrhea, headache, constipation, drowsiness	*Entamoeba hystolytica*
	hunger, insomnia, nervousness, weight loss, abdominal pain, gastroenteritis	*Taenia saginata* and other tapeworms

NEW DEVELOPMENTS IN DIAGNOSIS

The ever-escalating concerns about food-borne diseases have spawned the proliferation of rapid techniques for the detection of microbial contamination of foods and food-processing operations. Several new methods have been developed utilizing the biochemical, chemical and physical properties of microorganisms. Kits are currently available that can give extremely rapid (less than one minute) indications of the level of contamination of working surfaces, such as counters and cutting boards. Other techniques quickly differentiate between various strains of the same bacteria. Immunological tests and analyses based on the identification of specific DNA fragments have proven to be very accurate. Considerable progress has also been achieved in the development of unique biosensors for the detection of specific microorganisms.

In the future, the low cost and general availability of these techniques may result in home-testing kits, much along the same lines as those currently available for diabetes. These will allow consumers to monitor the sanitary state of their food preparation area. It will also keep the fast food, restaurant and food industries on their toes, knowing that their customers are able to monitor the hygienic quality of their products. Although such devices may seem excessive at this time, the worldwide increase in food-borne diseases, the globalization of our food supply and the proliferation of antibiotic-resistant microorganisms may well make inexpensive and rapid detection methods of this type a boon to future consumers.

SAFE EATING WHILE TRAVELING

What can be more exciting than travel? The lure of the open road, sparkling seas, exotic isles, the thrill of adventure—it is a temptation that very few of us can resist. Aside from the mystique of visiting different places and people, we have the possibility of tasting intriguing new foods. It was not always this way. In fact, the main preoccupation of ancient travelers was whether or not food would be available at all either on the road or at their final destinations. Indeed, significant risks were always associated with being away from the home environment where some degree of strict control occurred over the quality of food and water. A century ago, the major military campaigns were considered to be great heroic adventures for young men—a chance to experience the world. However, reviewing the risks and seeing the figures of comparative losses endured during these campaigns is interesting.[214]

			CAUSES OF CASUALTIES		
CAMPAIGN	YEAR	FORCES	Died of Disease	Killed in Battles	RATIO
Walcheren	1809	British	347 out of 1,000	17 out of 1,000	20 to 1
Russo-Turkish	1828	Combined	80,000	20,000	4 to 1
Russo-Turkish	1878	Russian	86,000	16,000	5.4 to 1
Crimean War	1853	French	75,000	20,000	3.75 to 1
U.S. Civil War	1861	Combined	335,000	145,000	2.3 to 1

Obviously, eating vile food, drinking bad water and living under atrocious hygienic conditions was far more hazardous than being in the front line of fire.

Fortunately, this situation has changed radically during the last century. Most travelers look forward to trying different foods and enjoying the comforts of different countries to which they travel. In fact, the possibility of trying new dishes is often a major highlight on any travel itinerary. Food ranks high among the subjects that all travelers describe upon returning home.

Sportsmen of the British Raj used to boast of eating some blazing hot new Indian curry as proudly as they would describe the ferocious tiger that they bagged. Explorers would talk of discovering some succulent callaloo pepper pot in the same wistful tones they used when describing their first encounter with the source of the Blue Nile. I have even heard seasoned international diplomats talk with far greater passion about a goulash they had just tried in Budapest than the signing of the nuclear test ban treaty.

With no doubt, trying new foods greatly adds to our experiences of the international world in which we live. Unfortunately, all too often, tourists end up with digestive disorders because the food or drink they consumed was contaminated and posed a serious risk to their health. Traveler's diarrhea is a major problem in the tourist industry. All too often, what was to be a pleasant adventure can end up with physical pain, discomfort and a forlorn wish to be back in the comfort of home.

The purpose of this section is to provide some simple practical advice about some of the risks that are faced while traveling, how to eat safely and what to do if you get sick. While the average person may suffer some fairly simple symptoms, as with so many other pathogenic risks, the old, the young, pregnant women and the immuno-compromised are particularly vulnerable to food-borne diseases encountered while traveling.

The current World Tourism Organization's figures estimate that over 800 million tourists travel yearly, with annual receipts approaching $700 billion. According to their latest forecasts, this annual figure will surge to 1.6 billion tourists visiting foreign countries by the year 2020, spending in excess of $2 trillion.[215] Tourists of the 21st century will be traveling further afield with the percentage of long-haul trips to foreign countries increasing from 18 percent in 1995 to 24 percent by the year 2020. Although the major proportion of holiday-taking tourists will come from industrialized countries, a significant proportion of this projected figure will be made up of travelers from developing countries. China will lead as the world's top tourist destination, with North America and Europe lagging far behind.

This phenomenal growth in travel has significant implications upon our health. On the one hand, international travel to countries with poor sanitation systems routinely results in exposure to much higher risks of food-borne diseases than at home. Returning tourists or travelers coming from such countries often bring these risks back. Even people who travel from one industrialized country to another face much higher risks of developing food-borne diseases than they would in their country of residence. An estimated 20–60 percent of all travelers run the risk of contracting diarrhea.

Seeing some of the results of a study carried out with the cooperation of a large British tour operator who surveyed clients on their satisfaction upon returning is interesting. Over 1 million data sets were analyzed annually. Included was a subjective questionnaire regarding health. The following table shows an example of this data.

Understanding some of the reasons why certain travelers are more sensitive to the risks of food-borne diseases than others is not difficult. General fatigue and discomfort experienced during long voyages, jet lag, lowered immunity, different climates or altitudes and a general change in diet reduce the travelers' resistance, making them far more susceptible to food-borne diseases. While most people know many of the simple precautions to take while traveling, it is difficult to be on

INCIDENCE OF SUBJECTIVE TRAVELER'S DIARRHEA IN BRITISH PACKAGE HOLIDAY TOURISTS—SUMMER 1996	
HOLIDAY DESTINATION	% TRAVELER'S DIARRHEA
Egypt	63
Dominican Republic	57
Kenya	56
Mexico	49
Tunisia	37
Jamaica	30
Antigua	22
Barbados	12
Greece—mainland	12
Majorca	11
Cyprus	9
Florida	7
Austria	5
Switzerland	3

guard constantly, and the temptations that abound in foreign lands are difficult to resist. Tourists generally take most of their meals in restaurants or from street vendors. In fact, the more ethnic a food appears, the more desirable it is to the adventurous traveler who wishes to experience everything in the new environment to the full. Unfortunately, in many such establishments, the rules of hygiene are not always adhered to, and many tourists end up experiencing far more than they bargained for.

FOOD-BORNE DISEASE RISKS TO TOURISTS

The major intestinal risks to tourists come from the food and beverages they consume. Water is well-known as a vehicle for certain infectious diseases such as cholera, typhoid fever, dysentery and others that have their primary seat in the digestive tract. Yet, water is our most important nutrient. Therefore, we must be particularly sensitive to water when we travel. Countries with poor sanitation often have unsafe water supplies. All the products washed, dipped, cooled or sprayed with this water assume a similar risk. Likewise, the ice made from this water poses similar or even greater risks, particularly if the producer does not employ proper manufacturing practices.

Foods that have been rinsed in unsafe water, such as salads and uncooked vegetables, are high-risk items, as is unpasteurized milk or cheeses made from it, raw meat, shellfish and seafood. Wild mushrooms and fish from tropical reefs can also be risky as are fish harvested from waters close to municipal sewage outlets.

TRAVELER'S DIARRHEA

The most common syndrome faced by tourists is traveler's diarrhea. This is typically characterized by frequent, loose bowel movements that are often accompanied by cramps, urgency, bloating, nausea and prostration. The degree of severity is closely linked to the area visited. The developing regions of Africa, Latin America, Asia and the Middle East top the high-risk rankings. The southern European countries bordering on the Mediterranean as well as some of the Caribbean Islands come next on the list with the United States, Canada, northern Europe, Australia and New Zealand generally considered as the lowest risk destinations. The location where food is prepared is also important. Meals from street vendors and restaurants pose a higher risk than those prepared in private homes.

Normally, traveler's diarrhea lasts three to four days during which the victim has four or five loose bowel movements a day. It usually begins during travels but can occasionally occur soon after returning home. The condition is typically self-limiting but can occasionally last up to a week or even more. If the fluids and salts lost during the episodes of diarrhea are regularly replaced, then traveler's diarrhea is very seldom a life-threatening condition.

Traveler's diarrhea is not due to one microorganism in particular. It can result from any number of infectious organisms to which insufficient resistance has been developed. Thus, any one of the entire range of enteric pathogens described in this book can be implicated. The most common microorganisms encountered are:

COMMON CAUSES OF TRAVELER'S DIARRHEA	
ORGANISM	DESCRIPTION (PAGE NO.)
Enterotoxigenic *Escherichia coli* (ETEC)	218
Salmonella (including *S. typhosa*)	225
Shigella (including *S. dysenteriae*)	229
Campylobacter	210
Vibrio	231
Viruses	273
Entamoeba	270
Giardia	270
Cryptosporidium	267

SHIPBOARD FOOD POISONING

For decades, cruise ships have been a popular vacation destination for anyone seeking a reprieve from the wintertime blues. Over 10 million people traveled on cruise ships in 2000 and that number is expected to double by 2010. But some vacationers have recently found themselves wishing they had never taken a cruise.

In 2002, a wave of gastroenteritis occurred aboard several international cruise ships, turning the vacations of many sea-bound sun seekers into the sort of trips they would most likely want to forget. In February 2004, more than 300 Carnival Cruise Lines passengers were stricken with stomach distress while on a Valentine's cruise in Mexico. Such outbreaks are not new to the industry. According to a 2003 World Health Organization (WHO) study "Emerging Issues in Water and Infectious Disease," since 1970 over 100 disease outbreaks associated with cruise ships have been documented. The WHO considers this figure low because many such illnesses go unreported.

In November 2006, more than 700 passengers and crew members aboard a transatlantic cruise fell ill with vomiting and diarrhea. The outbreak, believed to be from the *norovirus* group, struck people aboard the Carnival Cruise Lines' *Liberty,* one of the world's largest cruise ships.

In December 2006, 384 passengers of *Freedom of the Seas,* the largest cruise ship in the world, contracted a *norovirus.* At the same time, 97 passengers and six crew members of *Sun Princess,* another cruise ship, were struck with *norovirus* symptoms. Weeks earlier, 97 passengers of the same *Freedom of the Seas* had also contracted the virus.

In January 2007, several cases were discovered aboard the *Queen Elizabeth 2* in what the CDC called an "unusually large outbreak." Nearly 17 percent (276 out of 1,652) of the passengers reportedly fell ill and 28 crew members were also ill. The ship was boarded and investigated by members of the CDC while it was docked in Acapulco, Mexico. On its April 1, 2007, voyage, the Princess Cruises–owned ship *Caribbean Princess* had at least 79 passengers and four crew members sick with *norovirus.*

It is obvious that special measures involving updated technologies will have to be put in place to limit these outbreaks.

PREVENTATIVE MEASURES

Fortunately, most episodes of traveler's diarrhea can be prevented. The first line of defense is the information the traveler has about the country of destination. This is usually available from reputable travel agents or the local public health authorities. Information may also be accessed from the Internet home page of the Centers for Disease Control and Prevention (http://www.cdc.gov/travel/). If in doubt about the hygiene state of a country's food and water supplies, erring on the side of caution is best. Although most large, modern hotels in developing countries do their best to insure the health of their clients, it is not always possible despite the efforts made. Until travelers can be assured that the risks of contracting traveler's diarrhea in the country of destination has been reduced to a very low point, they must be prepared to depend largely upon their own efforts to avoid it.

In the past, the general practice existed of taking antimicrobial agents as prophylactics against the range of food-borne infections and traveler's diarrhea. However, these preparations killed all the beneficial microorganisms in the gut as well as the bad ones. Current thinking advises against this practice. Other agents, which slow the peristaltic (pumping) activity of the intestine, such as Imodium, are also considered to be ineffective as preventatives.

Certain antibiotic preparations, including ciprofloxacin or other fluoroquinolones, are effective in particularly hazardous parts of the world but should never be taken casually. These are strong antibiotics and are effective only when the organisms involved are not resistant. They should be taken only after consultation with a physician and when the circumstances are severe enough to warrant them. While they may be effective against the bacteria involved in traveler's diarrhea, they will not work with many parasites commonly found in the food and water of certain countries.

When appraising the most sensible and reliable prophylactic measures to consider when traveling, the disciplined adherence to a few simple dietary precautions can go a very long way in preventing the occurrence of traveler's diarrhea. The following discusses the major precautions to follow.

Water Treatment

- Always drink bottled beverages. Bottled beer and soft drinks are normally safe, and bottled water is a must. Anything that is carbonated is more reliable, because it is difficult for someone to tamper with before you purchase it. It is not unknown for local people to fill water bottles with any source of water, twist on a cap and sell it as purified water. Use properly sealed, bottled water—this means all water that goes into your digestive system, including the water that you use to brush your teeth. (Do not forget to keep your mouth closed while taking a shower.)
- When bottled water is unavailable, drink only water that has been boiled or beverages made with water that has been boiled, i.e., tea or coffee. Water should be boiled for at least one minute at sea level and for three or four minutes at high altitudes (because of the lower boiling temperature).
- When bottled or boiled water is unavailable, the only choice is to treat water with chemical disinfectants such as a standard tincture of iodine or iodine-based tablets specifically made for the purpose. Both

these products are usually available in pharmacies. Tincture of iodine (2 percent solution) should be used by adding five to seven drops into a liter or quart of water. If the water is cold or a little cloudy, this amount should be increased to 10 drops. Shake and let stand for about 30 minutes before drinking. (Triple this time for cold or cloudy water.) Use tablets according to package directions. After the water is treated, you can add some fresh lemon or lime juice just before drinking. This removes much of the iodine taste.

- Researchers from Los Alamos Technical Associates and MIOX Corporation of Albuquerque have developed a battery-powered disinfecting "pen." The device electrochemically generates mixed oxidants from a salt solution that individuals can use to purify drinking water. There was dramatic 99.99 percent reduction of all test bacteria and viruses within one to 10 minutes. Experiments demonstrated that the miniature pen cell electrochemically generated a mixture of oxidants from a salt solution that was able to inactivate *C. parvum* eggs, as well as bacterial spores, bacteria and viruses to produce safer drinking water in minutes. One day it may be cheap enough for tourists to take backpacking with them.
- Needless to say, avoid ice made from questionable water at all costs. Several portable filters available on the market claim to remove all offensive microorganisms, but health authorities have not fully verified their effectiveness. However, they are extremely convenient, not very expensive and definitely worthwhile to take along if you expect to be in a difficult situation for some time. Try and get a filter that guarantees a pore size of 0.1 microns—this will get rid of all parasites and bacteria. You can even get some that are silver impregnated and claim to get rid of viruses as well. Follow directions carefully.

Foods

It does not take a genius to understand that foods rinsed with contaminated water pose the same risks as the water itself. The major problems faced are with raw foods, particularly fruits and uncooked vegetables such as salads. (Take along vitamin supplements in the event that raw fruit and vegetables pose too great a risk.) If you have an opportunity to purchase fresh fruit you can peel yourself, take advantage of it. Other foods to watch out for are unpasteurized milk and dairy products, poor-quality seafood, reef fish (particularly barracuda) and raw meat.

Some feel a great temptation to be adventurous in foreign lands, but caution is always in order. Most large restaurants and hotels qualify as safe places to eat. They may not be the most ethnic or exciting, but the food is generally prepared under strict supervision. The fare in small, local restaurants and street foods can be extremely tasty. However, you must make sure that the operations are clean, and the food is freshly made and served very hot. (A conscientious street food vendor is always looking after his or her products and fanning away dust and flies.) In the rural areas of some countries such as Indonesia, it is a common tradition to place several bowls of different foods out on the table and to be charged only for that amount consumed. Whatever remains is kept in the bowls, which are then topped up and offered to the next guest that wanders in. When considering that all the food is selected and eaten with fingers, some of which may not have been washed, this epicurean adventure is one that should be weighed very carefully. I speak from bitter experience.

WHAT IF YOU GET SICK

Although the symptoms of traveler's diarrhea are uncomfortable and inconvenient, they are easily managed and are not life threatening. The routine symptoms of cramps and diarrhea are usually self-limiting and over within three or four days. A number of treatments can reduce the symptoms and even the length of their duration. However, if a high fever develops or if signs of blood appear in the stool, this is indicative of a serious infection. Seek medical help immediately. The following applies only to routine traveler's diarrhea.

Fluid Replacement

The most important thing in any prolonged episode of diarrhea is to ensure that lost fluids and salts are replaced. In adults this is important, but in infants and children, it is critical. Ideally, you should replace lost fluids by drinking a solution of salts such as those specifically recommended by the World Health Organization (WHO) for this purpose. Packets of these salts, which are commonly known as oral rehydration solution (ORS) salts, are usually available in pharmacies or outdoor sports stores. The ORS salts should be dissolved in clean, reliable water as recommended on the package. The resultant rehydration solution to be used for traveler's diarrhea contains the following ingredients:

INGREDIENTS OF ORAL REHYDRATION SOLUTION	
INGREDIENT	AMOUNT IN FINAL ORS SOLUTION (GRAMS/LITER)
Glucose	20.0
Sodium chloride	3.5
Trisodium citrate	2.9
Potassium chloride	1.5

If you are not able to obtain ORS packets, then get hold of the local equivalent of an isotonic sports beverage (Gatorade type) and add one-half teaspoon of table salt to every liter. You can also use the water from freshly opened young coconuts—it is both sterile and isotonic. (It will probably taste better than the ORS solutions.) Failing that, add three teaspoons of sugar and one level teaspoon of table salt to a liter or quart of clean, reliable water. You can also drink fruit juice diluted with clean water. (Milk is not a good idea as it will only make things worse.)

If children get severe diarrhea, make sure they drink ORS or a substitute, and get them to a qualified physician. Kids do not complain about dehydration until they are very ill.

Absorbents

Various fiber supplements (Metamucil, Citrucel, Fiber Lax and so on) are bulk-producing laxatives that absorb water in the intestine. Other preparations such as kaolin/pectin suspensions (Kaopectate, Ka-Pec and others) absorb a considerable amount of water and give firmer stools, but they are not very useful at the initial stages of traveler's diarrhea. They can be used successfully once the acute phase has passed. They can also shorten the duration of the remaining symptoms. As with all other medicines, prescription or over-the-counter, never exceed recommended doses.

Bismuth subsalicylate preparations (Bismatrol, Pepto-Bismol, Stomach Relief Formula and so on) can decrease the rate of diarrhea and, in some cases, can shorten the duration of or even prevent the illness. However, do not take these products for extended periods—the side effects can be quite dramatic. Reading and following the label directions carefully is essential.

Many people swear by products such as charcoal capsules, gelatin capsules containing activated charcoal to rid the stomach of toxins, and a variety of local preparations, but their effectiveness has not been authoritatively confirmed. In fact, avoiding the use of indigenous products is usually best because some may have pharmacological properties that aggravate the situation. If they result in problems or side effects that only show up after you return home, pinpointing the cause and proposing a solution may be difficult or impossible.

Antidiarrheal Drugs

A number of preparations are available on the market that can significantly relieve the symptoms of diarrhea. They reduce the number of stools and lessen much of the discomfort of traveler's diarrhea. The most common of these are loperamide hydrochloride preparations such as Imodium, Lomotil, Pepto Diarrhea Control, Maalox Anti-Diarrheal and so on. Some of these may require a prescription. If you have a high fever or any signs of blood in the stool, do not take these preparations. They are likely to slow the course of a serious infection and result in further complications. See a physician.

Another effective drug is codeine, a derivative of opium. This has long been used for the treatment of diarrhea and reducing the pain of cramps. Codeine requires a prescription and should be used only with the advice of a physician. It can also cause severe constipation in some people, so it should be taken only in very difficult circumstances. It should be kept in reserve as a last resort.

Antibiotic Treatment

The most effective tool against traveler's diarrhea is proper antibiotic treatment if it is available. Most large hotels have competent physicians on staff who will have access to effective antibiotic treatment. A very wide range of antibiotics are recommended, including tetracyclines, fluoroquinolone-based preparations such as ciprofloxacin, or preparations containing sulfamethoxazole and trimethoprim such as Bactrim or Trisulfam. These should be taken only under the supervision of a physician and will normally clear up the condition within two to four days.

Yogurt

Natural yogurt has often been recommended to relieve the symptoms of traveler's diarrhea. This idea is based upon the presumption that healthy, live lactobacillus bacteria will successfully compete with and displace the pathogenic bacteria causing the intestinal problems. In fact, some studies with Finnish travelers have found that "probiotic" lactobacilli can decrease the incidence of traveler's diarrhea.[216]

I have often employed this practice myself but only after the acute symptoms of traveler's diarrhea have passed. I went on the premise that at that point, my intestine would be ready to host a load of fresh lactobacilli since most of my normal intestinal bacteria either were lost as a result of the diarrhea or were killed along with the pathogens by any antibiotic treatment taken afterward.

I have not relied on yogurt available in most developing countries. I usually use the newer live, probiotic yogurt available in most supermarkets. It is a highly controlled culture and seems to help get things back to normal.

A Note of Caution for Pregnant Women

Pregnant women are at a particular risk while traveling to countries with poor sanitation. Pregnant women should not use many of the common medicines used to treat or relieve the symptoms of traveler's diarrhea. If they must be employed, it should be only under the advice or supervision of a physician. The same goes for standard antibiotic treatment, because many such as ciprofloxacin or sulfamethoxazole are not advised for pregnant women.

In fact, pregnant women should avoid all travel to developing countries if possible. The decreased immunity associated with pregnancy greatly increases risks to both woman and unborn child.

WHAT TO TAKE WITH YOU ON YOUR TRAVELS

The following is a list of some of the more common items you should try and take with you when you travel to countries where you may encounter traveler's diarrhea. (It does not include standard first aid items.)

Pepto-Bismol (bismuth subsalicylate)

Fiber supplements

Kaolin/pectin preparations

Oral rehydration solution (ORS) salts

Tincture of iodine or water purification tablets

Portable water filter

Antimotility agents (such as loperamide or codeine preparations)

Antibiotics such as ciprofloxacin or sulfamethoxazole

As strange as it may sound, you should also take laxative preparations because constipation very commonly occurs while traveling.

SOURCES OF INFORMATION*

Aside from the public health authorities in your locality, the best sources of information can be found on the Internet. The most reliable site is the Centers for Disease Control and Prevention Travel Page (http://www.cdc.gov/travel/). Here you will find all sorts of information about the countries you plan to visit along with expert advice about dealing with the problems you might encounter. The site named, appropriately, Travelers' Health is really quite excellent. Here there is a wealth of information pertinent to traveling abroad, starting with a list of all the countries you might want to visit. There are health alerts for most of the countries that even include warnings about the air quality in certain cities. There are tips about general travel that include information on insects, weather exposure and infectious diseases. It is one of the most comprehensive sites available for travel warnings.

Another site that can be helpful to travelers is the home page of the World Health Organization, listed on the Web (http://www.who.org/). This site lists all countries that are members of the United Nations and details any health issues in them.

Travel Health Online is an excellent Web site that has information about general travel health issues, preventative medicines and other related information. One of the most important features of this site is the list of travel medicine providers in several countries. This could save people a lot of grief if they do get sick in the countries listed. It also has excellent articles about specific topics, including traveler's diarrhea. This site can be found on the Internet at http://www.tripprep.com.

The Medical College of Wisconsin has an excellent site, which is located at http://healthlink.mcw.edu/travel-medicine/index.html. Other sites to visit include the International Society of Travel Medicine, Travel Health Online, the International Association for Medical Assistance to Travelers, Global Emergency Medical Services, the U.S. State Department travel warnings—it even has the CIA World Factbook.

In summary, travel can be one of the most enjoyable experiences we can have in this diverse world. Staying healthy while traveling makes the experience even more enjoyable, but much will depend upon you.

Bon voyage!

---

* Please note that Internet addresses can change at short notice. Be prepared to look up the site on one of the available search facilities such as Google in order to find the latest addresses.

PROBLEMS COMING
DOWN THE ROAD

As noted earlier in this book, in mid-September 2006, newspaper head-lines announced a major national outbreak of illness due to contamination of bagged spinach: deadly *Escherichia coli* O157:H7 bacteria. Consumers were warned not to eat bagged spinach, and grocery stores and restaurants immediately got rid of all bagged spinach from their shelves and menus. In California, spinach harvesting, sales and marketing came to an abrupt halt. By the time the outbreak was over, 204 people had become ill across 26 states and Canada. More than 100 individuals had been hospitalized, 31 had developed hemolytic uremic syndrome (HUS) and three had died.

Of all fruits and vegetables, leafy greens are the most likely to be associated with a food-borne disease outbreak. Leafy greens account for more than 30 percent of outbreaks, 10 percent of illnesses and 33 percent of deaths traced back to fruits and vegetables.[217]

The extent of the 2006 outbreak caused many people to consider our modern horticultural production and distribution system to determine if risk levels had changed. Was the system up to the task?

In the last decade there have been many developments in the hor-ticultural sector, particularly the supply chain dynamics. The introduc-tion and acceptance of bagged salads, greens and beans has resulted in a marked increase in the consumption of fresh produce in the United States. Spinach consumption alone is up 90 percent since 1992! Since consumers are eating more produce fresh, production and distribution require more care. It is estimated that 75–90 percent of fresh spinach is processed into bagged salads.

A second significant factor affecting produce is the increasing con-centration of ownership within the industry. The nationwide outbreak could be traced back to one supplier even though there were 30 different national "brands" involved. In the bagged salad business, two processing firms account for about 90 percent of the U.S. retail market. It's not dif-ficult to see how risky this can be under the best of circumstances. When the threat of sabotage or bioterrorism is factored in, production control mechanisms must be in place and up to any challenge.

Produce is grown in a natural environment and routinely exposed to all the microorganisms in soil. Currently, the technology to "pasteurize" fresh produce has not been perfected, although it may be possible one day to greatly reduce the bacterial load with a mild form of irradiation. Until that happens, however, we have to ensure a production system that minimizes the risk of microbial contamination. In all likelihood this will require the incorporation of a Hazard Analysis of Critical Control Points (HACCP) system specifically engineered to produce operations. While most large commercial growers have adopted food safety programs and use third-party audits to reduce risks, the fact that outbreaks continue to occur only shows that these programs are not up to the task.

Three separate outbreaks of *Salmonella* infections associated with eating Roma tomatoes were detected in the United States and Canada in the summer of 2004. In one multistate outbreak from June 25 to July 18, different strains of *Salmonella* were isolated. When the three outbreaks were totaled, 561 cases from 18 states and one province in Canada were identified, but the source was never found. In 2008 another national *Salmonella* outbreak with Roma, plum, and round varieties of tomatoes occurred. The earliest report of illness came on April 16 and by mid-June, the source had not been found. Of the 167 cases that had been reported during that period, 23 resulted in hospitalization. The growing number of horticultural products found infected with animal pathogens points to the critical need of changing our quality control procedures.

In the 2006 spinach *E. coli* outbreak, the contamination was traced back to spinach from a 2.8-acre field that had been packed at one processing facility. This small field was part of a 50.9-acre piece of land leased for leafy green production; the rest of the property was devoted to cattle grazing. Potential risk factors at or near the particular production field included the presence of wild pigs and irrigation wells exposed to feces from cattle and wildlife. The strain of *E. coli* responsible for the outbreak was identified in samples of river water, cattle feces and wild pig feces on the ranch.

This set of circumstances is not unique. There are no laws or regulations preventing large-scale production of produce close or even adjacent to cattle operations. The products of cattle production go through the most rigorous hygienic and inspection protocols, but that is not the case for produce. What is more significant is that meat is cooked before consumption, while produce, with very few exceptions, is not. Until the produce sector can demonstrate that their goods do not pose a high risk to consumers, they should be subject to rigorous government inspection.

IS THE THREAT FROM BIOTERRORISM REAL?

In a post–9/11 world, it would not be appropriate to avoid the subject of bioterrorism in any book on food-borne diseases. We all must eat to survive, and food or beverages are natural vehicles for agents of bioterrorism.

Terrorism generally refers to premeditated and politically motivated violence, usually with the intent to gain some sort of influence. The Federal Emergency Management Agency (FEMA) defines terrorism as "the use of force or violence against persons or property in violation of the criminal laws of the United States for purposes of intimidation, coercion, or ransom."[218] Bioterrorism involves the actual or threatened use of biological agents by individuals or groups with ideological goals. Some terrorists are attracted to any weapons that can cause massive casualties, simply because they want to cause death on an unprecedented scale. Bioterrorism relies on biological organisms, or their toxins, that are effective in harming people, animals or plants. Chemical agents are poisonous substances made by man, which are often lumped under the bioterrorism label.

There are hundreds of organisms that can do us harm, including bacteria, viruses, fungi and parasites. Among the pathogens often considered as possible bioterror agents are *Bacillus anthracis,* the anthrax bacteria, and *Yersinia pestis,* the bacteria that caused the Black Plague. Other frightening organisms include *Mycobacterium leprae,* the bacteria responsible for leprosy, and *Wuchereria bancrofti,* the microscopic filarial worm that causes elephantiasis—diseases that result in such dreadful disfiguration they could easily terrorize a population.

The poisonous toxins produced by living organisms include those derived from plants, animals and microorganisms. Among the best-known are the deadly toxin from the bacteria *Clostridium botulinum,* ricin, a toxin extracted from castor beans, and tetrodotoxin from fugu (puffer) fish. Of course, there are hundreds of others derived from roots, beans, flowers, mushrooms, sea creatures, snakes, frogs, not to mention other microorganisms. Although it is a little more difficult to gain access to purified biological agents than it was in the very recent past, it is not impossible. All varieties of organisms, including some very pathogenic ones, are stored in academic or commercial culture collections in various countries around the world and, in the past, have served as preferred sources of materials for terrorists.

There is also the possibility of culturing pathogenic organisms from any number of sources—the soil, human or animal waste, garbage or any other putrefying mess. Pathogens exist everywhere. The problem with this final approach is that you really have to know what you're doing, and this knowledge is usually beyond the abilities of most terrorists—so far.

THE DALLES INCIDENT

The best-known case of bioterrorism to occur on U.S. soil involved the use of biological agents by a religious cult, the Rajneeshees, in a small town in Oregon called The Dalles in 1984. When this case was over, almost 800 people had been poisoned, the cult escaped to more sympathetic environs and the town's economy was left in shambles.

The cult founder, Bhagwan Shree Rajneesh (1931–90), was a complex man who may have originally started out with good intentions but ultimately drifted to the dark side in a desire to acquire riches and enjoy the lifestyle of the wealthy. He graduated from high school in 1951 and began to study philosophy at college, but had a great deal of difficulty keeping his mental faculties intact. He tried to manage this problem with steady meditation.

He eventually graduated from college in 1955 with an M.A. in philosophy and became an assistant professor at the University of Jabalpur in 1960. Rajneesh started giving public lectures about the divine energy of sex and, predictably, began to attract a great many followers.

By fall 1970, he started the Neo-Sannyas International Movement and in the following year he changed his name to Bhagwan (the Blessed One) Shree Rajneesh. The Blessed One started to gain a great many Western followers.

He set up his first ashram in the city of Poona, India, with a few fellow Indian disciples. Rajneesh steadily became better known and, by 1976, he was one of the main attractions on the guru circuit frequented by many Westerners searching for a greater meaning in their lives. Because of his beliefs, he encountered opposition in India so he decided to move his ashram. One of his more aggressive Indian followers, Ma Anand Sheela, convinced Rajneesh to move his operation to the United States in 1981 where the pickings would be much better since the majority of the Rajneeshees were Westerners.

In short order, Ma Anand Sheela bought a 64,000-acre Oregon property known as the Big Muddy Ranch for $5.6 million, even though it was evaluated for tax purposes at only $200,000. A large part of the ranch was located in Wasco County, a rural area with a population of about 20,000. The seat of Wasco County was a small town called The Dalles, which had a population of around 10,000 people. Little did these townsfolk know what was about to descend on them.

After the Rajneeshees purchased the Big Muddy Ranch, they set about building their new ashram and, under Ma Anand Sheela's growing influence, the focus of the Rajneeshees shifted from leading a highly spiritual life to making money. There was great pressure to work and an even greater pressure to transfer all earnings to the ashram. To reflect the growing wealth, Rajneesh began driving around the commune in one of his growing fleet of Rolls-Royce automobiles.

Right from the start, trouble began to brew between the ashram and Wasco County. The most contentious problems between the Rajneeshees and the surrounding community resulted from Oregon's tough land use laws, which greatly limited development in rural areas—not very convenient for an ambitious ashram. In order to continue their expansion of Rajneeshpuram (the new name of their ashram), the cult decided to work around the laws. Using the state's own liberal voter registration laws, they decided to grab control of a nearby town of only 40 residents called Antelope. They accomplished this by building several housing units to supplement the ones on the ashram and then proposing to build a large office facility and several other new buildings there. The horrified Antelope city council refused to give them building permits on the grounds that there was not enough water to support all this new construction.

The Rajneeshees decided to pursue legal action and eventually were permitted to develop their current properties, but not any future development. The agreement did not last long, and the irrepressible Rajneeshees took full control of the city council, running out the remaining older residents. This was the turning point in relations between the Rajneeshees and the other inhabitants of Wasco County, because it offended many people who normally would not have given the group a second thought. The Rajneeshees then took over the Antelope school board and became known in the greater Oregon political scene as a genuine threat to rural community life.

By the beginning of 1984, the cult was under considerable pressure from the U.S. attorney's office in Portland. The office started an immigration investigation that could have led to the deportation of many Rajneeshees, including the Bhagwan. Even the state's attorney general was investigating the legal status of Rajneeshpuram.

Tensions were growing in response to all the legal actions and a number of inflammatory television appearances by Sheela. By 1984 the ashram had acquired an arsenal of semiautomatic weapons and handguns for its new police force, known as the Peace Force. As a result of Sheela's manipulations, the ashram started to take on characteristics of George Orwell's *Animal Farm*. All power may have derived from the Bhagwan's authority, but he had no involvement in the daily operations of the organization other than his daily Rolls Royce cruise through the ashram. Sheela ran the cult, controlled the finances and directed all the operations of Rajneeshpuram through her small inner circle of trusted women, referred to as the "moms."

Because Sheela was accountable only to the Blessed One, everyone had to toe the line or risk being "turfed out" of Rajneeshpuram. The ashram became more militant and built a large fence around the Bhagwan's residence, complete with sentry posts. One member of the ashram told of a conversation she had with one of the armed sentries, who had previously been a close friend of hers. She asked why the man's attitude toward her had grown so distant. He replied, "Sheela's orders, she says it isn't good to get friendly with people you might have to shoot." The ashram had made the transition from spirituality and enlightenment to greed and violence.

Sheela lost patience and, in consort with her inner circle, decided that the Wasco County court was a problem that had to be dealt with. The county court controlled the permits that the Rajneeshees needed and the court's growing truculence was proving to be a major impediment to the cult's ambitions.

The Wasco County Court was made up of three elected commissioners. As it happened, two of them were up for reelection in November 1984. Sheela, with the Bhagwan's approval, decided to gain control of the Wasco County court by manipulating the election. She did this by bringing thousands of homeless people to Rajneeshpuram. Once they were considered to be local, they would be eligible to vote in the November election. In order to put the finishing touches to this plan, Sheela came up with an additional strategy. To ensure victory for the Rajneeshees, Sheela decided to poison the local water supply in order to make the Wasco County voters so sick they wouldn't be able to vote. Thus was hatched the first plan for large-scale bioterrorism in the United States.

As a result of the FBI investigation that followed the incident, a great deal about how the Rajneeshees executed the plan has come to light. Much of the information came from Krishna Diva (David Berry Knapp)—the former mayor of Rajneeshpuram—and was expertly documented by Dr. Seth Carus in his working paper "Bioterrorism and Biocrimes."[219]

According to the testimony of Krishna Diva, Sheela hatched the idea and, together with her close associate Ma Anand Puja, began looking into the possibility of using biological agents in a serious way. Ma Anand Puja (Dianne Onang) is considered the person most directly involved in obtaining and developing the biological agents used by the Rajneeshees. Born in the Philippines and brought up in California, Ma Anand Puja took up nursing and was registered in 1997. She then left the United States to work in clinics throughout the Philippines and Indonesia. She traveled to India and, after hearing the Bhagwan speak, decided to join his ashram in Poona. Because of her background, she became the director of the ashram's health center and soon became very close to Sheela.

Once the cult moved to the United States, Puja had full control over all of Rajneeshpuram's medical facilities. However, her real power, which extended far beyond the medical arena, came from her close association with Sheela. Her tyrannical behavior made her unpopular with other ashram members, who sometimes referred to her as "Dr. Mengele" (the infamous Nazi doctor). In subsequent interrogations, Krishna Diva described Puja as someone who delighted in death and savored the idea of carrying out plots involving poisons. He even suggested that some people thought that Puja was involved in the mysterious death of Sheela's first husband in 1980.

In preparing to execute Sheela's plans, Puja looked at several different biological agents. To avoid suspicion, she selected an organism that is commonly found in cases of food poisoning, *Salmonella typhimurium*. Puja considered several other biological agents, including *Salmonella typhi*, the organism that causes typhoid fever. Puja liked the idea of using typhoid bacteria, as it was likely to cause several weeks of debilitating fever. Fortunately, because of the risk that ashram members themselves could become infected, this organism was eventually abandoned.

Based on further testimony from Krishna Diva, it appears that Puja had seriously contemplated infecting people with the AIDS virus. Apparently, the Rajneeshees purchased a freeze-dried sample of the virus specifically for that purpose. But other than an unconfirmed report that Puja deliberately infected one individual with HIV, there is no indication that this lethal organism was used.

As unbelievable as it may sound, the Rajneeshees obtained their pathogenic strain of *Salmonella typhimurium* simply by ordering it from a commercial supplier. The cultures are delivered as purified disks containing the freeze-dried bacteria. It is a simple matter to grow these in sterile culture media if you have the required equipment—which is also easy to obtain. It appears that the cultures of *S. typhimurium* were produced in a secret laboratory located directly on the grounds of Rajneeshpuram.

Everything was now in place for Sheela and her cohorts to start doing their dirty work. The first opportunity came on August 29, 1984, when three of the Wasco County commissioners came to Rajneeshpuram for a routine fact-finding visit. Two of the commissioners, Judge William Hulse and Commissioner Ray Matthew, were kindly offered glasses of water, which the Rajneeshees had previously contaminated with *S. typhimurium.* Both men became very sick, and Judge Hulse ended up in the hospital.

Apparently, the Rajneeshees tried going after a larger swath of people at the Wasco County courthouse by spreading some of the liquid *S. typhimurium* culture throughout the building on doorknobs and flush knobs of toilets, but this did not have the desired effect, since no one became ill. It is likely that the organisms did not survive when exposed to the air.

Armed with the knowledge that the best way to make people sick was to contaminate the foods they were eating and drinking, the cult went about sprinkling liquid culture on salads at a local supermarket with the goal of giving the local people the "runs." It is not known what the effects of these small individual tests were, but, regardless of the outcome, by early September 1984 Sheela and her merry band of poisoners were now ready to do some serious testing.

Armed with a considerable amount of *S. typhimurium,* the cult members began pouring vials of culture into food products at various restaurants throughout The Dalles. Their favorite targets were the attractive salad bars found in so many restaurants. People naturally gravitate to the salad bar because of its variety and healthy reputation. Dressed in civilian clothes rather than their traditional orange ashram garb, the Rajneeshees added their poisonous *S. typhimurium* brew to the salads, the salad dressing and other condiments at the salad bar. Not satisfied with that, they added it to the coffee creamers as well. They were successful beyond their wildest dreams!

In a publication titled "A Large Community Outbreak of Salmonellosis Caused by Intentional Contamination of Restaurant Salad Bars," staff members of the National Center for Infectious Diseases and Epidemiology at the Centers for Disease Control and Prevention in Atlanta describe how 751 people became ill after eating at salad bars in several restaurants.[220] The investigators had systematically ruled out all the possibilities of accidental contamination occurring as a result of poor practices or unhygienic sanitation habits on the part of employees at the various restaurants. The inescapable conclusion was that the poisonings were the result of a number of deliberate acts. There is little doubt that the actual number of victims was considerably higher than the 751 reported because The Dalles is located by an interstate highway and any number of unsuspecting travelers passing through town may have been infected. However, as is often the case in food-borne disease outbreaks, their cases were not reported.

After their success at the restaurants, the Rajneeshees ceased their attacks. The enormous publicity generated by the epidemic made it evident that their plot to poison the water supply would fail. The Rajneeshees abandoned their efforts to take over Wasco County.

Bioterrorism was initially considered only a remote explanation for the outbreak. In 1984 no one imagined that such a thing could be possible. It was only after the FBI began investigating the cult for other criminal violations that the source of the attack surfaced. A vial of S. typhimurium, identical to the particular strain responsible for the outbreak, was found in the laboratory at Rajneeshpuram. Then members of the ashram began spilling the beans. It was not long before they admitted to contaminating the salad bars and planning to contaminate the city's water supply.

In November, hearings were held on the use of federal land in and around the ashram by the Rajneeshees and bills were introduced to repeal the charter of Rajneeshpuram. In March 1985, the state superintendent of schools threatened to cut off aid to the Rajneeshee school. The Rajneeshees succeeded no further in their political ambitions. Federal investigations into their operations progressed. Even though Sheela had destroyed a great deal of information, there was enough evidence for a federal grand jury to issue a 35-count indictment charging the Bhagwan, Sheela and six others with conspiracy to evade the immigration laws.[221]

The Blessed One attempted to flee from the law, but his private jet was intercepted in North Carolina, where he was seized and incarcerated. Despite his lawyer's pleas that the Bhagwan was too ill to be kept in jail, he was soon returned to Oregon. He pled guilty to concealing his intent to remain in the United States and lying to immigration officials in 1981. He agreed to pay $400,000 in fines and court costs—not a particularly difficult setback. He was also handed a 10-year suspended prison sentence and ordered to leave the country within five days.

The Bhagwan left the United States for refuge in the Himalayas. He was not well received by the Indian public. He tried to reestablish his community but was met with hostility and opposition. He died in Poona in 1990 at the age of 59.

Sheela did manage to flee the country but was soon arrested in Germany. She was returned for trial in the United States and indicted on charges of attempted murder, conspiracy to commit murder, assault, wiretapping, arson, burglary, and the poisoning of two county commissioners—not bad for the manager of a commune devoted to love and revelation. She was fined almost $500,000 and ordered to give up her permanent resident status in the United States. Apparently, she did not pay this. She was also given concurrent prison terms but, incredibly, was released for good behavior after serving only two and a half years of her sentence in a federal medium-security prison. She eventually ended up in Basel, Switzerland, under the name Sheela Birnstiel and opened two nursing homes where she looks after Alzheimer's patients.

THE 2007 CHINESE PET FOOD RECALL

The following example illustrates what we may encounter on a regular basis in the future. After more than three weeks of complaints from consumers, on March 15, 2007, the FDA learned that certain pet foods were making a great many cats and dogs ill and even killing some of them. After a rapid investigation, the FDA found that contaminated vegetable proteins imported into the United States from China had been used as ingredients in pet food. The recalls began voluntarily with the Canadian company Menu Foods on March 16, 2007, when company tests showed sickness and death in some of the test animals. The poisoning manifested itself as renal failure and was mostly associated with the consumption of wet pet foods made with wheat gluten from a single Chinese company.

In the ensuing weeks, several other companies that had received the contaminated gluten also voluntarily recalled dozens of pet food brands. Soon after the initial recall, contaminated rice protein from a different source in China was also identified as being associated with kidney failure in pets in the United States, while contaminated Chinese corn gluten was associated with kidney failure with pets in South Africa. As a result of investigating the pet food crisis, a broader Chinese protein export scandal unfolded, raising concerns about the safety of human food as well.

This scandal demonstrates how difficult it is to provide a safe food supply. In 2007, the United States imported more than $7 billion of agricultural products from China. The government should manage this level of exports with high regulations to ensure quality and reliability. Canada, traditionally the largest exporter to the United States, is known for the quality of its agricultural products, as are Australia and New Zealand, two other top agricultural exporters. This is not the case with China, which continually tops the list of foods retained and rejected by the FDA.

Regulations in the United States still leave many gaps. For example, when protein content is measured, protein as such is not analyzed. Instead the nitrogen content is measured by a method called Kjeldahl analysis. This method determines total nitrogen in a substance by digesting it with sulphuric acid and a catalyst; the nitrogen is converted to ammonia, which is then measured by titration. In foods most of the nitrogen is protein, and the term *crude protein* is the total "Kjeldahl nitrogen" multiplied by a factor of 6.25 in the case of animal proteins and 5.7 in the case of plant proteins. This is an open invitation for any criminal to adulterate a protein source with a nitrogen-bearing compound to bring up the Kjeldahl value and make the protein level appear higher.

In the 2007 pet food scandal, both the wheat gluten and rice protein concentrates were mislabeled and found to be nothing more than

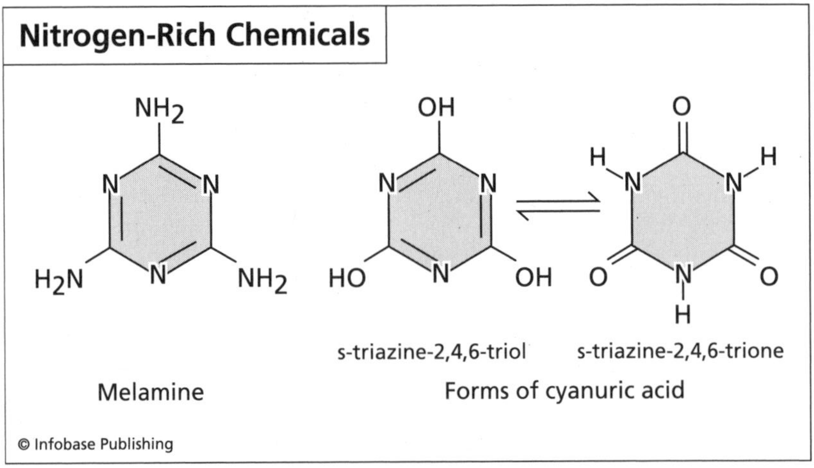

Figure 20A.

wheat flour. Wheat flour does produce wheat gluten, but to separate it out is an expensive process. To mimic the high protein levels of real wheat gluten, the chemicals melamine and cyanuric acid were added to bring up the nitrogen content so the Kjeldahl analysis would make the protein level appear high. One look at melamine and cyanuric acid says it all. Both chemicals are packed with nitrogen that would be considered protein after a Kjeldahl analysis. With a nitrogen content of 66 percent, if melamine alone went through a Kjeldahl analysis, it would come out as 380 percent protein.

In China, illegally adding melamine to animal feed is nothing new. An April 30, 2007, *New York Times* story said that using melamine to adulterate feed has been an "open secret" in China for years. The general manager of one melamine-producing chemical company stated, "Many companies buy melamine scrap to make animal feed, such as fish feed. . . . I don't know if there's a regulation on it. Probably not. No law or regulation says 'don't do it,' so everyone's doing it. The laws in China are like that, aren't they? If there's no accident, there won't be any regulation."[222]

A portion of the tainted pet food was used for farm animal feed and fish feed. The FDA and the U.S. Department of Agriculture discovered that some animals that ate the tainted feed had been processed into human food. In this incident, government scientists have determined that there was a low risk to human health from consuming food from animals that ate tainted feed.

This terrible incident highlights what can happen in a food system where all the participants do not share a common goal. It can take years of interaction to know your trading partners and to be able to gauge whether they understand the rules. Until that time, you must have every possible safety precaution in place.

WHERE DO WE GO FROM HERE?

Fear and resentment of what is new is really a lament for the memories of our childhood.

Sir Peter Medawar (1915–87), British immunologist (1982)*

CAVEAT EMPTOR

Caveat emptor is the Latin maxim "let the buyer beware!" In the case of foods that can transmit food-borne diseases, it is a particularly fitting remark. We are confronted with dangers and hazards that are thoroughly hidden from us. When faced with weekly headlines describing one food-poisoning outbreak after another, you would think that most consumers would be more cautious about what they eat. Yet, we naively go on eating and treating foods as if we are all immune to the effects of the diseases that so many of them carry. No wonder that a distraught father can utter the words, "I don't care how long I live, I will never believe that my son died from eating a cheeseburger. Never."[223] Today, despite the fact that food-borne diseases rank very high on the list of consumer concerns, most people still do not believe that they will be the ones to get sick as a result of eating ordinary foods.

The supermarket chains, the food and food service industry and the government all boast that America has the best and safest food supply in the world, but it is difficult to see exactly what they are referring to. Yes, the food generally available in America is safer to eat than most foods available in poor, underdeveloped countries. However, this does not mean that the food supply is safe. If anyone doubts this, then one look at the number of cases of food-borne diseases that occur annually should be enough to convince anyone how unsafe our food really is. Researchers have estimated that somewhere between 10 and 30 million cases take place each year—in the region of a half-million Americans every week! Somewhere in the vicinity of 10,000 people a year die from food-borne diseases and their effects. Burying our heads in the sand and continuing to believe that all is well in the food supply will not make us any less liable to be struck down by food-borne diseases. It is time for everyone involved in bringing food to the consumer to face up to their responsibilities and come clean. Consumers deserve to know the risks they face from the hazards in the foods they desire *before* they put down the money to buy them.

A NEW GOVERNMENT INITIATIVE

On May 12, 1997, Vice President Al Gore announced a comprehensive $43 million plan to increase the overall safety of the American food supply. The plan was dubbed "Food Safety from Farm to Table" and specified improved inspections, more public education and increased use of the latest scientific developments to dramatically reduce food-borne illnesses.

This program grew out of increased efforts to modernize the nation's food safety following a number of tragic and well-publicized food-borne disease outbreaks. A major part of this effort was focused on encouraging the adoption of Hazard Analysis and Critical Control Point (HACCP) systems. Although HACCP was required by the FDA for seafood and by the USDA for meat and poultry, the new measures would apply to fruit and vegetables.

A national early warning system was announced to track and combat outbreaks of food-borne illness. This surveillance system was maintained by the Centers for Disease Control and Prevention (CDC), the FDA and the USDA, working together with state authorities. In addition, work commenced on a national public education campaign on safe food handling.

In order to improve overall risk-assessment capabilities, government agencies established an interagency risk assessment group to coordinate federal risk-related research applicable to food safety. They also developed improved modeling techniques to estimate the impact of consumer exposure to pathogenic microorganisms. The agencies focused research on the development of rapid tests to detect pathogens such as salmonella, *cryptosporidium, E. coli* and hepatitis A virus in foods. They also studied how these pathogens became resistant to antibiotics and traditional food-preservation techniques. They sought to develop new technologies for prevention and control of pathogens in meat, poultry, seafood, eggs and fresh produce and to better educate physicians on how to diagnose and treat food-borne diseases.

Under this initiative, the federal government, together with state and local governments, industry and academia, conducted research, risk assessments and cost-benefit analyses to determine how food-borne diseases occur and how they might be prevented, in the most cost-effective manner. They also improved surveillance and investigative efforts to locate and monitor disease outbreaks through intensified inspection of food processors. Existing state health department sites charged with tracking cases of food-borne infections were strengthened. Together with federal food-safety agencies, they were electronically linked to create a powerful new network to detect and prevent outbreaks of food-borne illness. To further strengthen this outbreak-response system, an intergovernmental group, the Food-borne Outbreak Response Coordinating Group (FORCG), was established to deal with interstate outbreaks of food-borne disease. FORCG's role was to review outbreak responses in consultation with industry and consumer groups and then make recommendations to improve the system.

Representation on FORCG includes

- U.S. Department of Agriculture (USDA)
- Department of Health and Human Services (DHHS)
- Food and Drug Administration (FDA)
- Centers for Disease Control and Prevention (CDC)
- Department of Defense (DOD)
- Environmental Protection Agency (EPA)
- Council of State and Territorial Epidemiologists (CSTE)
- Association of Food and Drug Officials (AFDO)
- Association of Public Health Laboratories (APHL)
- National Association of City and County Health Officers (NACCHO)
- Association of State and Territorial Health Officials (ASTHO)
- National Association of State Departments of Agriculture (NASDA)

The FDA developed several approaches to deals with the scope and magnitude of food-safety issues. The Farm to Table concept recognized that food safety starts at production and that all steps in the process between the farm and the consumer's table can contribute to a food-safety problem. Another program involved a national consumer and food-handler education campaign, based on work started by the Partnership for Food Safety Education in 1997 (Fight BAC!), comprising specific activities designed to modify unsafe practices in the home and in retail and cafeteria operations. At long last, the more vulnerable groups received special food safety information.

Fight BAC! was intended for consumer education in the safe handling of foods after purchase. The FDA recognized that a seamless interagency approach to food-safety was essential to the success of the program. Meanwhile, the Association of Food and Drug Officials called for a vertically integrated national enterprise food safety program that would be inclusive across all barriers between federal and state agencies, professional associations, industry and consumer advocacy groups. Key components of this vision included

- Science and risk-based control methodologies
- Public and private partnerships
- Seamless integrated system from farm to table

The goal was a single food-safety system that used all existing government resources to improve the reliability of surveillance and enforcement activities, thereby increasing the level of food safety and the level of consumer confidence.

A collaborative stakeholders' meeting was sponsored by the FDA, USDA, CDC and EPA in Kansas City, Missouri in September 1998, where state and county government representatives and industry and consumer groups were charged with devising a plan for addressing the nation's food-safety needs. Among the major objectives were the creation of an early alert system for reporting cases of food-borne disease outbreaks, a national database for food storage and safety information, a system to trace contaminated products back to their source, rapid laboratory tests to recognize food-borne illnesses and a simplified interagency outbreak response system. In addition, working groups in Kansas City identified six areas for improvement

- Data collection and sharing
- Roles and responsibilities–capacity and resource needs
- Communications
- Coordinating outbreak responses and investigations
- Minimum uniform standards
- Laboratory operations and coordination

Selected participants at the meeting were assigned to one of these workgroups, which met a few months later in Baltimore, Maryland, to develop strategies to meet the needs of the stated areas for improvement and to set a time line and budget for their completion.

The laboratory operations and coordination group worked to harmonize methods used for investigation of food-borne outbreaks and selected rapid and sensitive methods for detection of *E. coli* O157:H7 as a pilot program for interagency cooperation. The same group joined with the data collection and sharing group to develop eLEXNET, a rapid-alert network for interstate recognition of food-borne outbreaks. The outbreak coordination and response group published the document "Multistate Foodborne Outbreak Investigations: Guidelines for Improving Coordination and Communication," which was made available on the Internet.

Many of the groups' activities have been curtailed or suspended as a result of a review by the Bush administration, which seems to believe that placing responsibility for food safety largely in the hands of the USDA is the best route to follow. The Bush administration wants to improve the federal government's ability to rapidly identify and characterize a bioterriorist attack. As a result, the USDA budget was adjusted to support a new Food and Agriculture Defense Initiative to enhance monitoring and surveillance of pests and diseases in plants and animals, conduct research on emerging animal diseases, increase the availability of vaccines, establish a system to track selected plant disease agents and complete the National Centers for Animal Health in Ames, Iowa.

This approach is vehemently opposed by groups such as the Center for Science in the Public Interest. Because of the USDA's mission to promote agricultural interests, Caroline Smith DeWaal, CSPI's food safety director, does not believe they can develop an uncompromising public health mission. In a May 8, 2007, letter to the Committee on Agriculture, she stated

> It does not make sense to greatly increase responsibilities at USDA
> when the agency has such a poor record of performance in recent

years. The Food Safety and Inspection Service (FSIS) at USDA manages a meat inspection program established over 100 years ago with twice the resources of FDA's food program. Even with its huge budget, the products FSIS regulates cause many outbreaks and illnesses each year. In fact, while USDA regulates only 20 percent of the food supply, these products caused 27 percent of outbreaks tracked by CSPI using CDC data. While improvements made in the 1990s showed initial declines in pathogen levels, those declines were not sustained. In fact, salmonella rates in poultry increased from 9 to 16 percent between 2000 and 2005. Human illnesses linked to *E. coli* O157:H7 also increased between 2003 and 2006 according to CDC data, following several years of decline.

Consumers cannot trust the USDA to take on the huge responsibility of managing the entire food safety system, when that agency lacks a public health mission and a consistent record of improvement for the meat and poultry products it currently regulates.[224]

It is difficult to predict where the issue of food safety will go in the future. There are a great many political imperatives at play that have little to do with fighting food-borne diseases. Placing so much responsibility for food safety into the hands of the agency whose primary mandate is the support of the agricultural sector does not comply with any traditional understanding of what arm's-length independence should be in a regulatory agency. Politics has no place in this process. Until food safety is placed on a solid independent regulatory foundation, food-borne diseases will never be controlled.

Starting in December 1997, a Food and Drug Administration program based on HACCP principles went into effect in the seafood industry. It required domestic and foreign seafood processors and distributors to focus on identifying and removing all hazards within the production and distribution system that could result in food-borne disease outbreaks. This systematic approach is considered to be far more effective in providing consumers with safe food products than the old system of occasional spot-checks and random sampling. The same program started in January 1998 for the country's meat and poultry plants. Although the largest plants were targeted initially, by January 2000 even the smallest operations were covered.

There has also been significant progress in the important area of fruits and vegetables that are sold and often consumed raw or minimally processed. Guidelines aimed at promoting good agricultural practices throughout the production and post-production system were prepared, and producers encouraged to follow them. It is likely that these guidelines will be very influential in other countries as well, since they apply across a very wide spectrum of fruit and vegetable production. Processors of packaged fruit and vegetable juices have also been required to implement comprehensive HACCP programs in order to eliminate the significant problems involving pathogenic microorganisms that have cropped up over the past few years.

Products that have received particular attention recently are eggs and ground beef patties. A major attempt was made to reduce the problem of *Salmonella enteritidis* in fresh shell eggs, a major cause of food-borne illness in the United States. Aside from improvements in egg production, demands have been made to improve the handling and storage of eggs to upgrade their overall safety. Improvements in the cooking procedures of hamburgers to reduce the possibility of selling undercooked products in food service establishments and fast-food outlets have been put in place. Considering the potential for harm caused by the recent Topps ground beef contamination, it makes the need to ensure effective HAACP all the more urgent.

In addition, significant new information is being exchanged on the new national computer network of public health laboratories (PulseNet). The goal is to quickly locate and identify food-borne disease outbreaks in order to bring them to a quick end. Response times are reported to be up to five times faster than was previously possible.

For 1999, the administration proposed an increase of 101 million dollars for the National Food Safety Initiative. The 1999 National Food Safety Initiative builds on the successes of the 1998 initiative as well as fills the gaps identified during 1998. The focus of the initiative was on enhancing the safety of imported and domestic fruits and vegetables, targeting food safety education and also implementing of HACCP systems in designated sectors of the food supply.

Specifically, this involved the chief agencies in identifying potential food safety threats, enlarging their capacities with the FoodNet early-warning surveillance system and supporting improved information sharing among themselves and with the public. The Economic Research Service (ERS) is involved in measuring the effectiveness of food safety measures by thoroughly analyzing food-borne illness surveillance data.

A program of research for accurate risk assessment of microbial hazards for the general population and high-risk groups was initiated along with assessments to identify food safety hazards so that more accurate regulatory decisions could be taken. The inspection function was expanded to implement new preventive measures. It emphasized domestic and imported produce as well as the comprehensive implementation of HACCP programs.

In January 2000, the Department of Health and Human Services launched Healthy People 2010, a comprehensive, nationwide health promotion and disease prevention agenda. Healthy People 2010 includes close to 500 objectives designed to serve as a road map for improving the health of everyone in the United States during the first decade of the 21st century.

Healthy People 2010 builds on the original initiative and stresses two goals: (1) to increase quality and years of healthy life and (2) to eliminate disparities. The objectives are organized in 28 focus areas with each objective stipulating a target for improvements to be achieved by the year 2010. A limited set of objectives, known as the leading health indicators, is intended to help everyone more easily understand the importance of health promotion and disease prevention and to encourage wide participation in improving health. These indicators were chosen based on their ability to motivate action, the availability of data to measure their progress and their relevance as broad public health issues.

The National Center for Health Statistics (NCHS) is responsible for coordinating the effort to monitor the nation's progress toward these objectives. National data are gathered from more than 190 different data sources, from more than seven federal government departments (Health and Human Services, Commerce, Education, Justice, Labor, Transportation and the Environmental Protection Agency) and from voluntary and private nongovernmental organizations.

FOOD SAFETY IN A POST–9/11 WORLD

The events of September 11, 2001, highlighted the need to enhance U.S. security. Congress responded by passing the Public Health Security and Bioterrorism Preparedness and Response Act of 2002 (more commonly known as the Bioterrorism Act), which was signed into law on June 12, 2002.

This act requires that the Food and Drug Administration (FDA) receive prior notice of food imported or offered for import into the United States beginning December 12, 2003. While most of the required information is the common invoice data normally provided by importers or brokers to customs when goods arrive in the United States, the act requires that the FDA now receive this information in advance of shipments. This allows the FDA time to review, evaluate and assess information before a food product arrives and to shift resources to target inspections, help intercept contaminated products and help ensure movement of safe food to market. This summary is taken from the FDA's Center for Food Safety and Applied Nutrition. The full document, "Protecting the Food Supply" is available online at http://www.cfsan.fda.gov/~dms/fsbtact.html.

OUTBREAK ALERT!

The government is not the only source of information on food-borne diseases. *Outbreak Alert!* is perhaps the finest example of a consumer organization's effort to keep the public aware of the potential hazards that exist in our food supply.

Normally, food-borne disease outbreaks are investigated by state and local health officials. Occasionally, these officials call on the Centers for Disease Control and Prevention (CDC) to help investigate larger or multistate outbreaks. However, because states are not required to report food-poisoning outbreaks to the CDC, many outbreaks go unreported. In *Outbreak Alert!* Caroline Smith DeWaal of the Center for Science in the Public Interest has filled the gap by researching state outbreak information, combing through scientific and medical journals and newspapers for outbreak reports and gathering information from the CDC in order to compile the most complete information available about outbreaks of food-borne illnesses linked to specific foods.

Aside from cataloging disease outbreaks, *Outbreak Alert!* also provides a unique view on policy issues of particular interest to consumers. The current edition of *Outbreak Alert!* is accessible online: http://www.cspinet.org/foodsafety/outbreak_alert.pdf.

S.T.O.P

Safe Tables Our Priority (S.T.O.P.) was formed in 1993 after the outbreak of *E. coli* associated with Jack-in-the-Box restaurants in the Pacific Northwest. Because of the magnitude of the outbreak, the threat of *E. coli* contamination garnered nationwide media attention for the first time. Victims and families who had lost or nearly lost their loved ones came together to form S.T.O.P., with its mission to prevent unnecessary illness and loss of life from pathogenic food-borne illnesses.

The S.T.O.P. program has three objectives:

1. To provide information and improve services to those made ill by food. S.T.O.P. provides information and support to victims and their families through a hotline, a Web site and an information clearinghouse.
2. To prevent food-borne diseases by building awareness of the causes and outcomes of these diseases and ways to prevent them through public education and media campaigns.
3. To reform government and industry practices to reduce pathogenic contamination of food before it reaches consumers. This includes animal husbandry and slaughtering; processing; manure management and the exposure of produce to animal fecal matter; food service handling; and animal and food transportation.

This organization is one of the best for people seeking advice on procedures to follow to assess damages resulting from food-borne disease outbreaks.

THE GLOBAL FOOD SAFETY INITIATIVE

In April 2000, a group of international CEOs discussed the importance of improving food safety in order to ensure consumer protection, strengthen consumer confidence and set forth the requirements for rational food safety schemes throughout the food supply chain. Following this meeting, the Global Food Safety Initiative (GFSI) was launched in May 2000. The initiative is facilitated by the Comité International d'Entreprises à Succursales (CIES—the International Committee of Food Retail Chains) otherwise known as the Food Business Forum.

A key goal of the program was to monitor the issues surrounding the development of food safety standards (Global Standards Project). GFSI has developed a guidance document against which food safety standards for manufacturing could be benchmarked based on three key elements: food safety management systems, good practices for agriculture, manufacturing or distribution and hazard analysis and critical control point (HACCP).

A key issue in the benchmarking process was the recognition that different food safety standards existed. GFSI needed a process by which mutual recognition or equivalence could be achieved. Through this process of exchange of information on consumer safety needs, globally recognized improved standards were eventually developed. With the growing volume of agricultural products entering international trade, this private sector scheme is critical in assuring safe products for consumers.

RISKY BUSINESS

The world around us is laden with risks. We face them driving our roads and flying the skies. We confront risks while busy at work and others when enjoying ourselves at leisure. Eating and drinking also present a great variety of particular risks. Tap water contains toxic chlorine and fluorine compounds. Fermented alcoholic beverages all contain small amounts of toxic fusel oils. Legumes such as peas and beans contain several antinutritional toxins such as hemagglutinins, phytates and various enzyme inhibitors. Stored potatoes often contain the potent glycoalkaloid poison solanine, and akee fruit contain the hypoglycin toxin. Dangers are everywhere.

These and other risks have always been a fundamental aspect of life. Many people have a tendency to reminisce about the good old days when life was simpler and people had fewer challenges and risks to face. In fact, this sentimental vision is nothing more than sheer fantasy. Hindsight, experience and a longing for bygone romantic eras make them appear simple and uncomplicated. Every society has considered its own particular age fearful and complex but bygone days as splendid. Remember Vermeer's apprehension of van Leeuwenhoek's discovery of animalcules and his admonition that it was a Tower of Babel in the making if van Leeuwenhoek proceeded with the new discoveries?

The impression of reduced risk in former times is more a reflection of nostalgia than of fact. The levels of sickness and mortality in times past far exceeded those of our own lifetimes. The consequences of disease were so great that large segments of the world's population were literally wiped out. Epidemics toppled governments and wielded a far greater impact on the world's social and economic order than did all the famous battles and wars combined. *Yersinia pestis*, the bacteria responsible for the black plague, changed the social structure of Europe and its peoples for all times.

In truth, the good old days were not really so good. The practice of addressing contemporary risks and challenges through persistent reference to glorious bygone days can be misleading and counterproductive. Effectively dealing with today's risks requires all the advanced knowledge and technology we have at our disposal. Our greatest weapons in the ongoing battle against disease are our intelligence and wits, not our fears and emotions. Food-borne diseases are essentially biological problems requiring intelligent biological solutions. Succumbing to fears of the scientific unknown and feeding the ever-present phobia of technology helps no one, neither does pandering to politics or short-term expediency. The risks associated with foods must be managed in the same manner as other risks. The experience gained through years of scientific research must be actively applied to improve their safety. Unfortunately, the continued high incidence of food-borne disease outbreaks indicate that this is not happening to the extent it should.

Assessing risk is no easy matter. Like everything else in life, absolute freedom from risk of food-borne disease is not an achievable goal. In analyzing risks, it is normal to compare them with one another and to determine how they might affect our routine living conditions. We know that chlorine is toxic, but what is the risk of chlorinated water compared with contaminated water? Since, for all practical purposes, people living in the great urban centers have little opportunity to get pure crystal-clear water, what possible choices do we have? Often, the choice comes down to drinking contaminated water chlorinated by the municipal government or boiled by the consumer. Most cities opt for chlorinated water because it is more practical and provides a lower health risk than the alternative of consumer-boiled water.[225] If it were to be discovered in future that the consumption of chlorine-treated water might possibly shorten our lives by a few years, we would probably still choose to use it. The other alternative of drinking improperly boiled, contaminated water currently kills people in the millions without waiting until they reach a ripe old age. The goal of risk assessment is to provide the groundwork for selecting the best overall choice based on the evidence available. It is seldom easy or clear-cut.

The notion of degrees of risk is one of the most difficult concepts for consumers to accept. The assessment of food safety requires likely proof that the food under review will not cause consumers any harm. However, such determinations cannot guarantee that the same food will not cause harm under every possible circumstance. Absolute freedom from risk is simply not possible for any food or beverage, including water. Therefore, we must accept the fact that various degrees of risk are associated with the consumption of foods. We must have a food system that reliably supplies us with products that represent the lowest practical degree of risk.

The average consumer finds this a rather complicated and disturbing idea. Most people would much prefer to believe that something is either safe or unsafe—a clear and categorical statement. Something that is not safe in any way should not be on the market. Unfortunately, it is not as simple as that because degrees of risk are associated with the consumption of all foods. Assessing the risks of foods in an objective and quantitative manner is not an easy task. It is further complicated by the many different opinions of consumers, legislators and scientists. Consumers believe the determination of safety to be a simple, straightforward process, while scientists know how complicated it can be. Consumers consider the issue of safety very personally—how it affects them as individuals. Scientists must consider the population in its entirety when making judgments. Consumers look for unrealistic absolute guarantees. Scientists readily accept inevitable uncertainties and widely varying degrees of risk.

The supervision of risk consists of three major, integrated elements. The first is risk assessment—the process of evaluating the relative degree of the risk. The second element is risk management—the business of making the correct choices to control or minimize these risks. The final element of this trilogy is risk communication—making sure that consumers know and understand the risks they face when confronted with various food choices. This last element is by far the most difficult matter with which to deal.[226] Aside from the difficulty in communicating complex matters in a simple way, misinterpretation can have very significant commercial consequences. No one wants to tell consumers about the risks they face when eating foods for fear of losing them as customers. This is evidenced by the limited progress in this latter area, while work in the areas of risk assessment and risk management has advanced significantly. Unfortunately, until honest and effective risk communications directed at consumers are developed, the true value of risk assessment and management will never be realized. Given the frequency of food poisonings we read about weekly, consumers have little choice but to exercise great caution with all foods until verifiable risk information becomes more readily available.

During the past 25 years, the information available about consumer products has improved dramatically. Products that have the potential to cause harm to individuals or the general public are clearly labeled. Cigarettes have explicit warning labels, food ingredients and additives are clearly spelled out and hazards associated with electric products are conspicuously highlighted. Yet, foods that can and do make people very ill continue to be produced and sold to consumers without a proper indication of the potential threats they harbor. Such products must be treated like all other consumer products. A distinct label must inform consumers of the need to take proper steps and precautions in the handling and preparation of these products. Raw products such as chicken, meat, fish and seafood not specifically treated to reduce pathogenic microorganisms significantly should display a clear warning:

Warning: There is a strong statistical likelihood that this product contains disease-causing microorganisms. Exercise due caution in handling and cooking these products. Make certain that cross contamination with other products does not occur.

Of course, a more effective solution would be zero tolerance for all pathogens in food products, but this is not the case at the present time. The irony of the situation is that current standards permit the sale of contaminated foods that can endanger the public while, simultaneously, the same public pays taxes to employ an army of inspectors and technicians to enforce these standards. Surely, something is wrong with this.

The available data indicates that, at the present time, approximately 40–45 percent of the population is in an immunocompromised state of health. No one doubts that this figure will increase dramatically over the next two decades. The reasons for this are plain:

- The postwar baby boomers are currently more than 55 years old and are just beginning to experience the onset of a diminished immune capacity. This will create a boom of immunocompromised citizens.
- Modern therapies for life-threatening diseases are placing many more people under medical treatments (such as radiation or chemotherapy) powerful enough to reduce immune responses.
- An increased life expectancy is expected for the hundreds of thousands of HIV-positive patients due to new drug treatments that slow the course of the disease but fail to restore immunocompetence.
- The negative impact of the rapidly escalating level of environmental contaminants and allergens on the population's overtaxed immune system compromises the immune system.

Assuming that within the next decade the number of immunocompromised people in the United States will exceed more than 50 percent of the population would not be unreasonable. This means that another 60 million citizens will be at an increased risk. This comes to more than 150 million people! If the food supply does not improve dramatically, millions more will come down with food-borne diseases. Deaths will increase accordingly.

There can be no more convincing evidence of this than the major recall of processed meat products that occurred in January 1999 when the USDA ordered Thorn Apple Valley, Inc., to recall 30 million pounds of meat products produced in its Forrest City, Arkansas, processing plant. This included all the hot dog and luncheon meat produced between July 1998 and December 1998, products distributed nationwide and shipped to foreign countries, including Russia and South Korea. The concerns focused on possible contamination with *Listeria monocytogenes*—a gravely dangerous organism for immunocompromised consumers. To date, this has been the largest food product recall in history, exceeding the massive 25 million-pound recall of Hudson Foods in 1997.

On its Web site, Thorn Apple Valley, Inc., whose motto is "A New Generation of Quality," states that their products are sold under a number of well-established brandnames and private labels. Following another USDA public announcement of the recall on April 13, 1999, Thorn Apple Valley stated that all its products on store shelves or in distribution were produced under one of the most comprehensive food safety programs in the industry. They further stated that all those products were produced under inspection by the USDA and only products produced at the Forrest City plant before December 31, 1998, were subject to the January 22 recall. Thorn Apple Valley also noted that the USDA confirmed that no one became ill as a result of eating Thorn Apple Valley products identified in the press release.

How much of the 30 million pounds recalled was consumed? How effective can a recall of products shipped six months earlier be? How many of us remember what we ate two weeks ago, much less six months ago? Had the Forrest City Thorn Apple Valley plant been on an HACCP program, and if so, how effective was it, because the *listeria* contamination was only detected after USDA sampling and testing? Knowing the low level of food-borne disease incident reporting, it's nearly impossible to estimate the number of immunocompromised people who were exposed to these products.

Many companies, large and small, have encountered severe problems in the safe processing of foods. In October 2002, poultry giant Pilgrim's Pride launched another huge meat recall and halted production at its Pennsylvania plant because of possible contamination with *listeria*. The company recalled 27.4 million pounds of fresh and frozen ready-to-eat turkey and chicken products. As mentioned earlier, in September 2007, the Topps Meat Company recalled 21.7 million pounds of ground beef because of *E. coli* contamination.

At the present time, all the evidence we have indicates that the situation of food-borne diseases is not getting significantly better; in fact, some aspects are getting worse. Almost everyone responsible for bringing safe food to the consumer has opted to keep their head down and lie low in hopes that the problem will simply disappear. Unless a vast public outcry against the current state of our food occurs, this will most likely continue. Supermarkets and fast-food, food service and food companies will continue to quietly settle out of court all the food poisoning claims they are faced with. The garbage swept under the rug will pile higher and higher. Until the public raises a great commotion, nothing will change. It is time to come clean.

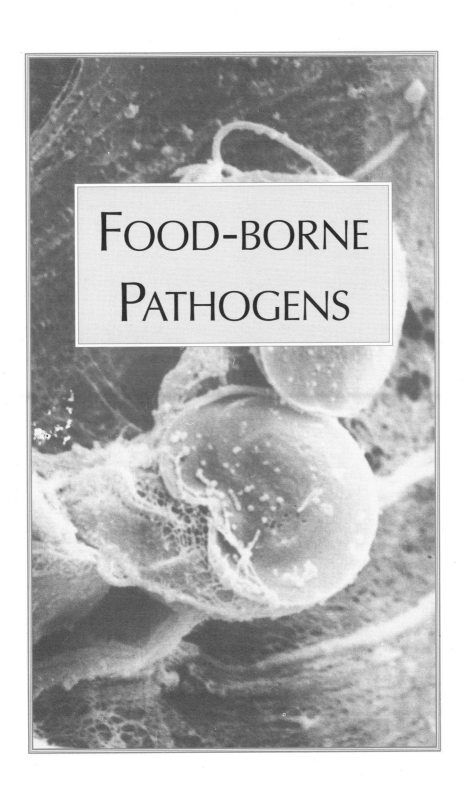

FOOD-BORNE
PATHOGENS

BACTERIAL DISEASES—
INFECTIVE FORMS

*Even while I protest the assembly-line production of our food, our songs,
our language, and eventually our souls, I know that it was a rare home
that baked good bread in the old days. Mother's cooking was with rare
exceptions poor, that good unpasteurized milk touched only by flies and
bits of manure crawled with bacteria, the healthy old-time life was riddled
with aches, sudden death from unknown causes, and that sweet local
speech I mourn was the child of illiteracy and ignorance. It is the nature of
a man as he grows older, a small bridge in time, to protest against change,
particularly change for the better.*

John Steinbeck (1902–68) *Travels with Charley:
In Search of America* (1962)*

INTRODUCTION TO BACTERIA

Bacteria are one of the oldest forms of life on earth. They comprise a large
group of microscopic, single-celled organisms characterized by a fully
developed cell wall but no clearly distinct nucleus (see figure 21). They
do have a sort of nuclear region that contains the mass of DNA,‡ but they
lack the typical nuclear membrane found in higher plants and animals.
Throughout the eons, we have seen great changes in the forms different
animals and plants have taken. This is not the case with bacteria. Evolution
in bacteria has expressed itself more in terms of highly adaptable metabolisms rather than in increasingly complex physical structures. This causes
their unmatched success. No other single biological group can exist and
flourish in as wide a range of living conditions nor can any other group
adapt itself so quickly to changing environmental circumstances.

Bacteria are extremely flexible in their manner of obtaining the
energy and nutrients they require to survive and flourish. They exist in
almost all possible environments—air, soil, water, rocks and wood. They
survive in temperatures ranging from the Antarctic cold to bubbling hot
springs and have even been found living in the hydrothermal vents on
the floor of the ocean. (One of the first jobs I ever had was to cultivate

---

* *The Columbia Dictionary of Quotations* is licensed from Columbia University Press.
  Copyright © 1993 by Columbia University Press. All rights reserved.
‡Deoxyribonucleic acid (DNA) is found in the nuclei of most cells, including all
  human, all animal, all plant and all bacterial cells. It is the principal material that
  transmits hereditary characteristics.

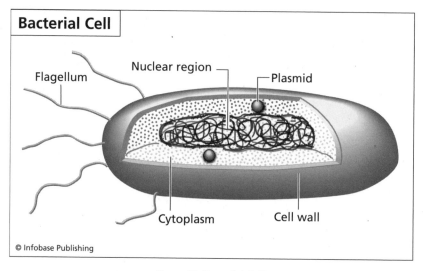

Bacterial Cell

Flagellum

Nuclear region

Plasmid

Cytoplasm

Cell wall

© Infobase Publishing

Figure 21. **Bacterial Cell**

bacteria found growing in jet engine fuel. The bacterial contamination of the fuel was thought to have been responsible for a number of fatal airline crashes.) Bacteria generally subsist on small organic materials such as acids or sugars. However, some are able to carry out photosynthesis much in the same way as plants do. Many bacteria also coexist in various forms of symbiosis with plants, animals and other forms of life. This exceptional adaptability has placed bacteria among the world's most successful biological species.

Bacteria reproduce by simple cell division. Once they find an environment that can supply them with the necessities of life, such as organic nutrients and a suitable temperature, they start to multiply. The first thing they do is duplicate the DNA that exists in their nuclear area. Once duplicated, each package of DNA migrates to the opposite ends of the cell. The cell then pinches itself together in the middle and completes the division into two small daughter cells. These then grow into adult cells and start the process all over again. If you use a typical division time of 30 minutes, you can figure out how quickly their numbers can increase. (To simplify matters, after 15 hours, a single cell will have produced roughly 1 billion offspring.)

The presence of large numbers of bacteria within a plant or animal does not necessarily signify disease. On the contrary, it may be essential or beneficial to a normal metabolism. Two examples are the colonization of our digestive system by lactic acid bacteria and the nitrogen-fixing, rhizobium bacteria associated with certain plants. However, when bacteria invade a plant or animal and interfere with normal metabolism or damage cells and tissues, they are considered pathogenic, and their presence constitutes an infection.

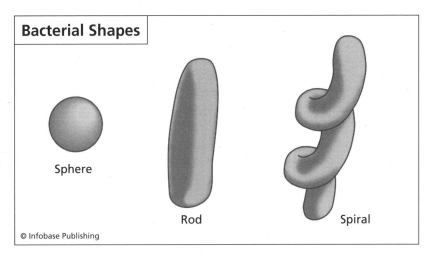

Figure 22. **Bacterial Shapes**

Bacteria are classified into species based on criteria such as shape—spheres (cocci), rods (bacilli) or spiral forms (vibrio or spirochetes) (see figure 22). They differ from one another in their ability to grow in either the presence or absence of air (aerobic and anaerobic, respectively) and in their ability to form tough, resistant spores when placed under particularly adverse conditions. They are even classified on the basis of how their cell walls absorb certain dyes. In 1884, Hans Christian Joachim Gram, a Danish physician, developed a method of staining bacteria in order to help identify them. The very same method is still used today. Bacteria on a microscope slide are first stained with a deep blue dye (gentian violet) and then dipped into a solution of iodine and potassium iodide in water. When the slide is subsequently rinsed with ethyl alcohol, the bacteria will either retain the strong blue color (referred to as Gram-positive) or will be completely decolorized (called Gram-negative). Sometimes a red stain is added later in order to give the decolorized bacteria a contrasting color that makes them more visible. Typical Gram-positive bacteria are small spheres (staphylococci) that produce boils or abscesses. Typical Gram-negative bacteria are the little rods (bacilli—*Bordetella pertussis*) that cause whooping cough.

Certain bacteria can actually move under their own power and are piloted around by hairlike appendages called "flagella" (see figure 23). These can arise from all parts of the cell surface or from either or both ends. The bacteria can move forward, backward or twirl around in one spot, depending on how the flagella propel it. This type of locomotion enables the bacteria to move toward attractants such as food and away from unfavorable elements such as toxic chemicals.

The hereditary material of bacteria is in the form of a very large, circular DNA molecule. Several bacteria carry smaller DNA inclusions located elsewhere in the cell, called "plasmids." These also carry genetic

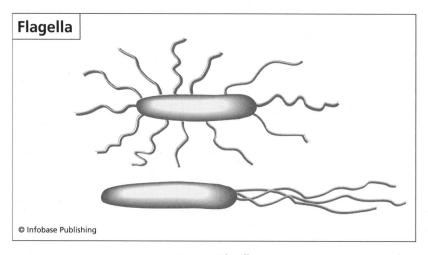

Figure 23. **Flagella**

information but are not necessary for the function of reproduction. These plasmids and the information contained in their DNA can be transferred to other bacteria by a simple exchange mechanism. This ability to exchange DNA easily can have very positive consequences for bacteria and very negative repercussions for us. For instance, a bacterium's resistance to certain antibiotics, which may have taken thousands of generations to evolve, is often encoded and kept in the plasmid DNA. Once formed, these plasmids can be quickly and efficiently transferred among different bacteria of the same species and even among different species of bacteria. Thus, beef or poultry bacteria, which have developed resistance to the antibiotics routinely added to animal feed, can quickly transfer this resistance to bacteria pathogenic to humans. The pathogens immediately become much more difficult to control because our primary weapons of defense against them—antibiotics—have been rendered quite useless.

Plasmids often contain DNA that controls the very characteristics that make bacteria pathogenic. Certain nonpathogenic strains can become pathogenic just by accepting a plasmid from a pathogenic strain with which it comes into contact. This becomes a major concern when plasmids that contain the DNA for high virulence characteristics transfer between species. When referring to the recent origin of the new and dangerous pathogen enterohemorrhagic *E. coli* O157:H7, one scientist stated that the bacteria, "Is a messenger, bringing an unwelcome message that in mankind's battle to conquer infectious diseases, the opposing army is being replenished with fresh replacements."[227]

Bacteria can also be categorized according to their lifestyles. Those that live on dead animal and vegetable matter are called "saprophytes." These bacteria play a critical role in the environment by decomposing and recycling dead animals and plants back into their original elements, thereby making them available once more as elements or nutrients for new growth. Bacte-

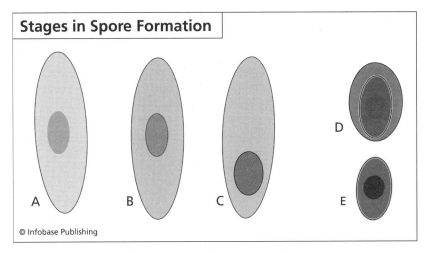

Stages in Spore Formation

© Infobase Publishing

Figure 24. **Stages in Spore Formation**

ria that live on or within living animals or plants are called "symbionts." Several are a normal part of various animal and human tissues, including the digestive tract and the skin, where they play a fundamental role in life's everyday processes. The bacteria benefit from this relationship, but so does their host. Therefore, the process is dubbed "mutualistic." Other types of symbionts called "commensals" do not particularly benefit their host but do not cause them particular harm either. A third type of symbiont, "parasitic" bacteria, provides no advantages at all. On the contrary, they are harmful and can destroy the plants and animals on which they live.

Many bacteria are capable of forming highly resistant spores. Spores are not really considered to be a part of the bacteria's normal life cycle. They are generally formed in response to some environmental challenge, such as a lack of food or inadequate moisture (see figure 24). Spore formation becomes a sort of hibernating mechanism where the bacterium goes into suspended animation until favorable conditions return. Once this happens, the bacterial spore germinates into a fresh bacterial cell and is ready to reproduce in the usual way all over again.

In the spore-forming process, the bacteria's genetic material (DNA) in the nuclear region condenses and migrates toward the area where the spore will eventually develop. Very soon after, a thin membrane forms around this DNA and begins to transform itself into a resistant wall. The remainder of the bacterial cell coalesces and adds to the formation of this wall, then it dries out. Once this wall is fully formed, bacterial spores are extremely durable and resistant to all sorts of challenges such as heat, cold, acids and even toxins. As a result, viable spores are very common in all soil and dust, where they can survive in this state for many years until activated once again by conditions favorable for growth.

As described above, researchers have long known that microorganisms are intimately involved in the spoilage of a wide range of food and beverage products such as meat, fruits, vegetables and milk, among others. On the other hand, the importance of microbes in the effective production of other foods and beverages is equally well-known. Without working yeasts, molds and bacteria, we would not have cheeses, sauerkraut, dill pickles, yogurt, beer, wine or countless other products. In yet another role, certain bacteria exist symbiotically with leguminous plants such as beans and are critical to agriculture because they enrich our soils with nitrogen.

Within the family of bacteria, more than 200 different species are officially considered to be pathogenic toward humans. The most infamous of these are responsible for cholera, typhoid fever, dysentery, tuberculosis, diphtheria, leprosy, syphilis, pneumonia and plague. The extent of their pathogenicity varies depending upon the particular species or strain as well as the overall condition of the infected victim. The full range of pathogenic effects exerted by bacteria is beyond the scope of this book, which will focus only on those concerned with food-borne diseases.

A final concept to consider is the one of offending microorganisms. Offending organisms are simply defined as those that cause us harm or damage. None of the technologies currently used to control these microorganisms actually removes them from solid foods. Removal is physically impossible, unless you can filter them out, as is the case of certain liquids passing through specially designed filters. All other technologies simply seek to remove the organism's offensiveness rather than the organism itself. As an example, pasteurization does not remove any bacteria, it simply kills enough of them to make milk safe to consume and to give it a suitable shelf life. This makes perfect sense because if infectious bacteria are no longer able to infect, they are no longer considered offensive. The concept of an offending or nonoffending microorganism should be clearly understood in relation to food-borne disease. Once destroyed or rendered totally inoffensive, one bacteria is much the same as another. Pathogens treated in this way are no worse than the masses of lactobacilli found in all that natural yogurt we love to eat. This is not the case with bacterial or fungal toxins, some of which cannot be made inoffensive through heat or any other means.

CAMPYLOBACTER

When first studied at the beginning of this century, the bacteria we know today as *Campylobacter* was originally thought to be a pathogen of only animals. The name *Campylobacter* simply means "curved rod" (a *cam* + a *bacillus*). In fact, this bacterium was originally considered to be a vibrio because of its spiral-type shape. Theobald Smith, who studied *Salmonella* with D. E. Salmon, found what he characterized as a spirillum-type bacterium associated with disease-induced abortions in cattle. The organism was subsequently dubbed *Vibrio fetus* in recognition of its microscopic appearance and its pathological effects. Because of their close connection with animals, only a restricted amount of research was carried out on these bacteria. The first association of these bacteria with human illness occurred after World War II when one scientist ascribed a large outbreak of milk-borne diarrhea to a bacterium (*Vibrio jejuni*) known to be responsible for dysentery in calves.[228]

Scientists determined only in the 1960s that distinct molecular differences existed between the DNA of classical vibrio, which are responsible for certain severe human diseases, and that of the spiral-shaped bacterium associated with calf and human diarrhea. Thus, the new name *Campylobacter* was coined to account for this difference.

From relatively humble beginnings, the small, Gram-negative *Campylobacter jejuni* has, for more than a decade, become the organism most commonly found in food-borne diarrhea and gastroenteritis incidents. Despite the fact that very little was published about this bacteria before 1980, the recoveries of *Campylobacter* quickly began to exceed those of salmonella in a wide range of gastroenteritis victims.[229] Recent figures estimate incidents of campylobacteriosis to be more than double those of salmonellosis. Typical symptoms include diarrhea, cramps, vomiting, fever and headache. These effects may linger for more than two weeks but are usually over within six days. *Campylobacter* infections can also become life threatening if they enter the circulatory system (a condition called campylobacter bacteremia).[230]

Longer-term complications can be very serious and include appendicitis, cholecystitis (gallbladder inflammation), pancreatic inflammation and enlargement of the colon to a point where it can no longer move the feces. *Campylobacter jejuni* has also been very closely linked to Guillain-Barré syndrome, a serious neurological disorder characterized by extensive nervous tissue damage. Some scientists consider this bacteria to be a major cause of this condition,[231] particularly since more than 50 percent of Guillain-Barré syndrome patients have evidence of prior *Campylobacter* infections. The severe nature of this debilitating disease and its close linkage to the bacteria add a note of great concern for the very common occurrence of campylobacteriosis.

Because the routine symptoms of campylobacteriosis are similar to the stomach flu, an episode can be easily mistaken for the flu. Recent estimates indicate that only about 5 percent of victims have severe enough symptoms to visit a doctor. The number of physicians who go through the trouble of obtaining stool cultures and then reporting the outcome to national authorities continues to be a question. As a result, the full extent of this disease is still to be determined. Apparently, however, the peak occurrence of incidents normally falls between May and December, with the zenith taking place during the month of July.

Campylobacter is a commensal bacterium in a great many animal species, particularly those used for human foods. Cattle, pigs, goats, sheep and poultry all test positive for *Campylobacter* and represent the main animal reservoirs of concern to us. Tests have shown that from 50–100 percent of poultry products sold on the retail market are contaminated with *C. jejuni*. As high as 60–80 percent of cattle and swine have been found to harbor this pathogen. *Campylobacter* is often found in unpasteurized milk and the products made from it. A wide variety of shellfish and seafood can be infected as well. This makes *Campylobacter* one of the most widely spread agents of food-borne disease in our food system. Not only domestic poultry but wild birds can also carry this bacterium. They were found to be responsible for fouling (no pun intended) a Florida community water system, causing almost 900 cases of *Campylobacter* gastroenteritis. The transmission of *Campylobacter* in milk has even been attributed to wild birds, such as jackdaws, as a result of their aggressive habit of pecking through the tops of milk bottles.[232] In 2006, more than 5,700 laboratory-confirmed cases of *Campylobacter* were recorded.

CLOSTRIDIUM PERFRINGENS

Clostridium perfringens is closely related to its more famous relative *Clostridium botulinum* but does not work in quite the same way. The mode of action of this disease is a classic toxicoinfection. First described in 1895, the organism was only characterized as being of food-borne origin in 1943. *Clostridium* is a Gram-positive anaerobic bacteria[233] (see figure 25). Anaerobic organisms, as their name suggests, do not require free air or oxygen to survive. They were first discovered by Pasteur while he was studying the fermentation of butyric acid. Despite the apparent anomaly, his research conclusively demonstrated that some microorganisms did not need oxygen to live and grow. They are able to derive their energy requirements through the fermentation process rather than from typical oxygen metabolism. He introduced the terms aerobic and anaerobic to describe life in either the presence or absence of oxygen, respectively.

Clostridium perfringens is also a spore-forming bacterium. Once they form, *Clostridium* spores are very resistant and capable of withstanding five hours of constant boiling. As a result, *Clostridium* spores can be found everywhere in the soil and dust and in the intestinal tracts of a wide variety of animals. Food poisoning caused by *Clostridium* is very often linked to food prepared in institutions, restaurants, cafeterias and any other place where food is made well in advance of serving.[234]

Victims usually ingest foods containing large amounts of bacteria, which then colonize and flourish in the intestine. When the bacteria form spores, they release an enterotoxin that causes intense stomachache and diarrhea. (It has also been reported that certain strains do not have to undergo sporulation in order to form the toxin.) The onset of disease, which can range from eight to 22 hours, depends upon the ingestion of a heavy load of bacteria to initiate growth in the intestine. The symptoms are usually over within 24 hours, but fatalities have occurred as a result of severe dehydration following diarrhea. Another form of *C. perfringens* dis-

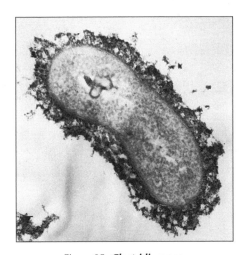

Figure 25. **Clostridium spp.**
Courtesy Istituto Superiore di Sanità, Rome, Italy.

ease is called necrotic enteritis or pigbel (pidgin English for pig belly). Although it can be fatal, this disease occurs extremely rarely and is more a problem in developing countries, such as Papua New Guinea, where gluttonous feasts (usually involving pigs) often follow periods of famine. The sudden mass of food overloads the system and makes individuals very susceptible to disease.

The foods most frequently implicated with *C. perfringens* poisoning are beef, chicken, turkey and pork. Spices used in conjunction with these foods are also excellent sources of *C. perfringens*. A recent study of fresh sausages (chorizos) in Argentina revealed that 110 out of 136 samples were positive for *C. perfringens*.[235] Dairy products are another good carrier for this bacteria. During the St. Patrick's Day festivities in 1993, *Clostridium* in corned beef caused two totally unrelated incidents, one in Virginia and another in Ohio.[236] *Clostridium perfringens* has also been found in the newer generation of vacuum-packed pouch products (also called *sous-vide*—French for "under vacuum"), which have become so popular in the retail and restaurant trade.[237] It is also a concern for all caterers, because heat-shocked clostridium spores can germinate and rapidly multiply in foods if they are not cooled quickly enough.[238, 239]

ESCHERICHIA COLI

Escherichia coli was first described by the German physician Dr. Theodore Escherich in 1885.[240] He called this Gram-negative bacteria *Bacterium coli commune* to indicate that it occurred in the intestines (colons) and was extremely common in humans and animals. In fact, the ubiquitous presence of *E. coli* in the human intestine long obscured its role as an agent of food-borne disease.[241] For the greater part of this century, the food industry did not consider the detection of fecal *E. coli* in food samples as anything more than an indication of poor sanitary practices. More recent data have proven that although these bacteria normally reside in the human intestinal tract, many types can be pathogenic, and some can be dangerous to the extreme. The most well-known symptoms of this type of bacteria are known to us as traveler's diarrhea, tourista, or Montezuma's revenge. This commonly occurs in people who travel from a relatively uncontaminated

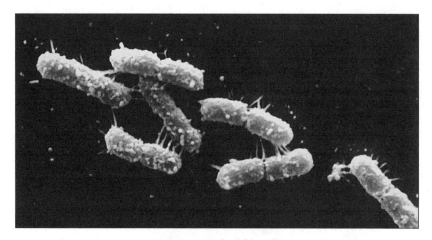

Figure 26. *Escherichia coli*
Courtesy Istituto Superiore di Sanità, Rome, Italy.

environment, where most foods are prepared in a controlled and sanitary manner, to locations where hygienic practices barely exist at all.

We now know that four main forms of disease are associated with the *E. coli* bacteria—enterohemorrhagic (bloody diarrhea), enteroinvasive (damages the intestinal tissue), enteropathogenic (severe diarrhea), and enterotoxigenic (traveler's diarrhea). Because the true significance of *E. coli*'s role in food-borne diseases has come to light only recently, examining all four forms of the bacteria is worthwhile. As with *Salmonella*, different forms of *E. coli* are also characterized by the specific antigens from both the body (O-type) and flagella (H-type). As an example, one of the most dangerous of the coliform bacteria is the enterohemorrhagic type called *E. coli* O157:H7, which causes severe hemorrhagic colitis and kidney failure in children. It is a life-threatening form of *E. coli* that must be avoided at all costs. It can generally be controlled through good hygiene and thorough cooking of meat products, although it is beginning to turn up in other foods and beverages. Unfortunately, this is the very same organism that keeps cropping up in recent news reports. Another type, *E. coli* O27:H20, exerts its effect through toxicoinfection.

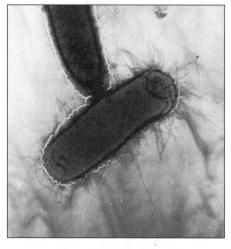

Figure 27. *Escherichia coli*
Courtesy Istituto Superiore di Sanità, Rome, Italy.

It has caused disease outbreaks following the consumption of soft cheeses made from unpasteurized milk such as Brie and Camembert.

Enterohemorrhagic E. coli (EHEC)

It is thought that the *E. coli* O157:H7 originally evolved as early as 1955 because hemolytic uremic syndrome (HUS)—a typical characteristic of *E. coli* O157:H7—was first described by a Swiss pediatrician while examining a dairy-related outbreak. HUS is characterized by sudden gastrointestinal bleeding, anemia, blood in the urine and renal failure. It occurred again in 1975, when doctors took a stool sample from a California-based female naval officer who had a severe case of bloody diarrhea. They cultured a rare form of *E. coli* and sent it to the Centers for Disease Control (CDC) in Atlanta where it was promptly placed in storage.

In December 1981, a severe outbreak of hemorrhagic diarrhea occurred in White City, Oregon. Local physicians were unable to identify the responsible organism and called Dr. Lee Riley, a California-based epidemiologist who was associated with the CDC. No specific microbial agent was immediately found, but shortly thereafter there was another outbreak in Michigan. As was the case in the Oregon outbreak, a McDonald's restaurant was implicated.

By this time, Joy Wells, a microbiologist at the CDC, had isolated *E. coli* O157:H7 from stool samples of the victims. However, it was not until two months later that investigators discovered the same *E. coli* O157:H7 in a processing plant that had supplied the suspected burgers to McDonald's. It was then that Dr. Wells took it one step further and canvassed the thousands of *E. coli* samples maintained at the CDC and found the one that had been responsible for the hemorrhagic diarrhea episode that took place in 1975. They were finally on to something conclusive and in 1982 they published the results in the *New England Journal of Medicine*.[242]

When *E. coli* O157:H7 was first discovered, it was a true rarity among pathogenic bacteria because no one could accurately estimate the minimum infectious dose (the minimum number of organisms required to cause an infection). For most bacteria, the average infectious dose ranged from 100 to 1,000,000,000. However, for *E. coli* O157:H7, its pathogenicity was so great that the ingestion of one single cell was thought to be sufficient to cause an infection. Even then, its true potential could not be fully known because the outbreaks of it had been so limited.

A decade after its conclusive discovery, I recall bringing up the subject of *E. coli* O157:H7 pathogenicity at an international meeting on food safety in Orlando, Florida.[243] I was so impressed with its high potential for infectivity as well as its severe symptoms that I felt obliged to ask one of the senior government speakers what the government was doing about *E. coli* O157:H7. The reply I got was that little was being done since it was very uncommon and, as a result, was not considered to be a major problem. Few food safety regulators understood the seriousness of its threat. As its name suggests, the enterohemorrhagic type has particularly alarming symptoms. It is typically characterized by a very bloody diarrhea and painful abdominal cramps that can be very severe. The amounts of blood in the discharges have been so great that this infection has often been mistaken for other severe intestinal injuries. ECO157 may also cause hemolytic uremic syndrome (HUS), a condition that destroys red blood cells and causes acute kidney failure. Frequently, these symptoms are followed by strokes or seizures and may require long-term or even lifelong kidney dialysis. All of these effects were featured in the 1993 Jack-in-the-Box restaurant incident—one of the most dangerous food-borne disease outbreaks recorded in the United States.

ECO157 produces an extremely potent toxin very similar to that of the dysentery bacteria *Shigella dysenteriae*. In a scenario that seems to repeat itself all too often, the deadly ECO157 apparently originated from a much less dangerous enteropathogenic *E. coli* but may have picked up the shigella-like toxin through a plasmid transfer from another strain of bacteria.[244] The toxin exerts its effect by interfering with the cells' normal protein metabolism. Both intestinal and kidney cells are severely affected.

The animals most often implicated with ECO157 are beef cattle. Hamburgers are the form of food that serves as the most common vehicle for the bacteria's transmission. Raw milk seems to be another frequent route of infection. ECO157 has been isolated from cattle with diarrhea but also from cattle, pigs and chickens that appeared to be perfectly healthy. This poses an extremely difficult problem for animal health inspectors. Without the ability to distinguish and separate ECO157 carriers from other animals, the risk of slaughterhouse cross contamination multiplies astronomically. Even very minor amounts of cross contamination can be critical, because the number of consumed ECO157 cells required to cause a full-blown infection is very small, perhaps as low as a single cell. This combination of extreme virulence, difficulty of detection in the host animals, low intakes required for infection and recurrent presence in the most popular foods available makes ECO157 a truly dangerous threat. Little wonder that the American Gastroenterological Association considers *E. coli* O157:H7 infection a serious national problem in terms of severity of illness, medical costs, lost productivity and epidemic potential.[245]

Vegetarians can also be victims of this pathogen. In 1992, a small but lethal ECO157 outbreak occurred in Maine.[246] The source of infection was traced to a garden fertilized with unsterilized manure from the family cow and calf. In 1991, a serious outbreak of diarrhea and hemolytic uremic syndrome due to the presence of ECO157 in apple cider occurred in Massachusetts.[247]

Aside from the risks of eating contaminated food, simply touching animals can result in serious illness, as evidenced by the case of a 13-month-old farm infant who became infected after coming in close contact with some calves.[248] Because ECO157 appears to be so common in farm animals, the potential risks for children posed by petting zoos should be reevaluated.

In mid-July 1996, one of Japan's largest outbreaks of food poisoning this century occurred involving approximately 10,000 victims, most of them schoolchildren from the Osaka and Sakai areas. Eleven people died.[249] The episode was so serious that the Japanese Government invoked an old law in order to designate the outbreak as an epidemic. The organism found to be responsible was *E. coli* O157. Although sushi was originally thought to be the carrier food, roast pork and raw liver were also implicated. The famous daikon radishes were eventually suspected, which brought howls of protest from Japanese vegetable farmers. More than 500 children were hospitalized, with more than 50 showing signs of very serious illness. The incident took more than three months to come to an end and sadly concluded with the suicide of the managing director of the Sakai School Lunch Program Association, who felt personally responsible for the whole tragic affair.[250]

On September 13, 2006, CDC officials were alerted by epidemiologists in Wisconsin and Oregon that fresh spinach was the suspected source of small clusters of *E. coli* serotype O157:H7 infections in those states. On the same day, New Mexico epidemiologists contacted their Wisconsin and Oregon counterparts about a cluster of *E. coli* O157:H7 infections found in New Mexico and associated with fresh spinach. Wisconsin public health officials had previously reported a cluster of *E. coli* O157:H7 infections to the CDC on September 8, and four days later the CDC confirmed that the *E. coli* O157:H7 from infected patients in Wisconsin matched patient isolates from other states.

By September 26, a total of 183 persons infected with the outbreak strain of *E. coli* O157:H7 had been reported to the CDC from 26 states. Among them, 95 were hospitalized, 29 had hemolytic uremic syndrome (HUS) and one person died. The deaths of two other patients possibly related to this outbreak were under investigation.

Fresh spinach was identified as the source of the outbreak. One hundred twenty-three of 130 patients reported consuming uncooked fresh spinach during the 10 days before illness onset. In addition, *E. coli* O157:H7 matching the outbreak strain was isolated from three open packages of fresh spinach consumed by patients.

On September 14, the FDA advised consumers by press release not to eat bagged fresh spinach. On September 15, a California company that bags spinach under several brand names announced a voluntary recall of all fresh spinach–containing products. On September 16, the FDA expanded its warning and advised consumers not to eat fresh spinach or products containing fresh spinach. On September 21, the FDA informed consumers that only spinach grown in three California counties (Monterey, San Benito and Santa Clara) was implicated in the outbreak.

A short time later, during the months of November and December, more than 70 people became ill with *E. coli* O157:H7 associated with eating contaminated lettuce at Taco Bell restaurants in the northeastern United States. Cases were reported to the CDC from New Jersey, New York, Pennsylvania, Delaware and South Carolina. Among the people who were ill, 53 were hospitalized and 8 developed hemolytic uremic syndrome (HUS).

Both incidents highlighted the growing problem of *E. coli* O157:H7–infected horticultural products and the need to ensure that these products go through the same HACCP systems as other foods.

The repeated appearance of *E. coli* O157:H7 in acute outbreaks on a worldwide basis has prompted many health professionals to rank this dangerous type of bacteria uppermost among the list of menacing emerging pathogens.

Enteroinvasive E. coli (EIEC)

As their name suggests, EIEC bacteria can invade cells in the same way as shigella can. They exert their effects on the surface cells of the colon or small intestine. Symptoms usually include diarrhea, vomiting and fever. It is interesting to observe that the invasive characteristics of EIEC results from a plasmid identical to one found in *Shigella flexneri*, a bacteria that exhibits the very same traits. Two different species of bacteria have one identical type of virulent plasmid—a model example of two different bacteria sharing the same pathogenicity.

Enteropathogenic E. coli (EPEC)

EPEC is the most common type of pathogenic *E. coli* and is the one often implicated in infant diarrhea. Bottle-feeding of babies has been found to be an important risk factor in the manifestation of this problem. Reinfection by contact with baby feces is another common mode of transmission. Needless to say, scrupulous cleaning of bottles, linens, appliances, toys and anything else that the baby touches is the best way to prevent this.

This bacterium works by clinging to the inner surface of the intestines, causing the lining cells to perish. The phenomenon is officially termed "attaching and effacing." Once the intestine is damaged in this way, diarrhea quickly follows. This ability to adhere to the intestinal surface and destroy lining cells seems to be transmissible to other bacteria by the exchange of plasmids. Consequently, this type of pathogenicity has a strong potential to be transferred to nonpathogenic strains of *E. coli* with which EPEC occasionally comes in close contact. It is one of the reasons that we keep seeing new pathogenic varieties appearing.

A recently recognized subgroup of EPEC is called enteroadherent or enteroaggregative *E. coli* (EAEC). It has been implicated in serious and long-lasting bouts of diarrhea.[251] Although fever is seldom associated with this infection, the diarrhea is very serious and often bloody. EAEC has occasionally resulted in deaths.

Enterotoxigenic E. coli (ETEC)

ETEC is another group of *E. coli* known to cause distinct disease. It occurs much more commonly in developing countries where sanitation remains at a rudimentary level. ETEC works by producing toxins that interfere with the water- and electrolyte-absorbing mechanisms of the intestine and results in severe, watery diarrhea. It strikes down children as well as adults who have not developed any degree of immunity. Tourists or soldiers coming from a relatively clean environment (such as the United States troops in the Gulf War) are ideal potential victims. Diarrhea in children is often followed by severe dehydration and malnutrition and is a leading cause of infant mortality in the developing world. The World Health Organization (WHO) estimates that this type of diarrhea results in more than 3 million deaths annually in the age group comprising one to five year olds.

HELICOBACTER PYLORI

In 1983, Australian scientists Barry Marshall and Robin Warren stunned the world with their discovery of a strange bacterium called *Helicobacter pylori* (originally *Campylobacter pylori*) that was able to reside in the stomach of humans successfully. The concentrated acid and high concentration of digestive enzymes of the stomach make it a very inhospitable environment. Most were very surprised to learn that a bacterium had evolved a means of withstanding the stomach for long periods. What was even more surprising was that this microorganism was responsible for the majority of stomach ulcers from which such a large proportion of the population suffered.

In order to protect itself from its own digestive enzymes and corrosive acids, the stomach lining is covered by a thick layer of mucus. *Helicobacter pylori* safeguards itself by living within that same mucous layer. When the body responds to this threat of infection, the immune defense system is not capable of getting directly at the invading *Helicobacter* cells. Researchers have speculated that this continued, but unsuccessful, immune response may be the factor ultimately responsible for the creation of ulcers. Fortunately, specific antibiotic therapy has been incredibly successful at completely ridding long-term sufferers of this problem. Unfortunately, a very dramatic rise in therapy-resistant *Helicobacter pylori* bacteria has recently occurred and may be far more difficult to treat in the future.[252]

Because of the importance of sanitation, the rate of *Helicobacter* infection in developing countries is generally above 70 percent. In developed countries, the rate of infection varies from 30–70 percent, with approximately 50 percent of Americans over the age of 50 being infected. Scientists still do not know for certain whether *Helicobacter pylori* is actually a food-borne bacterium. It can be transmitted through the fecal-oral route when someone does not carefully adhere to personal hygienic practices. However, despite a considerable amount of work trying to determine if food animals are common reservoirs of these bacteria, results are inconclusive. Researchers know that prior *Helicobacter pylori* infections are linked to an increased risk of stomach cancer.[253]

LISTERIA MONOCYTOGENES

As with the other pathogens we have examined, *Listeria* was first discovered about a century ago. It is a small, Gram-positive, rod-shaped bacterium. Like *Campylobacter*, it was not originally thought to be a pathogen for humans since it was found only in the blood and livers of animals. The shape and typical place of recovery of the bacteria resulted in the name *Bacillus hepatitis*. This organism was soon found to be identical to another named *Listerella hepatolytica* after Joseph Lister, the famous British surgeon who first applied antiseptic procedures to the operating room. Since these bacteria have the very nasty habit of entering monocytes and neutrophils (white blood cells), it was agreed to call them *Listeria monocytogenes*.

Listeria monocytogenes has come into prominence recently as a serious element in food-borne disease. Some have speculated that it was the agent responsible for Queen Anne's 17 failed pregnancies in the 17th century.[254, 255] *Listeria monocytogenes* can be found everywhere we look in nature. Animals, fish, plants, water, soil and waste residues all harbor this microorganism. Within the group of domesticated food animals we are primarily concerned with, *Listeria* seems to favor the ruminants—cattle, sheep and goats. The symptoms of infection are often related to nervous system deterioration. In ruminants, they are characterized by the animals aimlessly and endlessly trudging around in circles. Many commonly believe that the occurrence of listeriosis in these animals may somehow be associated with the feeding of silage, the fermented fodder produced in the silos that we see on virtually every farm.

Although this bacterium was always associated with animal disease in the past, it has more recently been linked to serious diseases in humans. *Listeria* can cause meningitis and encephalitis as well as severe pregnancy and fetal infections. Victims are usually the very young or the very old, and the rate of fatalities is staggering—about 70 percent if the condition is left untreated.[256] Even when pregnant women are properly treated, a case fatality rate of 25–30 percent of fetuses occurs. Listeric abortions can occur during the last half of pregnancy and often result in stillborn or acutely ill babies. If born alive, babies often die shortly thereafter.[257] The disease can be transmitted in many ways, including mother to fetus, infant to infant and animal to human.[258] The central role of food in the transmission of this disease was discovered only in 1982.[259] This is apparently the most common cause of human listeriosis.

The impact of *Listeria* on humans has been the subject of fairly intense debate. Since first recorded in 1929, human listeriosis remains a fairly rare disease. For this reason, many people, particularly those representing certain segments of the food and beverage industry, feel that far too much attention is being paid to this microorganism. On the other hand, the very severe symptoms that accompany listeriosis have prompted others to raise a warning alarm regarding the serious threat *Listeria* poses. What are the issues and facts that back either point of view?

Listeria monocytogenes bacteria are almost unique in their ability to survive and grow at temperatures as low as 3°C (37°F). In fact, this ability to multiply at low temperatures allows microbiologists to enrich mixed bacterial cultures with *Listeria* cells because other species of bacteria die or remain dormant in the cold. Unfortunately, this low-temperature characteristic poses very significant problems for the food industry in general and the dairy business in particular. Refrigeration is the single most important weapon in the battery of technologies used by the food and beverage industry to combat the proliferation of spoilage and disease microorganisms. Refrigeration is so highly developed and so fully integrated into our food system that it is employed continually from the moment of harvest or collection right up until the moment of final preparation and consumption in the restaurant or home. Little wonder, then, that considerable concern exists about a virulent and potentially lethal microorganism that is not only invulnerable to refrigerated storage but actually thrives in it.

The relative rarity of human *Listeria monocytogenes* infections results from our natural immunity to monocyte invasion. Our white blood cells (lymphocytes) are the body's first line of defense against threats from harmful microorganisms. At the first signs of infection, these cells rush to the site of invasion and use a variety of chemical and biological means to destroy the foreign microbes, including consuming them whole, much in the same way as an ameba would eat its prey (phagocytosis). The forces on both sides of the infection become locked in deadly one-on-one combat. It is the equivalent of trench warfare at the cellular level. The retaliatory techniques employed by *Listeria* even include the equivalent of working behind enemy lines. *Listeria* are capable of avoiding lymphocyte attack by spreading from cell to cell within our tissues without ever entering the circulatory system, where they might be vulnerable.[260, 261]

When our natural immunity is operating properly, we are quite capable of withstanding the threatening attack of *Listeria monocytogenes*, and we do so every day. If we are perfectly fit and not suffering from any conditions that have weakened or overtaxed our immune system, we are not in the high-risk category. Therefore, this microorganism is unlikely to cause disease. Unfortunately, few of us are perpetually in a perfect state of health. If our immune systems are not up to the task, *Listeria* can quickly turn the tables on us with devastating consequences.

A great many factors and circumstances influence the functioning of our immune system. Environmental threats such as smog and pollution, mild illnesses such as colds or flu, and physical or even mental stresses can play havoc with our immune system. For the majority of people, however, these challenges do not weaken the system to the point where it cannot handle *Listeria monocytogenes*. Nevertheless, a significant proportion of society is at severe risk to listeric infections. In the case of senior citizens, it is a segment that is growing rapidly. Scientists have long known that pregnant women, newborns, senior citizens, people receiving radiation for cancer treatment or immunosuppressant therapy (transplant recipients), diabetics and AIDS patients all have a significantly reduced immune function. Not surprisingly, they are the very same groups most subject to listeriosis. Much of this reduced immunity is perfectly natural in the course of our lives and does not necessarily indicate any inherent weaknesses in our constitution. However, if the population of pregnant women, newborns, senior citizens (over 65) and cancer, organ transplant and AIDS patients were totaled, we would come up with a population of approximately 70–100 million immunocompromised people in the United States.[262, 263] This does not even include all those people whose immune systems are temporarily under challenge from colds, flus and other viruses.

Pregnant women experience reductions in their immune system in order to ensure that they do not reject the growing fetus. This is a natural defense mechanism to safeguard the baby's survival, and all pregnant women experience this phenomenon. An unfortunate side effect is the greatly increased susceptibility of pregnant women to *Listeria*. The potential results of listeriosis during pregnancy are very serious and generally result in extremely negative consequences. In the first instance, the mother may be affected mildly or will be without any apparent symptoms at all. However, the baby will be born severely ill and will frequently die. In another case, the mother experiences severe symptoms and prematurely delivers either a stillborn or a deathly ill baby. At other times, the mother dies, and the baby suffers no infection at all. Of course, variations occur in all three scenarios depending upon the severity and the onset of infection during the pregnancy cycle, among other factors. Fairly frequently, surviving babies have severe neurological symptoms, the most common of which is meningitis. Cases on record describe the mother of a neurologically affected child who did nothing more than eat a soft, well-ripened French cheese, traditionally made from raw milk, just a few weeks before giving birth.

In other segments of the population at risk of *Listeria monocytogenes*, the outcome can be just as severe. When these bacteria get around the defenses of the immune system, they have a propensity to kill and cripple people. The following table[264, 265] gives an idea of the shocking statistics this bacteria produces. Little doubt exists of *Listeria monocytogenes'* virulence.

CONSEQUENCES OF LISTERIA MONOCYTOGENES INFECTIONS	
CONDITION	RESULT
Listeria infection during late pregnancy	93% central nervous system infection of infants
Adult infections under age 40	11% case fatality
Adult infections over age 60	63% case fatality
Listeria meningitis in renal transplant patients	38% case fatality

Listeria monocytogenes has been found in a wide range of dairy products, raw vegetables and meat products in most countries. Several studies of meat products sampled in European supermarkets confirmed the recovery of *Listeria* to be as high as 80 percent.[266, 267] A 1991 Australian study of samples picked up at the retail level showed that over 42 percent tested positive for *Listeria*.[268] Raw, unpasteurized milk and the soft cheeses traditionally made from it are a major concern since *Listeria* continues to thrive at refrigeration temperatures. In a 1995 publication about the impact of *Listeria* in raw-milk cheeses in France, of the 11 cases reported among pregnant women, two had spontaneous abortions, four had premature births and two had stillbirths.[269] Of additional concern is an Australian study that recently demonstrated the relative ineffectiveness of microwave cooking in destroying *Listeria monocytogenes* in ground beef.[270] In another devastating incident in Canada, coleslaw made from cabbages naturally fertilized with manure from infected sheep resulted in stillbirths, abortions, meningitis and a mortality rate of 41 percent in those affected.[271] Poultry is also a significant source of *Listeria monocytogenes*. One study showed an incidence of 23 percent in broiler chickens.[272] Fish and seafood are yet another source of *Listeria*, which have been found in all forms of these foods, from the fresh, raw species to highly processed smoked and formulated products.

The problem of *Listeria* should not be taken out of its present context. According to current data, most people exposed to *L. monocytogenes* do not get sick. Normal, healthy individuals who possess no underlying illness are resistant to the bacteria. Our defense mechanisms handle the bacteria sufficiently to protect us. The actual incidence of reported disease outbreaks for *Listeria* is not very high. In fact, evidence has shown a decline in *Listeria* incidents in the United States from 1989–93, presumably the result of strict governmental policies and industry compliance. This had prompted the National Food Processors Association to demand the current zero tolerances set for *Listeria* in foods be moved upward to 2,800 bacteria per ounce.[273] This would be for foods not specifically directed at immunocompromised individuals. However, the number of people whose immune system is not operating perfectly (such as newborns, pregnant women, people with AIDS, immunosuppressed patients and the elderly) continues to grow rapidly. These individuals are at a much greater risk. For instance, AIDS patients are 300 times more susceptible than people whose immune system is working properly. This is definitely not a bacteria to take lightly. Current regulations for recall and seizure remain at a zero tolerance in the United States, but that is not the case for all European countries.

Listeria monocytogenes is a bacterium that bears close watching in future. It grows well in plants, animals, fish and all sorts of waste products. *Listeria* is therefore intimately associated with our entire food system. It is very resistant to the major bacterial control technology (refrigeration), and there has even been some debate as to its resistance to heat.

Although it does not appear to affect individuals whose immune system is operating properly, for all others it boasts a high degree of lethality. This fact alone requires that critical attention be paid to *Listeria monocytogenes*. When considering the aging population and the growing environmental challenges to the immune system of all individuals, a great many more people will likely fall into the susceptible, high-risk category.

Active surveillance for listeriosis has been conducted since 1996. In 2000, listeriosis surveillance was conducted in eight states (California, Connecticut, Georgia, Maryland, Minnesota, New York, Oregon and Tennessee) encompassing approximately 29.5 million people, or 11 percent of the U.S. population. Demographic data on all cases of culture-confirmed listeriosis identified were analyzed and revealed that the average incidence was 0.2 per 100,000 among non-Hispanics and 0.7 among Hispanics. Among non-Hispanics, the incidence was 0.2 in Native Americans, 0.2 in blacks, 0.2 in whites and 0.4 in Asians. Although the incidence remained higher in Hispanics across almost all age groups, the disparity between Hispanics and non-Hispanics appeared to be greatest among infants less than one year of age (11.9 per 100,000 v. 1.0 per 100,000 respectively) as well as among Hispanic women of childbearing age (15–39 years, 1.1 per 100,000 v. 0.1 per 100,000 respectively). The highest incidence of illness among Hispanic women of childbearing age was observed in the 30–34 age group (2.7 per 100,000).

The 12-fold greater incidence of listeriosis for Hispanic children and the 13-fold greater incidence for Hispanic women highlight the need to focus on these groups to determine the specific risk factors for infection. *Listeria* prevention strategies and educational campaigns on protecting infants and women of childbearing age should be targeted toward the Hispanic community.[274]

In contrast with other organisms, *Listeria monocytogenes* is a far more serious problem in developed countries than in poorer, developing countries, where it is seldom found. *Listeria* thus serves to highlight the issue of how our modern lifestyles contribute to the selection and development of certain pathogenic organisms.[275] Just as cold contributes to the selective enrichment of *Listeria* in bacterial cultures, so can the ubiquitous use of refrigeration selectively enhance *Listeria* numbers in the modern food systems of developed countries. In modern, developed countries, the percentage of immunocompromised individuals is far higher than in developing countries.[276] The use of low levels of antibiotics in animal feeds has resulted in a more widespread occurrence of antibiotic resistance in the developed world. The evidence clearly indicates that our acceptance of a particular lifestyle must be understood to include all its consequences. Such an understanding may then motivate us either to modify the way we live or to embrace procedures or technologies specifically suited to manage the new risks that have emerged.

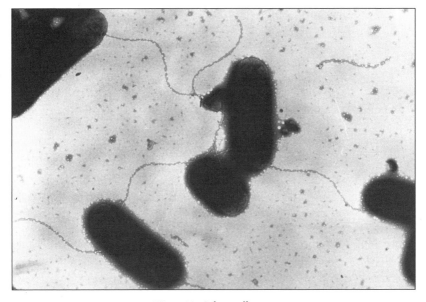

Figure 28. **Salmonella spp.**
Courtesy Istituto Superiore di Sanità, Rome, Italy.

SALMONELLA

Salmonellosis is one of the most frequent causes of recorded food-borne disease and probably the most well known. The salmonella bacteria do not owe their name to the fish but rather to the American bacteriologist D. E. Salmon who first characterized hog cholera disease more than 100 years ago. This erroneous association of the bacteria with the fish is so widespread that, at one point, a senator from the salmon-fishing state of Washington drafted a bill for Congress to change the name of the bacteria to Sanella and that of the disease to sanellosis.[277]

Salmonella has been implicated in food-borne diseases for a very long time[278] (see figure 28). Because of its rod-shaped structure, it was originally referred to as a bacillus. In 1888, the German scientist August Gärtner published definitive evidence linking this bacteria to food-borne disease. In the town of Frankenhausen, 57 individuals became ill after eating the flesh of a cow that had been slaughtered because it had a bad case of enteritis. One person died in the incident. August Gärtner isolated the bacillus from the spleen of the victim in question as well as from the organs remaining from the cow. It was an excellent example of thorough medical investigation. He subsequently dubbed the organism *Bacillus enteritidis*. Shortly thereafter, the bacterium was shown to be a common causative factor in many cases of food poisoning. In fact, well into this century, food-borne infections were routinely associated with "Gärtner's famous bacillus" (*Bacillus enteritidis*).[279]

The hog cholera bacillus (*Bacillus cholera suis*) was isolated by D. E. Salmon and Theobald Smith in 1885. For a long time, these bacteria were believed to be the cause of hog cholera. Researchers eventually found it to be a secondary invader, the real cause being attributed to a virus. This group of bacteria became variously known as the Gärtner group, the hog cholera group or the salmonella group. Ultimately, Gärtner lost the dubious honor of having his name attached to the most famous of food-borne diseases to D. E. Salmon. (This, of course, begs the question as to whether or not the American bacteriologist originally got his family name from the fish.)

The *Salmonella* group of bacteria is characterized as Gram-negative, rod-shaped microorganisms that generally have flagella. Early in this century, *Salmonella* was discovered to possess particular molecules called antigens that cause their host animals to produce specific antibodies. One type of antigen (the O-type) is closely associated with the cell body of the bacteria, while the other (the H-type) is associated with the flagella (see figure 29). These antigens eventually proved to be extremely valuable in characterizing the various types of *Salmonella* and other pathogenic bacteria that affect us.

Depending upon the type of *Salmonella* bacteria involved, the symptoms and severity of the disease varies greatly.[280] The most hazardous type, of course, is *Salmonella typhi,* the bacteria responsible for typhoid fever. In economically developed countries, this especially dangerous variety is not too common, and the incidence of typhoid fever is generally low. However, it still does occur occasionally. A very different story occurs in developing countries where the sanitation systems are not sufficient to prevent reinfection from human waste. In fact, the same can be said for any locale where the sanitation system breaks down, particularly after wars, earthquakes, hurricanes or other catastrophic events.

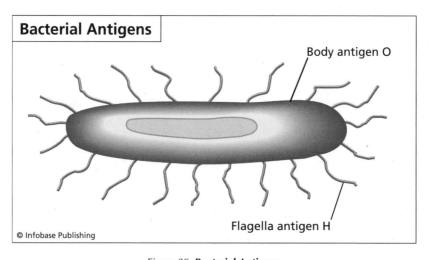

Bacterial Antigens

Body antigen O

Flagella antigen H

© Infobase Publishing

Figure 29. **Bacterial Antigens**

The spread of *S. typhi* is fairly straightforward and similar in many ways to other food-borne diseases. Infected people shed the typhoid bacteria in their feces. The *Salmonella* infiltrates the food and water system through direct contact with affected individuals or through untreated sewage wastewater. Reinfection is virtually guaranteed.

Typhoid fever is a very serious condition. It is an example of a rare circumstance where a food-borne pathogen can penetrate the intestine, enter the circulating bloodstream and commence multiplying. The symptoms include high fever, headache, vomiting and diarrhea. Typhoid bacteria can actually enter and hide in the very cells of the body (white blood cells—macrophages) that are supposed to defend us against them. Once the *S. typhi* enter these cells, they are very resistant to antibiotics, and repeated therapy is required. Just about any type of food or beverage can become the vehicle for transmission of this disease. One of the most infamous cases on medical record is Typhoid Mary, who was a chronic carrier of the typhoid bacteria although she herself did not experience obvious symptoms.[281] Mary was a carrier, she had poor personal hygiene habits and she worked as a cook in a food-catering establishment—a lethal combination of factors that resulted in multiple outbreaks of typhoid fever.

In another incident, an investigation worthy of an Agatha Christie mystery revealed that an extensive and fatal milk-borne typhoid outbreak in Dorset, England, was due to a disease carrier totally unconnected to the production of milk. The individual in question turned out to live in a house close to the farm. The inadequate plumbing and drainage system of this house occasionally overflowed into a common stream that fed local farms and deep wells. This overflow carried the typhoid bacteria to the cows and the local farm workers, causing tragic results. Fortunately, typhoid fever can be virtually eliminated through carefully applied sanitation practices and systems. Had the typhoid victims been in the habit of consuming pasteurized, rather than raw, milk, the incident would never have occurred. More recently, typhoid fever has been spread through salads, custards,[282] poultry, egg products[283] and other foods.

Under the right circumstances, other types of *Salmonella* bacteria can produce similar symptoms to *S. typhi,* a condition often referred to as paratyphoid fever. It is also generically referred to as enteric fever (because of the acute inflammation of the intestine). The two varieties of bacteria commonly involved are *S. paratyphi* and *S. hirschfeldii.*

By far the most prevalent form of *Salmonella* infection is caused by the great number of remaining types. They occur in all foods such as meat, seafood, dairy products and even fruits and vegetables.[284] Salmonella bacteria are so common on raw meat and poultry that some have suggested they be viewed as commensals or normal microorganisms naturally associated with these products.[285] Once ingested, the incubation period of the bacteria in the body is generally between 12 and 36 hours but can range from as early as six hours to as late as 72 hours. This variation in incubation period is due to factors such as the variety and amount of bacteria ingested, the state of the bacteria and the condition of the victim. The typical symptoms of salmonella infection include severe diarrhea, dehydration, fever, vomiting, headache and abdominal cramps. Depending upon the individual, the symptoms normally last from one to five days.

Occasionally, food-borne salmonella bacteria, which are normally limited to intestinal infections, will become a "sepsis." In other words, the microorganisms enter the body's circulatory system. When this happens, rather than being limited to a case of gastrointestinal infection, the victim goes through a full-blown case of "septicemia," or blood poisoning. Once in the bloodstream, the salmonella can invade many other tissues, causing severe consequences. The symptoms are akin to those of S. typhi. When my middle daughter was two years old, she contracted just such a condition.

In addition to the significant illnesses directly experienced by victims, the list of sequelae, or long-term aftereffects, to salmonellosis is of great concern. Various forms of arthritis; aneurisms; heart, spleen, liver and renal infections; meningitis; phlebitis; and abscesses of the pharynx and genitals are just a few examples from this list. All salmonella infections are to be taken very seriously.

Typical food-borne offenders are S. typhimurium, S. enteritidis, S. heidelberg, S. newport, S. montevideo, S. dublin, S. meunchen, S. manhattan, S. havana, S. orianenburg and S. saint paul. One look is enough to see that the various types of salmonella read as if they were an airline travel guide. It reflects the discouraging fact that salmonella is ubiquitous in nature and leaves countless victims in its globe-trotting wake.

The majority of salmonella infections is derived from the consumption of food and beverages. Beef, chicken, turkey, pork, fish, seafood, unpasteurized fruit juice, tomatoes, dairy products and eggs have all been identified as prime carriers of this pathogen. Prepared products, such as cream-filled baked goods, and popular ethnic foods, such as Chinese and Mexican dishes, have also been involved in salmonella outbreaks. In a 1995 United States survey, about half of the animal feed meals tested proved to be positive for salmonella.[286] Even fruits and vegetables can harbor salmonella, particularly when the practice of using natural, unsterilized manure as a fertilizer is employed. In this case, the spread of infection does not even go through the process of dilution through streams or groundwater if the manure is directly applied to the cultivation fields. The spread of salmonella bacteria has been so great that it is considered a geonosis, which simply means that it can come from all natural sources such as soil and water as well as animals. However, the foods most commonly recognized as major sources of this particular pathogen are poultry and eggs.

One of the largest outbreaks of salmonella food poisoning occurred in 1994 when an estimated 224,000 people fell ill after consuming Schwan's ice cream.[287] No particular problems were found in the dairy-processing plant itself. It was later discovered that the premix used for production was transported to the plant in tanker trucks that had been previously used to transport unpasteurized liquid eggs. The standing orders had been to clean and sanitize the tankers after every delivery of liquid eggs, but close inspection revealed outlet valves that were not clean. Since the premix did not receive any additional pasteurization prior to being used for making ice cream, any contamination that took place in the tankers was carried into the final consumer product. The net result was a massive national outbreak of food poisoning from *Salmonella enteritidis*—gastroenteritis infections characterized by high fever (91 percent of cases), chills (77 percent) and bloody stools (42 percent). A few unsanitary valves made almost a quarter of a million people very sick.

Three outbreaks of *Salmonella* infections associated with eating Roma tomatoes were detected in the United States and Canada in the summer of 2004. In one multistate outbreak that occurred from June 25 to July 18, multiple *Salmonella* types were isolated, resulting from exposure to Roma tomatoes from different locations of a chain delicatessen.[288] Each of the other two outbreaks was characterized by a single *Salmonella* serotype: Braenderup in one multistate outbreak and Javiana in a Canadian outbreak. In total, the three outbreaks resulted in 561 illnesses from 18 states and one province in Canada. A single tomato-packing house in Florida was common to all three outbreaks. Because current knowledge of the mechanism of tomato contamination and the current means of eradication of *Salmonella* in fruit are inadequate, further research is necessary for this sector of the agricultural industry.

SHIGELLA

The *Shigella* are an important group of bacteria that cause shigellosis or bacillary dysentery. This is one of the earliest recorded illnesses of mankind and is characterized by abdominal cramps, diarrhea and bloody stools. The microorganism responsible is a small, Gram-negative bacillus originally called *Bacillus dysenteriae* but renamed *Shigella dysenteriae* in 1950 after the Japanese scientist, Shiga, who first associated it with dysentery. Four different species of *Shigella* exist (*S. dysenteriae, S. flexneri, S. boydii* and *S. sonnei*), each differing in virulence and geographic distribution. *S. dysenteriae* is the most virulent species and is commonly found in developing countries. *S. sonnei* causes the mildest symptoms and is the variety found most frequently in developed countries.

Shigellosis is a very important disease in all developing countries as well as in those developed countries where crowded situations occur, such as in schools, nursing homes and mental institutions. During the exodus of hundreds of thousands of Rwandan refugees into the Northern Kivu area of Zaire in mid-1994, almost 50,000 died during the first month in the overcrowded camps. This tragedy was due to epidemics of diarrhea initially caused by *Vibrio cholera* followed by *Shigella dysenteriae*[289] a few weeks later. *S. dysenteriae* causes an extremely harsh form of diarrhea. For infants in developing countries, fatality rates as high as 25 percent have been recorded. In most developed country cases, the symptoms are usually over in a week or two. Because humans are the principal carriers of the bacteria, infected food handlers are considered to be the primary vehicles of transmission.

Almost all foods are susceptible, particularly if they are not cooked just before eating. Example are raw vegetables, a wide variety of salads (chicken, potato, macaroni and so on), dairy products and poultry and also sandwiches made from those ingredients. Outbreaks have occurred on airline flights and have often occurred on cruise ships.[290]

Shigella is almost indistinguishable from its very close *E. coli* relatives. In fact, the idea of merging shigella into the *E. coli* family has been considered but rejected primarily because the name has become so well established. Shigella behave very much like the enteroinvasive *E. coli* (EIEC), which makes sense because they both share the same virulent plasmids. Shigella multiplies rapidly and results in a full-blown invasion of the epithelial lining of the large bowel, resulting in inflammation and ulceration of the surface layer. Together with *Listeria monocytogenes,* it also shares the ability to spread infection within tissues by moving from cell to cell. *Shigella* has all the characteristics necessary to pose a major food-borne threat to humans. However, shigellosis is not considered to be a major disease in developed countries chiefly because the most common variety has limited virulence. However, if ECO157 can be taken as an example, only one plasmid transfer may turn this bacterium into a far more formidable enemy.

STREPTOCOCCUS

Streptococci are small, round, Gram-positive bacteria that usually appear like a chain of miniature beads under the microscope. Many types of *Streptococcus* bacteria are capable of producing a wide range of illnesses. The two main types of food-borne streptococcus are classified as groups A and D. Group A consists of one species, *Streptococcus pyogenes,* which can cause sore throat, scarlet fever and all the attendant complications. Group D has five different species, *Streptococcus faecalis, S. faecium, S. durans, S. avium* and *S. bovis,* which are responsible for various gastrointestinal problems very similar to those found with *Staphylococcus.* Food-related outbreaks due to *Streptococcus* are not very numerous, particularly since milk pasteurization has become virtually mandatory.

Symptoms associated with *S. pyogenes (pyo* is Greek for "pus") are sore throat, acute swallowing pain, tonsillitis, fever, headache and general malaise. The typical strep throat is characteristic of this disease. It usually takes from one to three days to develop and can last for more than a week. Although the prime source of this bacterium, unpasteurized milk, has practically been eliminated from the food supply, poor or unsanitary handling of other foods still results in occasional outbreaks. Food sources implicated are egg, potato, shrimp and pasta salads, steamed lobster, rice pudding, custard and eggs.

The typical symptoms of Group D organisms are diarrhea, vomiting, abdominal cramps, fever and dizziness. The symptom onset time is between two and 36 hours and may persist for several days. Food sources connected with these organisms are processed meat products, powdered milk and cheese. The incidence of outbreaks is very low and is usually associated with unsanitary handling.

VIBRIO

Vibrio bacteria are small, curved or comma-shaped Gram-negative rods[291] responsible for rather infamous diseases. The first of these was discovered by Robert Koch in 1883. *Vibrio cholerae* is responsible for cholera, a disease of pandemic (worldwide epidemic) proportions, which has ravaged the globe at least seven times during the last two centuries. In 1832, cholera entered the United States by way of New York and spread as far as the military outposts of the upper Mississippi. It entered the country again in 1848 through the gulf port of New Orleans, wound its way up the Mississippi River, and eventually spread across the continent to California along with the rush of gold seekers. Although several other incidents were recorded in the United States to coincide with large outbreaks elsewhere, aggressive preventative measures have kept cholera under close control.[292]

In some regions, notably the Indian subcontinent, cholera has become as feared as the plague and has been characterized by fatality rates in the 20–30 percent range. The symptoms are characterized by violent vomiting, severe diarrhea, thirst, cramps, weakness and, if not quickly and properly

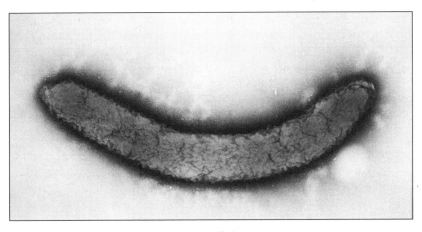

Figure 30. *Vibrio* **spp.**
Courtesy Istituto Superiore di Sanità, Rome, Italy.

treated, death. The tremendous loss of body fluids that accompanies the diarrhea not only results in acute dehydration but also serves to spread the bacteria in the sewage. Cholera is therefore much more prevalent in developing countries, where the lack of water treatment allows continuing cycles of reinfection to occur. Although water is the most important factor in spreading the disease, foods also bear a heavy responsibility. More recently, as evidenced by the outbreak of cholera in Peru in 1991, the consumption of shellfish and raw fish taken from water contaminated with vibrio proved to be the chief vector in the spread of this disease.

Another virulent form of this microorganism is *Vibrio parahaemolyticus*. It is similar to *V. cholerae* except that it specifically requires a marine environment for its survival. This *Vibrio* species is therefore a problem with all fish and seafood. It is most troublesome where fish are eaten raw, as in Japan and Korea. In fact, *V. parahaemolyticus* is the most common food-borne disease microorganism found in Japan. It is not as common in the United States. However, as the habit of consuming seafood and marine finfish expands, so will the incidents associated with this disease. Symptoms are similar to those of other gastric toxicoinfections—watery diarrhea, abdominal cramps, nausea, headaches and, occasionally, vomiting. Although some deaths have occurred due to this bacterium, they are usually limited to older people. The normal symptoms are generally moderate, and most victims recover in less than a week. As with all diarrheal episodes, care must be taken to replace lost water and electrolytes.

Vibrio vulnificus is yet another in this class of bacteria. Like *V. parahaemolyticus*, it requires seawater for its survival and is thus found in seafood and marine finfish. It commonly occurs in the warmer waters of the gulf states.[293] When ingested with food, it is responsible for a condition called fulminating or explosive septicemia, which is often a fatal disease. Again, this is associated with the consumption of raw shellfish such as oysters and clams. Test have shown that Tabasco sauce (not ordinary cocktail sauce) could reduce the number of *Vibrio vulnificus* cells on the surface but not in the flesh of oysters and, consequently, provides little margin of safety for habitual patrons of the raw oyster bar.[294]

Vibrio vulnificus has been earmarked as a cause of critical seafood-related illness for all people who suffer from some form of liver dysfunction. These particular individuals face a mortality rate of over 40 percent.[295] *Vibrio vulnificus* can also cause severe infections through wounds from cleaning shellfish or crabs, often resulting in the need for amputation of affected limbs. Several other marine species of vibrio have been implicated in food-borne diseases, but their rate of occurrence and the amount of evidence accumulated thus far preclude a definite link to human gastroenteritis.

When envisioning the devastation caused by Hurricane Katrina, which struck Louisiana on August 29, 2005, and was followed by Hurricane Rita less than a month later, the increased risk of food-borne diseases does not come to mind. Yet, food-borne diseases exploded in the aftermath of 2005's destruction.

The unprecedented damage caused to the Louisiana Gulf Coast by the two hurricanes resulted in the flooding of large residential areas in and around New Orleans. With the flooding came an immediate public health concern for outbreaks of infectious diseases, including cholera. Normally, all *Vibrio* infections in the United States are caused by noncholeragenic species such as *Vibrio parahaemolyticus* and *Vibrio vulnificus*. Cholera rarely occurs in the United States, and cholera epidemics are highly unlikely, even with extreme flooding such as that caused by the two hurricanes. Despite this, two cases of toxigenic *V. cholerae* were discovered in a Louisiana couple as a result of eating undercooked, contaminated seafood. Fortunately, no epidemic of cholera was ever identified.

On October 15, 2005, in southeastern Louisiana, a man (age 43) and his wife (age 46) had onset of diarrhea. The husband had a history of high blood pressure, alcoholism, diabetes and chronic renal failure that required dialysis three times a week. On October 16, 2005, he was hospitalized for fever, muscle pains, nausea, vomiting, abdominal cramps and severe diarrhea and dehydration; subsequently he experienced complete loss of renal function and respiratory and cardiac failure. However, after treatment with ciprofloxacin and aggressive rehydration therapy, the man recovered to his previous state of health. His wife had mild diarrhea and was treated as an outpatient with ciprofloxacin and extra fluids.

Because the couple's residence had been severely damaged and flooded by Hurricane Rita, both patients had waded in coastal floodwaters in late September, two to three weeks before the onset of their illness. Five days before onset, both had eaten locally caught crabs. On October 14, the day preceding onset, both had eaten shrimp purchased from a local fisherman. The shrimp had been boiled for five minutes; however, at least some of the boiled shrimp were returned to a cooler containing raw shrimp and were eaten later.[296] It is possible that this was the origin of the contamination.

YERSINIA

Yersinia enterocolitica is a small, fat, rod-shaped, Gram-negative bacterium that belongs to a rather small family of bacteria among whose ranks resides the most infamous disease microbe of all times and one that continues to strike terror into the hearts of all—bubonic plague. The bubonic or black plague bacterium, long known as *Pasteurella pestis*, has recently been renamed *Yersinia pestis* in honor of the Swiss-born, French scientist Alexandre Yersin. He discovered it in 1894 during the midst of the Hong Kong outbreak, the last bubonic plague pandemic, which resulted in more than a million deaths throughout Asia. *Yersinia pestis* is spread by the fleas of infected rats and is extremely rare at the present time, mainly as a result of improved housing and sanitary conditions. Nevertheless, public health surveillance continues to ensure that the sporadic outbreaks that occur in endemic areas do not spread further.

Another member of this group is *Yersinia pseudotuberculosis,* which, like *Y. enterocolitica,* is a food-borne pathogen. While *Y. enterocolitica* appears to be the prevalent form in northern Europe and North America, *Y. pseudotuberculosis* is the predominant form found in Asia. These two forms of *Yersinia* have been identified as food-borne organisms only during the last 20 years.

The virulence of *Y. enterocolitica* is associated with its basic ability to invade mammalian cells, a characteristic inherited along with the nuclear genetic material, not the plasmids. *Yersinia* does, however, have several plasmids that, cumulatively, confer additional virulence to the organism. The symptoms of yersiniosis are agonizing abdominal pain, diarrhea, headaches and nausea. The pain associated with *Yersinia* infections can be so intense that the symptoms are often associated with appendicitis. Appendectomies have needlessly been performed in several mistaken cases. The disease is self-limiting, with symptoms disappearing within two to three days. As with other diseases, certain individuals are more susceptible and will have symptoms for a much longer period after which serious complications can set in, including severe inflammation of the skin, nervous system and gastrointestinal tract as well as arthritis. *Yersinia* seems to favor the very young and the old with a peak preference for infants less than one year old.

Yersinia occurs in a very wide variety of animals. However, most organisms found are variants that show very little virulence. The one exception is pigs, which have been shown to be reservoirs of the same varieties of *Yersinia* that are virulent to humans. Milk has also been a source of several yersiniosis outbreaks, but it has also been found in raw vegetables, soy products, seafood and poultry. It also occurs commonly throughout the environment, in the soils and in the waters. It occurs in a wide variety of wild and domesticated animals, birds and aquatic species. *Yersinia enterocolitica* shares a love of the cold with *Listeria.* As is the case with *Listeria,* refrigeration is an effective means of enriching mixed bacterial cultures with *Yersinia* cells. This widespread occurrence of *Yersinia* and its tolerance to the cold requires that proper control and sanitation be exercised in food-processing operations to ensure that it is eliminated prior to refrigerated storage. A zero-tolerance approach has been suggested for this organism.

MISCELLANEOUS BACTERIA

Other types of pathogenic food-borne bacteria include *Klebsiella, Citrobacter, Aeromonas* and *Plesiomonas.* Symptoms resulting from these bacteria range from mild in the case of *Plesiomonas shigelloides* to fairly serious in the case of enterotoxigenic *Citrobacter freundii.* The outbreaks of disease resulting from these bacteria are quite sporadic and, in certain cases, a link between these bacteria and human disease has yet to be definitively established (e.g., *Plesiomonas* and *Aeromonas*).

Klebsiella is a coliform bacteria that has been implicated in some pretty serious conditions, including pneumonia, infantile meningitis and urinary infections. It has also been associated with ankylosing spondylitis because people with this condition have high blood levels of antibodies that are specific to *Klebsiella*. *Klebsiella* bacteria are widely distributed in nature and are regularly found in soil, water and even in the sawdust that is spread out on the milking floors of dairy operations. Because of its common occurrence in soil, *Klebsiella* can be carried on seeds that are further processed for food products such as sprouts.

Citrobacter is a Gram-negative bacillus that is found in a wide range of animals as well as in the soil and water. It has also been recovered from farm products such as vegetables. Most species of *Citrobacter* appear to be non-pathogenic, but some are, and their effects can be very disagreeable. *Citrobacter freundii* is one such variation that produces a toxin identical to the heat-stable toxin of enterotoxigenic *E. coli* (ETEC). This toxin interferes with the water and electrolyte absorbing mechanisms of the intestine and results in acute gastroenteritis, vomiting, nausea, fever, pain and severe, watery diarrhea within 12–24 hours of consuming the contaminated food.

Citrobacter has been recovered from raw vegetables, dairy products and shellfish. In the District of Columbia, during the fall of 1983, *Citrobacter* was implicated in an outbreak of gastrointestinal disease associated with the consumption of imported Brie cheese. At the time, *Citrobacter* had not been generally recognized as an enteric pathogen, but the opinion in this matter has since changed.

Aeromonas hydrophilia is a Gram-negative anaerobic bacillus that is found in a variety of animals as well as in fresh and brackish waters. It is pathogenic to humans and can cause infections when ingested with the food or water. Its exact role in gastrointestinal illness still remains to be worked out, but it is found in the stools of those with diarrheal disease. Two types of diarrheal disease have been associated with *Aeromonas hydrophilia*: the first is a diarrhea somewhat similar to cholera and the other is characterized by the bloody stool symptoms of dysentery. If the victim has an existing precondition or some underlying illness, a potentially dangerous general septicemia can result.

Plesiomonas shigelloides is a Gram-negative bacillus that is found in many animals as well as in freshwater. Most infections of *Plesiomonas* are considered to be waterborne, but when contaminated water is used anywhere within the food system, it can quickly become food-borne. The bacteria causes a mild gastroenteritis with typical symptoms of abdominal pain, nausea, vomiting and diarrhea, starting about a full day after the original consumption of the contaminated food.

TOXIN-PRODUCING FORMS

Something of vengeance I had tasted for the first time; as aromatic wine it seemed, on swallowing, warm and racy: its after-flavor, metallic and corroding, gave me a sensation as if I had been poisoned.

—Charlotte Brontë (1816–55), English novelist. *Jane Eyre,* ch. 4 (1847)*

BACILLUS CEREUS

Vague references to this disease were made on several occasions during the first half of this century. It was not until 1950 that any definitive accounts of *Bacillus cereus* food poisoning were made. The four separate incidents described involved a total of 600 Norwegian victims who had consumed a vanilla sauce made with contaminated corn starch. Since that time, *B. cereus* poisoning has been reported in all other countries that keep food-poisoning statistics and has involved a great many natural and prepared food products.

Bacillus cereus is a large, rod-shaped, Gram-positive, spore-forming bacteria. It is unusual in that it actually causes two distinct types of food poisoning depending upon the metabolic route it takes. The first disease is a diarrheal type of food poisoning and is brought on by the production of a very large protein toxin. This toxin is not very resistant to heat, and any proper cooking or reheating of food will usually destroy most of it. The symptoms of this type are very similar to those of *Clostridium perfringens* poisoning and consist of watery diarrhea, cramps and abdominal pain. The onset of symptoms is usually within six to 15 hours after food consumption.

The other form of the disease involves vomiting or emetic symptoms caused by a very small but very heat-resistant protein. Once formed in the food, no level of cooking or reheating will destroy it. The onset of symptoms is very rapid (one-half to five hours). In this way, it is very similar to staphylococcal food poisoning, for which it is often mistaken. Although vomiting is the chief symptom, it is occasionally accompanied by severe abdominal cramps. Fortunately, both forms of the disease almost never occur in the same food at the same time. In both cases, the symptoms are usually gone within 24 hours.

A wide variety of foods such as meat, dairy products, fish and vegetables have been incriminated with the diarrheal type of disease. The vomiting type of disease seems to be more closely related to starchy foods such as rice, potatoes and pasta. Presumably, the type of food it contaminates influences the metabolism of *B. cereus,* which, in turn, influences the form of disease it produces. In a recent outbreak at two child care centers in Virginia, chicken fried rice turned out to be the food responsible.[297] Scientists believe that *B. cereus* spores in the rice may survive cooking. If the rice is then kept at room temperature, the cells can begin to multiply rapidly and form a heat-stable toxin capable of surviving high heat such as stir-frying. This makes products such as fried rice the leading causes of *B. cereus* emetic food poisoning.

CLOSTRIDIUM BOTULINUM

With little doubt, if the subject of food-borne diseases ever comes up in conversation, most, if not all, people will immediately think of botulism. This is not too surprising because *Clostridium botulinum,* the Gram-positive, rod-shaped organism responsible for this disease, produces one of the most potent biological toxins known. What most people do not know is that botulism occurs very rarely and, in most cases, is easily preventable. However, when it does rear its ugly head, it is usually the subject of much sensational publicity.

Botulism has been recognized as a food-borne disease for over 250 years. It attracted widespread attention in the German medical community in 1793 after several people died from eating sausages that had been stuffed in a casing of hog's stomach. The condition quickly became identified as botulism after the Latin word for sausage—*botulus.* Once it became more widely known, the number of botulism cases grew steadily as an increasing number of physicians in Germany and other countries began reporting it. Botulism was of particular concern because of the unusually high rate of case fatalities. All this reporting was done without ever having the slightest idea of what actually caused the disease.

In 1895, the Belgian bacteriologist Emile Van Ermengem isolated the botulism bacterium after an outbreak involving a large group of musicians attending a funeral. He named the rod-shaped organism *Bacillus botulinum* to describe its shape and the symptoms consistent with botulism. Despite the relative rarity of its occurrence, botulism's high mortality rate, its frightening symptoms and its clear relationship to food always made this disease a sensational subject of the popular press out of all proportion to its actual importance—a situation that continues to exist to this day.

The poison *C. botulinum* produces is more than 10 times deadlier than rattlesnake venom, with as little as a tenth of a gram of tainted food capable of causing botulism. One confirmed case on record describes someone simply dipping a fork into a suspected bottle of eggplant under oil. Although the victim actually consumed none of the product, that person then used the same fork to eat other food items. The victim soon began vomiting and developed dysphagia (difficulty in swallowing) and double vision. Although the victim survived, little doubt exists as to the potency of the botulism toxin. Toxic doses are measured in a few nanograms (which come to about a billionth of an ounce). Botulism toxin is so toxic that, over the years, it has been used in biological warfare programs.

The toxin is classified as a very effective neurotoxin (nerve poison). Like other similar poisons, it causes severe muscle paralysis. It works by irreversibly blocking the nerve endings that send signals to the muscles. The resultant paralysis progresses downward, starting from the eyes and face, to the neck, throat, chest and extremities. Death often results because the respiratory muscles of the diaphragm no longer function, and the victim literally suffocates. Complete return of functions requires the generation of new nerve endings and therefore involves long recovery times.

Clostridium botulinum, along with several other Gram-positive bacteria, is a classic spore-forming organism. Botulinum spores are particularly resistant and, as a result, are ubiquitous in the global environment. Soil samples taken from every spot on the world map will yield botulinum spores. These spores occur so commonly that it is surprising more outbreaks of botulism do not occur. The main reason for this is the very specific requirements *C. botulinum* has for growth and toxin production. *Clostridium botulinum* is very sensitive to acidity. Even the small amounts found in tomatoes are often sufficient to prevent the formation of toxin. *Clostridium botulinum* is also an anaerobic bacterium, which means that it can grow and form toxin only in the absence of air.

Because of the anaerobic requirements of *C. botulinum,* the range of products implicated in food-borne outbreaks is limited. However, if the processing conditions are not vigorous enough to kill spores and the food is low in acid and devoid of oxygen, it is a good candidate for botulism. Canning and bottling are often implicated in outbreaks because they do not permit the entry of oxygen. Thick cuts of meats or fish that are fatty also prevent the penetration of oxygen into their interior regions and thus provide the environment necessary for *C. botulinum* to grow and produce toxin. Any products covered with oil or grease similarly exclude an exchange of air and promote the development of deadly toxin. One large Illinois outbreak in 1983 resulted from sautéed onions covered with margarine left on a grill overnight.[298] The commercial food industry in North America is generally well equipped to eliminate *C. botulinum.* All the processing conditions employed are directed at ensuring the destruction of spores and toxin. That is why so many canned foods seem overcooked. Whenever commercial foods are implicated in botulism incidents, it is usually the result of a breakdown in normal procedures.

Botulism cases generally fall into three distinct categories. The first is the conventional food-borne intoxication that results from the consumption of foods containing the toxin. A wide variety of foods are implicated in this type of botulism with home preservation responsible for the greatest number of outbreaks. Home-canned or bottled peppers, beans, spinach and asparagus have been particularly troublesome. Since spores of *C. botulinum* are found everywhere in the environment, particularly in the soil, it is not surprising that plant foods are a prime source. Other foods involved are canned fish, fish eggs, mushrooms, soups and various sauces. Home-processed ham, fish, liver paste and venison jerky have also been involved.[299] A few cases involving fatalities from the New York area were due to a type of salted whitefish called *kapchunka* or *ribyetz*, which is a much prized favorite of recent Russian immigrants. Some of this same fish was brought to Israel, where it managed to poison six additional people with one eventual fatality.[300] In another recent case in Oklahoma, beef cooked in a pot with a heavy lid and left for three days before being eaten cold resulted in the consumer being hospitalized for 49 days, 42 of which were on a mechanical respirator. The three days of standing unrefrigerated while covered by a heavy lid provided ideal anaerobic conditions for toxin production.[301] Proper heating before consumption would have destroyed the toxin. In the far northern areas, native foods such as parboiled, fatty whale and seal meats, eaten cold, have been implicated.

The second type of botulism, first identified in 1976 and now considered to be the most common type, is infant botulism. It affects children under 12 months of age and is caused by the ingestion of viable spores, which germinate, grow and produce toxin in the baby's intestinal tract. It is a classic toxicoinfection but is rarely fatal. Typical symptoms are constipation, weakness, poor feeding and a striking loss of head control. The one food implicated more than any other has been honey. However, scientists generally acknowledge that most incidents arise from the environment rather than from food. Infants are notorious for putting all matter of things into their mouths, dust and soil being on the top of the list. Since this form of botulism was first recognized, the number of confirmed cases has risen steadily all over the world because of the greater awareness and reporting by health and medical professionals.

A third and rather rare type of botulism is called wound botulism, which results when a wound is colonized by toxin-producing *C. botulinum*. This infection serves as a source of toxin that spreads out to other parts of the body through the circulatory system. Covering the wound with grease or an airtight bandage simply makes matters worse.

Yet another form of botulism exists, but its classification has not been clearly defined. It involves adults, but no apparent source of intoxication can be identified. Some researchers feel it may be an adult form of infant botulism brought on by changes in the normal population of intestinal bacteria, thus allowing *C. botulinum* to flourish.

In rapid-onset cases, the first symptoms are nausea or vomiting. The more typical symptoms follow—fatigue, headaches, swallowing difficulty, dizziness and muscular weakness. Visual impairment such as blurred or double vision and dilated pupils can also develop together with slurred speech. These are all classic symptoms of neurotoxins. In common with many other neurotoxins, death results from respiratory failure due to paralysis of the diaphragm and obstruction of airways. Whereas treatment was unavailable in the past, saving lives is now possible through the use of antitoxin serums and respiratory support systems.

Although *C. botulinum* spores are very heat resistant, the procedures for commercial canning were specifically designed to ensure their destruction. Cans must be processed to a so-called botch cook at the very geometric center of the can so that not a single spore can survive. If you consider the incredible volume of canned goods commercially produced on a daily basis, it is a testimony to the industry that so few botulism incidents have actually occurred. The rare incidents that have taken place in commercial canning resulted from accidents such as leakage of the can seams. These few commercial outbreaks have, naturally, received a good deal of publicity.

Acidic conditions prevent the germination of spores and the consequent production of toxin. The level of acidity is rather critical. During the period 1899–1975 in the United States, 34 out of the 35 botulism outbreaks that arose from supposedly high-acid foods involved homemade products (half of which were tomato based). When in doubt, it is best that the products be more acidic. Acids commonly used are acetic, lactic and citric acids.[302] While the spores of *C. botulinum* are very heat resistant, the botulism toxin itself is very heat sensitive. Thus, if a food is in any way suspect, boiling it for 10 minutes will inactivate the toxin. Never taste products from a swollen can or products with a poor odor before boiling.

In certain countries, such as Italy, where food is such a central aspect of culture, the conservative adherence to traditional methods of processing is a double-edged sword. While little doubt exists that the taste and quality of food in Italy are unsurpassed, the high proportion of foods produced by small, artisanal processors can present certain problems. In addition, a large variety of nonacidic foods are preserved under olive oil. These foods often find their way into the famous antipastos, which are a delight to behold and to eat. Unfortunately, they also provide ideal conditions for the development of botulism toxin.[303] A 1996 outbreak made national news with headlines crying out, "Mascarpone—The Killer Cheese!" Although botulism is still a relative rarity in Italy, it does occur about three times more frequently than in the United States, a country whose population is about four times greater.

The new generation of extended-life refrigerated foods may also pose a problem with *C. botulinum*. Such products include soups, sauces, salads, pasta, seafood and meat entrees. These products are usually hermetically sealed under a vacuum or under a specific atmosphere, both of which can result in ideal anaerobic conditions. Since clostridium can grow and produce toxin under refrigerated conditions, care must be taken to ensure the safety and wholesomeness of these products. Light cooking prior to refrigeration is not sufficient to kill botulinum spores. In fact, it could actually worsen the problem by killing other nonpathogenic bacteria that might have competed with and prevented the growth of *C. botulinum*.[304] The complete control of botulism in these types of foods depends upon the employment of a battery of preventative measures (such as increased acidity, proper heating and use of salt) that individually may not be sufficient but in combination work effectively.

On September 8, 2006, three patients from Washington County, Georgia, went to the hospital with cranial nerve palsies and progressive descending paralysis resulting in respiratory failure. The patients had shared meals on September 7. The following evening, physicians suspected food-borne botulism and notified the state health department after collecting specimens for testing at the CDC. On the same evening, the CDC dispatched botulinum antitoxin, which was administered to each of the patients the following morning. After receiving antitoxin, the patients had no progression of neurologic symptoms, but they remain hospitalized and on ventilators.

The following day, the Washington County Health Department and the Georgia Division of Public Health launched an investigation. The three patients had consumed several food items during their meals together on September 7, including juice from a single bottle of carrot juice. The bottle had a "best if used by" date of September 18, 2006, and was still well within its shelf life. Clinical specimens and leftover food and juice were collected and sent to the CDC for testing. On September 13, botulinum toxin type A was identified in the serum and stool of all three patients and on September 15 leftover carrot juice recovered from the home of one of the patients also tested positive for botulinum type A toxin.

Public health officials in all 50 states were notified of the outbreak and the implicated products. After these notifications, no additional cases of botulism were reported in Georgia or to the CDC. During this time, the FDA launched an investigation of the juice manufacturing plant in California. The FDA and the CDC tested other bottles of the implicated brand of carrot juice, including bottles from different lots, and all were negative for botulinum toxin. Because the toxin was found only in the bottle of carrot juice consumed by the three patients, a lapse in refrigeration of the carrot juice bottle during transport or storage was suspected, which would have allowed for growth of *Clostridium botulinum* and subsequent production of botulinum toxin.

On September 25, 2006, officials at the Florida Department of Health, the Hillsborough County Health Department and the CDC were notified that a patient had been hospitalized in Tampa, Florida, on September 16 with respiratory failure and descending paralysis. On September 28, botulinum toxin type A was identified in the patient's serum. Circulating toxin persisted more than 10 days after illness onset in this completely paralyzed patient, indicating ingestion of a massive toxin dose. The patient was treated with antitoxin, but remained hospitalized, paralyzed and on a ventilator. The Hillsborough County Health Department collected an open, one-liter bottle of carrot juice, which had been found by a family member in the hotel room where the patient had been staying during the month before being hospitalized. The hotel room had no refrigerator. The bottle, which had a "best if used by" date of September 19, 2006, had a different lot number than the bottle associated with the Georgia cases. On September 29, botulinum toxin type A was identified in carrot juice from the bottle found in the patient's hotel room. The FDA was notified and they in turn notified public health officials in all 50 states. The manufacturer provided the FDA with bottles of carrot juice from the same lot as the bottle found in the patient's room. The FDA tested juice from all of these bottles and found it negative for botulinum toxin. The carrot juice consumed by these four patients had been distributed in all 50 states, Mexico, Canada and Hong Kong, but fortunately no other cases were ever reported.

C. botulinum spores are found in the environment and can be present naturally in carrot juice and other foods that have not undergone the retort canning process, which involves high temperatures and high pressure. Acidification has been used as a solution to previous food-borne botulism outbreaks. In 1985, 36 patients in the United States and Canada were identified with botulism after eating at a restaurant in Vancouver, British Columbia. A case-control study implicated commercially produced, chopped garlic in soybean oil stored at room temperature as the source of the outbreak.[305] In 1989, a second outbreak of botulism associated with chopped garlic in oil occurred when three patients in New York were identified with botulism after consuming a meal containing unrefrigerated, commercially produced, chopped garlic in virgin olive oil.[306] After these outbreaks, FDA rules were altered to require that garlic-in-oil products contain an acidifying agent such as phosphoric or citric acid.

STAPHYLOCOCCUS AUREUS

As the name suggests, the causative factor in staphylococcal food poisoning is a stable toxin produced by the staphylococcus bacteria. Staphylococci are small, spherical, Gram-positive bacteria that, under the microscope, appear to aggregate into grapelike clusters[307] (see figure 31). (The ancient Greek word *staphule* means a "bunch of grapes.") Symptoms of staphylococcal poisoning were first recorded over 150 years ago. Both Robert Koch and Louis Pasteur described these microorganisms as early as 1878. A relationship between the disease and the bacterial toxin was not made until 1914. Although first demonstrated in milk, researchers soon found the toxin to occur in an extremely wide range of food products all over the world.

The most common type of *Staphylococcus* involved in food poisoning is *S. aureus*, better known as the common hospital "staph." The bacteria itself is quite sensitive to heat and other conventional means of control. As a general rule, fresh, unprepared foods are almost never a source of toxin, with the exception of unpasteurized milk from cows that have mastitis—an udder infection. This disease is most frequently introduced into food by the handling and preparation of foods by people who carry large numbers of the bacteria.

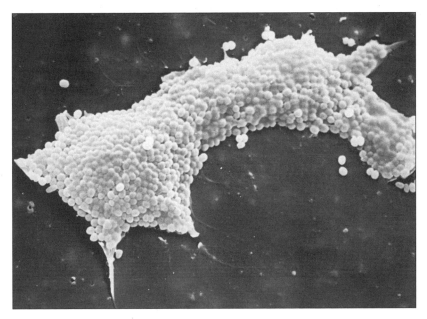

Figure 31. **Staphylococcus spp.**
Courtesy Istituto Superiore di Sanità, Rome, Italy.

Staphylococcus can be found everywhere in the environment. About 50 percent of all people carry *Staphylococcus*. When people handle food, infection comes from hand sores or by coughing and sneezing (high numbers of the bacteria are usually in the nasal passages). Once in the food, the *S. aureus* bacteria multiply and produce the enterotoxin (intestinal poison). Staphylococcal enterotoxin can withstand boiling for more than 30 minutes and resists freezing, dehydration and irradiation. It travels through our gastrointestinal system completely unaffected by the powerful digestive enzymes. Staphylococcal enterotoxin is a protein that is almost indestructible, and the ingestion of less than 1 microgram* of it is enough to cause severe illness. Individuals who eat the contaminated food are poisoned in the classical sense, and the symptoms become evident two to four hours after consumption.[308] These can be quite intense depending upon the individual's reaction and the amount of toxin ingested. Typical symptoms of the disease are nausea, vomiting, cramps and diarrhea. Recovery usually takes place in two to four days. More recently, it has become evident that *staphylococcal* food poisoning can exhibit the symptoms of toxic shock syndrome, a condition that can be fatal.[309] These symptoms include sudden high fever, vomiting, diarrhea, a drop in blood pressure, a rash on the palms and soles, confusion, headaches and seizures.

---

* 1 microgram = 0.000000035 oz.

S. aureus occurs in meat and meat products, poultry products, baked goods, cheese, eggs, fish, pasta, fruits and vegetables. Foods frequently implicated are the cream or custard fillings of pastries, sandwich fillings and prepared salads. The most common place where contamination occurs is in food service and catering establishments because foods receive the greatest amount of handling here. The incoming food may be clean, but contamination can result from poor practices. If hands or gloves are not disinfected before contact with foods or if foods are not refrigerated quickly after preparation, then an ideal situation for the growth of *Staphylococcus* and the production of toxin presents itself. Foods contaminated with staphylococcal enterotoxin cannot be decontaminated and simply await consumption by unsuspecting victims.

In the early 1990s, an outbreak involved almost 1,400 children who had eaten lunch served at several elementary schools in Texas. These lunches were routinely prepared in a central catering establishment and trucked to the various schools. Follow-up research pointed to contaminated chicken salad that had been prepared by boiling frozen chickens for three hours then cooling and deboning them. The meat was quickly cooled and then placed into 12-inch deep pans and stored in a refrigerator overnight. Health officials concluded that contamination probably occurred during deboning and that storage in deep containers prevented sufficient cooling to prevent the growth of staphylococcus and production of toxin. This incident served to highlight the critical importance of proper handling practices.[310]

Infections with methicillin-resistant *Staphylococcus aureus* (MRSA) have been reported in the United States for more than 30 years. At the outset, MRSA infections were primarily a problem of hospitals and nursing homes, but by 1997, half of health care–acquired *S. aureus* infections in the United States were methicillin resistant.[311] Shortly thereafter, community-acquired MRSA was described in both adults and children who did not have extensive exposure to hospitals or other apparent risk factors.[312] In 2002, the first report of a community-acquired outbreak of acute gastroenteritis caused by MRSA was reported.[313]

Shredded pork barbeque purchased from a delicatessen was reheated in a home microwave and three adults ate it less than 30 minutes after it was purchased. About 3 to 4 hours after eating, the three adults had nausea, vomiting and stomach cramps. The two children at the dinner, who did not eat the pork, did not become ill. Although MRSA toxin is not expected to be more virulent than nonresistant strains, it does point to the potential for ongoing intoxications that will be difficult to control.

DISEASES OF TOXIC SUBSTANCES

While most of us know that environmental pollutants, pesticides and radioisotopes from atomic tests can produce toxic effects, very few are aware of the potential threat posed by the wide range of natural toxins in foods. The one exception to this is, of course, poisonous mushrooms—a topic of which most of us have some minimal knowledge. However, a great many dangerous toxins naturally occur in foods. A rudimentary knowledge of their substance and nature is the best insurance to guard against them.

These toxins can be categorized as plant substances, marine substances and poisons that can develop in foods under special circumstances (acquired toxins). Livestock producers in the United States lose approximately 250 million dollars annually from animal deaths caused by poisonous plants.[314] Since we are mainly concerned with the foods we eat every day, the wide variety of natural substances consumed for their narcotic, hallucinogenic and other pharmacological effects will not be covered. The list is by no means complete. Some toxins, particularly in ethnic foods (e.g., akee poisoning), have not been included.

TOXIC PLANT SUBSTANCES

Unlike animals and insects, when faced with approaching danger, plants do not have the option of running away. Nature has therefore provided many of them with natural compounds to ward off different threats, such as hungry insects and animals or damaging attacks from various fungi. Recent research has proven that plants under attack by insects can produce higher levels of these toxins.[315] Some of these compounds can be quite toxic and cause illness in humans if consumed at a high concentration. Many scientists even consider these natural toxic compounds to pose a far greater risk to humans than pesticides and food additives and have asked that more attention be paid to this problem.[316] A few of the major groups are listed below.

Cyanogenic Glycosides

These compounds contain cyanide in a bound-up form and, under certain conditions (such as those in the digestive system), release this deadly poison. These compounds are found in cassava roots, lima beans and fava beans as well as in the seeds of almonds, peaches and apricots. The hundreds of millions of people living in the tropics, whose diet largely depends upon cassava, have developed simple processes to detoxify the flour and reduce the threat of cyanide poisoning. These include fermentation or grating and squeezing combined with heat. More recently, modern breeding techniques have reduced the levels of cyanide to a point where this special processing is no longer needed.

Goitrogens

These are among the most common toxins found in foods. Goitrogens occur in cabbages, rutabagas, rapeseed, mustard seed, brussels sprouts and cauliflower. If cows are fed the same plants, goitrogens can be detected in the milk. These substances act by preventing the thyroid gland from using iodine and, consequently, inhibit production of the thyroid hormones necessary for normal growth and metabolism. Anyone eating a balanced diet has little to fear. An amount far in excess of the normal intake of these foods is generally needed to cause problems. However, documented outbreaks of goiter have occurred in populations of poor people whose diet consisted mainly of rutabagas. Goitrogens are heat sensitive, so proper cooking destroys much of the activity of these toxins.

Hemagglutinins

Hemagglutinins are natural compounds that affect red blood cells and cause them to agglutinate or clump up. They can be found in many types of legumes such as soybeans, lima beans, lentils, kidney beans and peanuts. The hemagglutinin compound in castor beans (ricin) is so toxic, it has been used as an assassination agent and has potential as a biological warfare weapon. Fortunately, hemagglutinins are easily destroyed by the heat treatment used in routine processing. If raw beans are used, as long as they are properly cooked, there is little danger of intoxication.

The age-old tradition of assassinating political rivals or eliminating dissidents using poison continues unabated to modern times. Although it is an efficient means of getting rid of enemies, poison is often discovered. The end result is that the incident gains far more notoriety than other methods might, and the final outcome usually backfires. In fact, the only conceivable reason to use poison is as a weapon of revenge—to ensure that the victim suffers.

One well-known incident highlights the use of ricin for the purpose of political assassination. Georgi Ivanov Markov was born in 1929 in Sofia, Bulgaria. Trained as a chemical engineer, he started writing short stories after being hospitalized by an extended bout of tuberculosis. The quality of his work improved to the point where his 1962 novel *Men* won the Bulgarian Writers Annual Award. Not unexpectedly, as his reputation grew, both he and his work came under the close scrutiny of the Communist censors. Because his writing had become so popular, the Communist leader Todor Zhivkov tried to intimidate Markov into serving his regime, but Markov would not budge. The state apparatus turned against him, and his career took a decided turn for the worse. His 1969 play, *The Man Who Was Me,* was shown before an audience that included several Communist Party officials. They were very annoyed, and all further performances of the play were canceled. A close friend quietly warned Markov to leave Bulgaria, which he did.

After spending two years in Italy, Markov decided to move to England, and in 1972 he started working for the BBC. Because of his outspoken criticism of the Bulgarian government, all his written works were removed from Bulgarian bookshelves, and he was placed on trial and sentenced (in absentia) to six years and six months in prison for his original defection.

Nevertheless, Markov continued his public criticism of Bulgaria's Communist government and its leader Todor Zhivkov. These personal attacks against Zhivkov, the Communist Party strongman, made Georgi Ivanov Markov a marked man, and in July 1977 Zhivkov signed a politburo decree stating, "All measures should be used to neutralize enemy émigrés." Georgi Markov topped the enemies' list.

On September 7, 1978, Zhivkov's birthday, the assassin sent to kill Markov did his dirty work. Markov was in the queue at the Waterloo Bridge bus stop. He felt a sharp jab in his right thigh and turned around quickly to see a man stooping down to pick up an umbrella he had apparently dropped. The man mumbled an apology and quickly walked away.

Markov immediately felt a stinging sensation in the back of his right leg, but despite the pain he continued on his way to work. When he arrived at the office of the BBC World Service, he went to the washroom to look at his leg. He saw a small red spot that looked like a hive. The pain persisted, so he mentioned the incident to one of his colleagues. Later that evening, Markov developed a high fever and was taken to a hospital, where he was treated for blood poisoning. Unfortunately, the doctors did not have a clue as to what they were dealing with. Markov quickly went into shock and, after three days of utter agony, died.

Due to the statements Markov made to doctors concerning his suspicion that he was poisoned, Scotland Yard ordered a thorough forensic autopsy of Markov's body. The first thing the autopsy revealed was that his lungs were full of fluid and his liver showed signs of acute blood poisoning. His white blood cell count was extremely high and he had small hemorrhages all over his intestines, lymph nodes and heart. During the autopsy, tissue was cut from around the puncture wound on Markov's right thigh and sent to the Chemical Defense Laboratory at Porton Down. There, almost by accident, they discovered a tiny metal pellet—a jeweler's watch bearing—just a hair larger than the period at the end of this sentence.

The pellet measured 1.52 millimeters in diameter and was composed of 90 percent platinum and 10 percent iridium. It had two incredibly small cylinders with 0.35-millimeter diameters drilled through it in the shape of an X. The chemical experts found traces of ricin toxin in the X-shaped cavity. There is no known antidote to ricin poisoning, meaning that Markov was a dead man even while waiting for the bus.

Ricin has a structure similar to the botulinum toxin and works by entering the cells and shutting down protein synthesis. Without the required proteins, the cells die. Ricin is extremely toxic, with far less than a single milligram sufficient to kill a person.

In January 1979, after several months of investigation, the coroner's court in London ruled that Markov had been killed by 450 micrograms of lethal ricin toxin, contained in a miniature pellet injected with the aid of a specially designed umbrella that had been plunged into Markov's right thigh.

Despite the collapse of the Soviet Union, details of Markov's assassination and the link between the Bulgarian Secret Service and the Soviet KGB—which were thought to have supplied the toxin, the pellet and the umbrella—remain hidden but obvious. The epitaph on Georgi Markov's gravestone says it simply and elegantly: He died in the "cause of freedom."

Eight years earlier, Soviet dissident Aleksandr Solzhenitsyn had also suffered (but survived) ricin-like symptoms after a 1971 encounter with KGB agents. The seeming ease of access to this lethal poison has encouraged a gaggle of psychos to produce ricin for their own bioterrorist purposes.

In 2003, a group of six Algerian men were thought to be manufacturing ricin as part of a plot for a poison attack on the London Underground, but police were unable to recover any toxin during their raid.

In October 2003, an envelope with a threatening note and a sealed container was processed at a mail processing and distribution facility in Greenville, South Carolina. The note threatened to poison water supplies if certain demands were not met. The envelope was isolated from workers and other mail and removed from the facility. Laboratory testing at CDC confirmed that ricin was present in the container.

In November 2003, ricin was detected in the White House mail. The letter containing it was intercepted at a mail handling facility off the grounds of the White House and it never reached its intended destination. The powdery substance later tested positive for low potency ricin and was not considered a health risk.

In January 2006, ricin was found in a home in the suburbs of Richmond, Virginia. It was actually a mash of castor beans. The suspect, Yale-educated electrical engineer Chetanand Sewraz was supposedly isolating the toxin to kill his separated wife and not for bioterrorism purposes.

The examples above highlight the ease of making a highly toxic poison from fairly benign raw materials.

Oxalates

Over the years, a number of reports have concerned acute poisoning resulting from the ingestion of rhubarb and sorrel. The toxic agents thought to be responsible are oxalates. Oxalate poisoning from natural plants has always been a controversial issue. Some scientists claim that one would have to eat a minimum of 10 pounds of rhubarb leaves in order to get sick. Nevertheless, many medical reports have implicated oxalates ingested from natural plants. Symptoms of oxalate poisoning include ulcers of the mouth or gastrointestinal tract, gastric hemorrhaging and convulsions. Because of the high levels of oxalates in certain house plants, pediatricians often caution patients against having species such as *Dieffenbachia* in the house with young children around.

In December 2005, two individuals from Putnam County, New York, reported sensations of tingling, burning and stinging in their mouth after consuming taro root chips. Taro root naturally contains calcium oxalate, the agent responsible for the symptoms, but it is normally rendered harmless when properly prepared. In this particular case, the taro root chips were undercooked, and an unsafe level of calcium oxalate was present.

Pressor Amines

These compounds include potent biochemicals such as histamine, tyramine and tryptamine and their metabolites, such as serotonin and norepinephrine (powerful controllers of blood pressure). Although they are typical constituents of animal tissues, they are also found in many plants such as bananas, plantains and pineapples. Much higher levels are found in certain cheeses, the most notable of which is Camembert.

If an individual is exposed to a sufficient amount of pressor amines, severe headaches, perspiration, dilation of eye pupils, rigidity of the base of the neck, palpitations and blood pressure elevation can occur. On rare occasions, even cardiac failure can result.

For people who are sensitive, dietary restrictions are warranted to ensure that the intake of pressor amines is limited. The pressor amine content of foods can vary significantly depending on the way it was processed. Many foods naturally contain low levels of pressor amines, but if these products are aged, fermented or accidentally left to spoil, these levels can increase dramatically.

Foods to watch out for are fermented bean curd, fermented soya beans and sauce, fava beans, certain aged cheeses (not cream cheese or cottage cheese, which have no pressor amines), smoked, fermented or pickled fish and meat, sausages, pepperoni, salami, sauerkraut, shrimp paste and brewer's yeast extracts that are sometimes spread on bread as a snack.

Solanine

Solanine is a powerful inhibitor of cholinesterase, an enzyme necessary for the normal transmission of nerve impulses. Potatoes normally contain very small amounts of this material. However, when exposed to sunlight during storage, their concentration of solanine can increase very dramatically. Solanine is associated with the deep green-colored area often seen under the skin of these potatoes when they are peeled. It is a very toxic material and has been implicated in human fatalities. Solanine is not destroyed during cooking, so it is wise to exercise some caution. If the potato has an obvious deep green area, peel it all away before cooking.

Based on documents retrieved from terrorist training camps in Afghanistan, in September 2003, the FBI issued a warning that terrorists might attempt to use natural toxins, such as nicotine and solanine, to poison the nation's food and water. Fortunately, there is no evidence of this having taken place thus far.

TOXIC MARINE SUBSTANCES

Scuba divers know that if you approach any underwater marine creatures and they do not shy away from you quickly, then the chances of them carrying some toxic defense mechanism are quite good. However, encounters with marine toxins take place more often at the dinner table than under the sea. Food-borne marine toxins are quite serious and are responsible for a great many fatalities every year. The marine toxins of major concern are listed below.

Ciguatera Poisoning

This form of seafood poisoning has been known for more than four centuries. It is caused by a range of tropical and subtropical marine fish such as snappers, parrot fish (see figure 32) and other species that routinely feed on the poisonous algae (dinoflagellates) that occur near coral reefs. Symptoms usually consist of a combination of gastric, neurological and cardiac ailments. A poisoning episode usually begins with tingling of the lips and tongue, numbness, nausea, vomiting and diarrhea. This is followed by headaches, vertigo, paralysis, heart palpitations, respiratory paralysis and, occasionally, death. A variety of this disease is moray

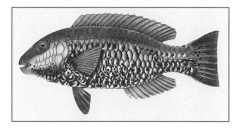

Figure 32. **Parrot Fish**

eel poisoning. Ciguatera poisonings have occurred all along the eastern seaboard of the United States and Hawaii. This has been mainly due to fish caught near coral reefs and then shipped to urban markets.

Puffer Fish Poisoning

Certain puffer fish (see figure 33), known as fugu fish in Japan, are considered a great delicacy. Fugu is highly toxic, but despite this the Japanese consider it a great delicacy and those who can afford to, continue to eat it. Lethal amounts of the poison tetrodotoxin are concentrated in the fugu's liver, gonads and skin. For a long time, the origin of the fugu's tetrodotoxin was a scientific mystery, with some scholars arguing that

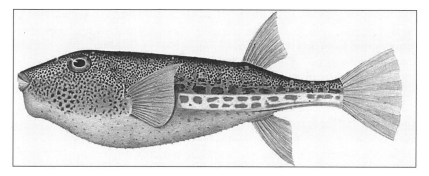

Figure 33. **Puffer Fish**

the poison was produced by the fish's body. However, it is now believed that the tetrodotoxin derives from bacteria associated with the fish and the marine organisms it eats.

Because fugu toxin is 1,000 times more poisonous than cyanide, only specially licensed chefs are allowed to prepare it. Obtaining a license to prepare fugu is a 10-year process, involving several varieties of puffer fish. It is such a stressful and exhausting process that chefs are supposedly able to hear the final lament of the puffer fish laid out on the chopping block.

From a taste and texture point of view, puffer fish is not exceptional; the real thrill of eating fugu is the chance to flirt with death. A well-trained fugu chef purposely includes a small amount of poisonous tissue in the serving so that the patrons experience limited symptoms. In medical terms, the first symptoms of the poisoning occur between 15 minutes and several hours after eating fugu.

Initial symptoms include tingling of tongue and lips, quickly followed by facial numbness. Salivation, nausea, vomiting and diarrhea with some abdominal pain develop early. Motor dysfunction with muscle weakness, hypoventilation and speech difficulties then develop. A rapid ascending paralysis occurs over four to 24 hours. Extremity paralysis is followed by respiratory muscle paralysis. Finally, the victim experiences cardiac dysfunction along with central nervous system dysfunction (e.g., coma), and seizures can develop. Patients with severe toxicity may have a deep coma, fixed nonreactive pupils, apnea and loss of all brain stem reflexes. In other cases, patients experience all the paralytic physical functions, yet can see and think very clearly. Death can occur within four to six hours as a result of respiratory muscle paralysis and respiratory failure.

Every year, because of miscalculations in the amount of poison left in the fugu fish, several hundred people are poisoned (with 20 to 100 fatalities) in Japan.[317] According to records, 1958 was a banner year with 176 fugu deaths occurring throughout Japan. The most famous victim was the Kabuki actor Mitsugora Bando VIII, who had achieved the status of a living national treasure. He expired in a Kyoto restaurant in 1975 after gorging himself on four bowls of chiri, a broth containing pieces of poisonous fugu liver. Considering that fugu consumption in Japan has been traced back to the Jomon period (c. 10,000–300 B.C.E.), Mitsugora Bando's death followed a long tradition.

Fugu consumption was largely banned in Japan from the 16th to the 19th centuries because of all the deaths related to it. However, Japan's first prime minister, Hirobumi Ito (1841–1909), the man responsible for the modernization of Japan, was also responsible for putting fugu back on the traditional Japanese menu. When he first tried it, Ito was so taken with its taste that he ordered the resumption of fugu preparation and sale.

Aside from puffer fish, tetrodotoxin is found in certain tree frogs and marine bacteria. In the hands of an experienced witch doctor, tetrodotoxin is the material responsible for turning people into zombies (the living dead) in countries like Benin and Haiti.

Scombroid Poisoning

This poison develops in tuna and mackerel that have not been quickly refrigerated or cooked right after being caught. It occurs due to the bacterial breakdown of the amino acid histidine into histamine—the identical compound released from our immune system as part of an allergic reaction. The same effects are occasionally encountered with products such as Swiss cheese. Symptoms include nausea, vomiting, headache, difficulty swallowing and itching of the skin. Death occurs quite rarely. Treatment, as one can guess, usually consists of antihistamine administration. Fish susceptible to scombroid poisoning must be frozen, canned, refrigerated or consumed as soon as possible after they are caught. Once fish develop scombrotoxin, neither cooking, canning nor freezing reduces toxicity. Scombroid poisoning is one of the most frequent forms of marine poisoning in North America and is often associated with canned tuna (domestic or imported) or frozen fish.

Shellfish Poisoning

Most of us are aware of the old rule of not eating shellfish during those warm months that do not contain the letter "R," i.e., May through August. During those months, mussels, clams, scallops and oysters can pick up poisons from certain blooms of planktonic algae (dinoflagellates) upon which they feed. Several forms of shellfish poisoning are known, such as paralytic shellfish poisoning (PSP), neurotoxic shellfish poisoning (NSP) and amnesic shellfish poisoning (ASP). The most serious form is PSP. It exhibits symptoms ranging from the tingling of lips, tongue and fingertips to vomiting, nausea, paralysis, respiratory failure and death. Amnesic shellfish poisoning results from a toxin called domoic acid. It can be very serious in elderly people since it is characterized by symptoms similar to Alzheimer's disease. More recently, it has been implicated in epileptic seizures.[318] Since consumers cannot tell the difference between normal and poisonous shellfish, the "R" rule should apply.

HONEY INTOXICATION

It is hard for most consumers to believe that a food as historically significant and as universally trusted as natural honey can have negative characteristics, but under certain conditions it can be toxic. In fact, in 410 B.C., Xenophon described one of the earliest recorded episodes of mass food poisoning—a result of honey intoxication.[319] Honey intoxication is caused by consuming honey that was produced by bees that selected rhododendrons as their main source of nectar. The actual toxin in the honey is called grayanotoxin and it comes in several forms, depending upon the particular plant variety in question. Honey intoxication is characterized by weakness, dizziness, nausea, perspiration and vomiting. This disease often results in dramatically reduced blood pressure and usually responds to the administration of fluids. Early chroniclers of various military expeditions tell of vast Roman legions being given honey by local tribesmen only to be slain later while under its paralyzing influence. Fortunately, this grim practice has gone out of fashion. However, the disease is still quite common in the area of the Black Sea and has also been found throughout North America. Honey intoxication is rarely fatal and usually lasts no more than one day. However, the increased demand and consumption of honey dictate that surveillance be maintained for this disease.

SUMMARY

Countless other toxins commonly occur in foods. However, generally speaking, they are not too great a concern for anyone eating a varied and balanced diet.

Even the way we prepare foods can have the effect of producing toxins. The high rates of stomach cancer found in populations that consume large amounts of smoked fish have been traced to the nitrosamines formed during the smoking process. Broiled meats such as steaks and hamburgers are another example. The coals in a normal outdoor barbecue are exceptionally hot. Whenever the fat from the foods drips down onto these hot coals, the intense heat does not simply evaporate them. The extreme heat pyrolyzes the fat and converts a small portion of it into carcinogenic compounds.[320] These carcinogens vaporize and then recondense on the meat waiting above. As long as consumers do not eat bottom-broiled steaks or hamburgers two to three times a day, this should not be a problem. Likewise, roasted products such as coffee have been shown to develop minute amounts of carcinogens during the roasting process.[321, 322] All this information merely reinforces the need to have a varied diet and refrain from consuming large quantities of the same foods constantly.

FUNGAL DISEASES

So by all means let's have a television show quick and long, even if the commercial has to be delivered by a man in a white coat with a stethoscope hanging around his neck, selling ergot pills. After all the public is entitled to what it wants, isn't it? The Romans knew that and even they lasted four hundred years after they started to putrefy.

Raymond Chandler (1888–1959), Letter, 15 Nov. 1951
(published in *Raymond Chandler Speaking*, 1962)*

Although more than 100,000 species of fungi are known, the ones of primary concern to us are the filamentous fungi or molds and mushrooms. Both of these forms of fungi have a very long history of human intoxication. In fact, fungi are responsible for some of the most potent toxins known.

MOLD TOXINS

Food intoxications can result from various molds. Mold spores are ubiquitous in the environment and many foods can become easily contaminated. The mold poisons are called mycotoxins from the Greek word for fungus. The most familiar of these toxins is aflatoxin produced by the mold *Aspergillus flavus*, a mold commonly found on peanuts and corn. Other toxins are produced by the molds *Fusarium* and *Claviceps*, which contaminate grains such as rye and wheat. Molds usually grow on damp grain or oilseeds (peanuts) where they excrete the toxin as a by-product of their metabolism. Unfortunately, most of these mycotoxins are very resistant to high heat and, as a result, cooking has very little effect on their harmfulness. Because these mycotoxins cannot be easily removed or destroyed, the only practical course of action is to ensure the prevention of mold contamination and growth throughout the entire chain of harvesting, drying, storage and processing.

Although only a small amount of material may be contaminated originally, an entire shipment of the product may have to be rejected, depending upon how it is processed. Certain products, such as peanut butter, can become uniformly contaminated with aflatoxin simply because the nuts are ground up and then homogenized. If two peanuts out of a large batch are heavily contaminated, whatever toxin is present

---

gets mixed in and evenly distributed throughout the entire lot. That is why peanut butter is very carefully controlled by both manufacturers' and government laboratories. On the other hand, because mold infection is often characterized by product discoloration, contaminated peanuts or grains can often be removed by modern electric eye sorters.

Aflatoxicosis

Aflatoxins are a group of toxic compounds produced by certain strains of the mold *Aspergillus flavus*. Aflatoxicosis results from the ingestion of aflatoxins contained in contaminated foods. It first came to light in 1960 when thousands of young turkeys, ducks and chickens died in England as a result of eating commercial feed contaminated with moldy peanut meal from Brazil. The cause of death was eventually traced to a highly potent and carcinogenic toxin from *A. flavus,* which was subsequently named aflatoxin.

Aflatoxins produce cirrhosis and cancer of the liver in a wide variety of different animal species. The regularity with which it causes these conditions makes it a toxin with great potential harm for humans. As a result, a considerable amount of attention has been paid to the elimination of this toxin from susceptible products in the commercial food industry. In developed countries, finding aflatoxins in foods at the levels that could cause significant disease occurs rarely. However, although acute aflatoxicosis is not a major concern, the long-term carcinogenic potential of low-level aflatoxin ingestion is still a preoccupation of medical research.

A major outbreak of aflatoxicosis occurred in India in 1974. People from more than 150 villages consumed contaminated corn for an extended period of time. Almost 400 people were affected, and 108 died. Typical symptoms included high fever, jaundice, edema, vomiting, pain and enlarged livers. In another outbreak in Kenya in 1982, 20 victims of aflatoxicosis were hospitalized and 12 died. A little more than 20 years later, in the spring of 2004, another widespread poisoning outbreak occurred in Kenya as a result of aflatoxin contamination of locally grown maize that had been stored in damp conditions. A total of 317 cases were reported, with 125 deaths. The government of Kenya worked quickly to replace food supplies in the most heavily affected districts. Without doubt, this is a very serious form of natural poisoning.

Aleukia

Alimentary toxic aleukia (ATA) is another serious and often fatal mold disease. It is caused when a toxic mold, called *Fusarium,* infects grain that has remained unharvested over winter. It was first recorded in Russia in 1913 and reached epidemic proportions during World War II when thousands of people died tragic and painful deaths as a result of ATA. Wheat and prosomillet, which traditionally form a major part of the meager diet of rural Russians, are particularly susceptible to *Fusarium* attack. Without proper storage, this continues to remain a threat.

ATA is characterized by pathological changes in the blood production and maintenance system and is reflected by a complete shrinkage of the bone marrow. The course of the disease is rather strange, starting with vomiting, gastroenteritis and throat inflammation. If ingestion of infected grain continues, this is followed by a period of two to eight weeks during which almost no overt symptoms are evident, but bone marrow destruction continues. The final stage results in alimentary tract ulcers and pulmonary hemorrhages. Mortality rates can be extremely high.

A recent epidemic of food poisoning occurred in Zhejiang Province, China after people ate moldy rice contaminated with *Fusarium* toxin. This was caused by the continuous rainfall that took place during the rice harvest season. Approximately 100 individuals were involved, and the onset of symptoms occurred within 10 to 30 minutes. Symptoms included dizziness, nausea, chills, vomiting, abdominal pain and diarrhea. Fortunately, no fatalities were reported.[323]

More recently, the Food and Drug Administration (FDA) has heightened its monitoring of a toxin called deoxynivalenol (DON), also known as vomitoxin, in wheat products as a result of the rainfall conditions favorable to *Fusarium* growth.[324] During a 1994 study, the FDA found samples of wheat containing levels of vomitoxin above the upper limit of one part per million (ppm). The industry was cautioned to exercise greater care in remaining below the advisory limit particularly when climatic conditions are favorable to mold growth. Vomitoxin has been linked to severe gastrointestinal problems in outbreaks in India and China.

Ergotism

Ergotism is probably the first recorded disease of a mold toxin, because it has been known for thousands of years. It results from eating rye and other cereals infected with the mold *Claviceps purpurea*. The ancient Greeks and Romans originally recognized it. Several major epidemics took place in Europe throughout the Middle Ages and beyond. This disease came to be known as St. Anthony's Fire because of the excruciating pain brought on by the severe muscle inflammation characteristically associated with it. A large outbreak that killed an estimated 40,000 people occurred in Limoges, France, in the year 943. Thereafter, major epidemics sporadically broke out in France, Spain and Germany, particularly during the 16th century. An interesting footnote in the history of ergotism was the cancellation of Peter the Great's plans to attack the Ottoman Empire in 1722. His Cossack troops and their horses had consumed infected rye, and hundreds had either died or gone mad, thereby causing Peter to abandon his plans.

Wherever it grows, rye is generally among the cheapest of grains. As a consequence, epidemics of ergotism usually affect the very poorest people in society. During the 20th century, two major outbreaks have occurred. The first was in the Soviet Union in 1926, where an untold number of the population was severely affected. The next large outbreak occurred in the south of France, near Avignon, in 1951. The outbreak occurred in the small French village of Pont-Saint-Esprit. This tiny town takes its name from the old bridge that spans the Rhône River.

That year, France experienced one of its wettest summers in a very long time. The conditions were ideal for the development of *Claviceps*, and in mid-August one of the town's two bakers noticed that the new batch of flour he used to make his baguettes was slightly grayer than the flour he normally received. Since flour distribution was a government monopoly at the time, he felt he had no choice but to use the flour he was given. Within a day, over 200 of the villagers, all of whom had purchased his baguettes, became very ill with what appeared to be food poisoning.

Several people began to complain of lightheadedness, nausea, vomiting, vertigo and diarrhea. In spite of the village's typical summer heat, people felt like they were freezing. Soon, people started going berserk, screaming through the night that they were being attacked by terrible apparitions. The hallucinations made people jump out of windows claiming that they were on fire or that they could fly like airplanes.

The likely cause of this was that the baguettes had been made with ergot-contaminated flour. Symptoms of both the gangrenous and convulsive forms of ergotism combined to produce an epidemic that was so bizarre and frightening that the outbreak captured the French newspaper headlines for weeks. It took some time before the consulting physicians brought in to analyze the problem noticed a resemblance between the ongoing difficulties in the town and epidemics of ergot poisoning that had occurred more than a century before. Others, including the police, thought that they were witnessing some form of mercury contamination—akin to Mad Hatter's disease—but the laboratory data eventually pointed to ergotism.

Before this incident ebbed, hundreds of villagers suffered weeks of unbearable sleeplessness and hallucinations. Four of them died agonizing deaths. It was months before the village of Pont-Saint-Esprit returned to a semblance of normal life. The memory of *le pain maudit* (the accursed bread) remains today.

The course of the disease is pretty grim. Once someone ingests the ergot toxin, he or she first experiences tiredness, muscular pain and a prickly sensation in the limbs. The limbs eventually become swollen and are subject to alternate sensations of intense heat and cold, hence the name St. Anthony's Fire. Eventually, gangrene sets in, and the affected limbs fall off. A second form of the disease, characterized by central nervous disorders, became more common after the 19th century. Ergotism occurs extremely rarely in the United States, the last major episode having occurred in 1825. The active component of ergot toxin, lysergic acid, received considerable publicity during the 1960s when one of its derivatives, LSD, became the product of choice for college students seeking mind-expanding, hallucinogenic experiences.

From June to August 2001, there were reports of a large number of cases of gangrene in Ethiopia. Barley samples were collected from the

affected areas, and they tested positive for ergot alkaloids. The back draft
of St. Anthony's Fire continues to
threaten us.

MUSHROOM TOXINS

Fatal poisoning of humans due to
the consumption of mushrooms has
been known for many centuries. The
common name toadstool has nothing to do with toads; it comes from
the German word *Todesstuhl,* which
means a stool of death. One of the
first recorded cases of mushroom poisoning involved the deaths of the wife
and children of the Greek poet Eurip-
ides in the fifth century B.C. Since
that time, hapless gourmands have
succumbed to these fungal delicacies
on a regular basis because without
prior experience, no easy way exists
of distinguishing edible mushrooms
from poisonous toadstools. In fact,
the only reason why relatively few fatalities occur is that the percentage
of mushrooms that are actually poisonous is really very small. However,
though their numbers may be limited, mushroom toxins make up for it
by their deadly nature. The popularity of natural foods has lead to an
increased incidence of mushroom poisoning among the general population. Mushroom poisoning continues to occur even with experienced
collectors. A recent report describes a person with over 30 years of expertise in collecting wild mushrooms who prepared a mushroom dish that
poisoned herself and family members, one of whom eventually died.[325]

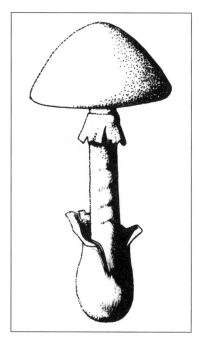

Figure 34. *Amanita*

Amatoxins

Among the most widely distributed fungus species are the *Amanita* (see
figure 34). The most famous member of them all is the death cap. Death
caps come in a variety of colors, which makes them difficult to distinguish
from other mushrooms. Other species of poisonous amanita include the
destroying angel and fool's mushroom. Amatoxin poisoning is characterized by a very long waiting period before the appearance of symptoms.
Usually, the victim has confidently discounted the possibility of poisoning
by the time the symptoms begin to show. After the initial waiting period,
the amatoxin strikes with a vengeance. The symptoms include sudden,
severe abdominal pains, vomiting, diarrhea and very restricted urine

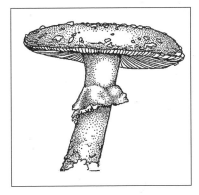

Figure 35. **Fly Agaric**

production. If the victim survives this first phase, it is still no indication of ultimate recovery. The death rate for amanita poisoning varies between 50 and 90 percent.

Muscimol Toxin

This potent neurotoxin is produced by the fly agaric (see figure 35) and panthercap mushrooms. This toxin has a rapid onset leading to tiredness, dizziness and abdominal pain. Shortly thereafter, victims experience spells of excitability and hyperactivity followed by delirium. Fatalities do not commonly occur among adults. However, children may experience convulsions and comas for up to 12 hours.

Psilocybin Toxin

Ingesting these toxins results more from deliberate intoxication than from accidental consumption. Several small, brown mushrooms of the genus *Psylocybe* have long been known for their ability to alter perception—their psychotropic properties. While in the past native American tribes used them in religious ceremonies, more recently people of all ages seeking hallucinogenic experiences have been the majority of victims. Poisonings by these mushrooms are seldom fatal, but small children have died from overdoses.

PARASITIC DISEASES

You had no right to be born; for you make no use of life. Instead of living for, in, and with yourself, as a reasonable being ought, you seek only to fasten your feebleness on some other person's strength.

Charlotte Brontë (1816–55), English novelist.
Eliza Reed to her sister Georgiana, in *Jane Eyre*, ch. 21 (1847)*

PARASITES

The last group of organisms associated with food-borne diseases are the parasites. Parasites are generally defined as organisms that obtain nourishment from other living organisms without providing any benefit in return. The parasite's unsuspecting victim is euphemistically called the host. Parasites are generally not classified as microorganisms since many can be seen without the help of a microscope. In fact, tapeworms, roundworms and flukes can be very large. The food-borne parasites with which we are concerned are those that use food animals as one of the hosts in their complex life cycles. In general, food-borne parasitic infections are not nearly as great a problem in well-developed countries as they are in developing countries. However, on a global scale, they are still considered to be extremely serious.

At one end of the parasite scale are the tiniest examples—the protozoa, which are simple, microscopic, single-celled organisms. The three most important ones found in foods are *Entamoeba hystolytica*, *Giardia lamblia (G. intestinalis)* and *Toxoplasma gondii*. At the other end of the scale are the flat tapeworms (cestodes), which can attain a length of 30 feet in the human intestine, and roundworms (nematodes), which can get as fat as two inches in diameter (see figure 36).

TAPEWORMS

When our primitive forebears first descended from the trees and developed the tools and weapons to kill animals and catch fish, they also assumed the risks of infection from a far wider range of parasites. The parasitization of humans by tapeworms has been known from the time ancient history began to be recorded. Tapeworms were once found in a 3,000-year-old Egyptian mummy. Early papyrus scripts recommended the

Different Parasitic Worms

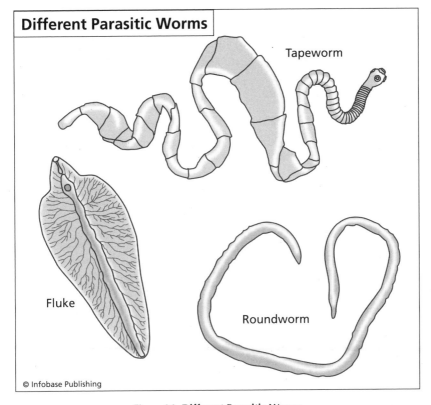

Tapeworm

Fluke

Roundworm

© Infobase Publishing

Figure 36. **Different Parasitic Worms**

use of garlic, honey and vinegar as a cure to get rid of them. With little doubt, tapeworms occurred commonly since they were often described in ancient Greek, Roman and Arabic medical texts. Despite our long historical knowledge of these organisms, only in the last century did researchers understand their parasitic nature, life cycles and mode of action.

The adult tapeworm is characterized by the presence of a small head, which has rows of tiny hooks for attaching to the intestine of the host. Right after the head is a narrow neck followed by flat, rectangular-shaped body segments. These segments contain both testes and ovaries and continually produce eggs. The body segments farthest from the head and closest to the end of the intestine develop most rapidly. Once they are fully mature, they separate from the rest of the worm and pass out with the feces of their host. These segments contain numerous eggs, which are simply encapsulated embryonic tapeworms waiting for a new host to release them.

If another animal or human host eats a detached segment, the segment regenerates a new head, complete with hooks, attaches itself to the host's intestine and recommences its growth. If, on the other hand, unhatched eggs are ingested, then they hatch in the intestine and bore their way into the tissues of the new host and form cysts known as cysticerci. The animal (or occasional human) harboring this stage of the parasite is known as an intermediate host in contrast with the primary host. This cysticercosis state is usually the most dangerous form of tapeworm disease, depending upon which tissues the larvae invade and damage. Once a primary host ingests the larvae, usually in the form of intermediate host cysticerci, contained in the food they eat, the larvae develop into adult tapeworms and attach themselves to the intestine. They maintain their nutrition by absorbing partially digested food through their surface skin.

The three tapeworms of greatest concern are the beef, pork and fish tapeworms of humans, called *Taenia saginata, Taenia solium* and *Diphyllobothrium latum,* respectively (see figure 37). Most often, they are acquired through the ingestion of larval cysts contained in meat and fish muscle. Where people routinely consume raw or partially cooked beef or pork, as with certain sausages for instance, the incidence of tapeworm infection can be very high. Asia, Africa, eastern Europe and Latin America continue to have a high incidence of these tapeworms as do recently arrived immigrants from these regions to North America. Both beef and pork tapeworms act in much the same way, that is, they cause abdominal discomfort, nervousness and, in some cases, loss of weight. This is understandable since the worms eat the food and essen-

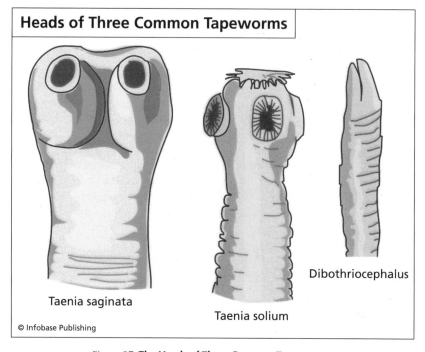

Heads of Three Common Tapeworms

Taenia saginata

Taenia solium

Dibothriocephalus

© Infobase Publishing

Figure 37. **The Heads of Three Common Tapeworms**

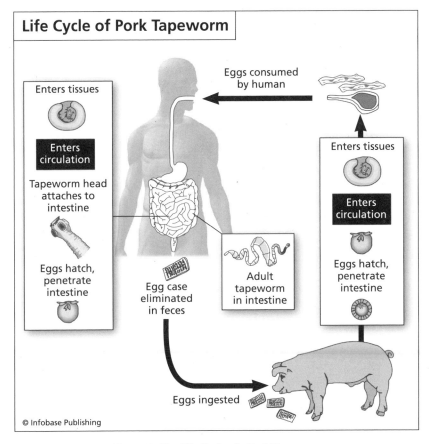

Life Cycle of Pork Tapeworm

Eggs consumed by human

Enters tissues

Enters circulation

Tapeworm head attaches to intestine

Eggs hatch, penetrate intestine

Egg case eliminated in feces

Adult tapeworm in intestine

Enters tissues

Enters circulation

Eggs hatch, penetrate intestine

Eggs ingested

© Infobase Publishing

Figure 38. **The Life Cycle of a Pork Tapeworm**

tial nutrients destined for their host. Some tapeworms grow to enormous lengths and can span the entire length of the intestine.

With the pork tapeworm, a much greater danger presents itself to humans when they happen to ingest the eggs and become the intermediate host (see figure 38). The hatched tapeworm embryos can burrow their way to the eyes, lung, liver, heart and brain of the victim, wreaking inflammatory havoc and infection all along the way. The most serious form of this disease experienced is cerebral (neurocysticercosis), which often leads to epilepsy and death.[326] It is now occurring more frequently in patients in the United States, but most of this disease was acquired out of the country.[327] Freezing of infected pork or beef can kill taenia cysticerci, but care should also be taken regarding the consumption of raw meat.

The consumption of raw, freshwater fish or even the tasting of minced fish and fish soup before it is fully cooked has resulted in widespread infection with fish tapeworms. Diphyllobothriasis was formerly known as Jewish or Scandinavian housewife's disease due to the habit of tasting gefilte fish (fish balls) before they are fully cooked. Fish tape-worms are, generally speaking, not too serious, but they are usually long lasting. For individuals genetically predisposed, a serious form of anemia can develop. In all cases, proper sanitation and inspection combined with sufficient cooking are a basis of prevention. These parasites are also susceptible to freezing.

ROUNDWORMS

Roundworms, or nematodes, are extremely numerous in nature—second only to insects in numbers. Many are free living, while others are parasitic upon plants and animals. The food-borne parasitic roundworms of particular interest to humans include *Ascaris lumbricoides, Trichuris trichiura, Trichinella spiralis* and *Anisakis simplex.*

Anisakids

Anisakids are small roundworms found in marine fish. The adult worms generally inhabit the intestines of fish-eating marine mammals and birds. The mammals shed eggs that hatch into larvae and are then consumed by different marine creatures until they reach fish to start the life cycle all over again. The chief source of human infection is the consumption of raw fish. Therefore, a greater incidence of disease occurs in Japan and Korea. Raw herring consumed in the Netherlands and Scandinavia are also sources of contamination. In recent years, the practice of keeping fish cold and in prime condition has also contributed to the good health and infectivity of the anisakids.

The symptoms of anisakid infection include fever and acute abdominal pains resembling appendicitis. The larval anisakids burrow their way into the wall of the digestive tract and cause local granulomas (inflamed masses of granular tissue). Generally, adult worms are eliminated in the

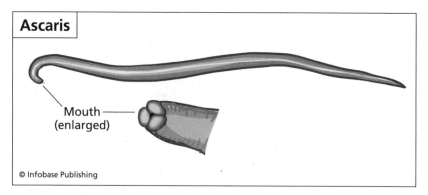

Figure 39. *Ascaris lumbricoides*

feces. However, serious infections can arise and have, at times, required the removal of affected stomach sections.

Disease incidences are directly related to the level of raw or lightly salted fish consumption. The more sashimi, sushi, seviche and raw herring eaten, the higher the frequency of anisakiasis. The potential for increased disease incidences has escalated in areas where the seal populations have swelled, such as along the California and Newfoundland coasts. Recent research in the Seattle area turned up anisakids in almost 10 percent of the salmon sushi.[328]

Ascaris

Ascaris is a genus of common, large roundworms found in humans, pigs and other animals (see figure 39). While they normally range from about six to 12 inches in length and are usually about one-fourth inch in diameter, specimens as large as 16 inches long by two inches in diameter are possible. The spread of ascaris occurs through the ingestion of their tiny eggs. Female Ascaris worms may contain as many as 25 million microscopic eggs at any time and can eliminate as many as 200,000 per day into the host's intestine. The eggs are then spread in human and animal waste. The use of unsterilized night soil, which contains Ascaris eggs, as a fertilizer is a definite cause of reinfection and the reason why this parasite is found on fresh vegetables. The worm is found in other animals, which can serve as alternate sources of infection. (As noted earlier, I even found one wrapped around the yolk of a fresh hen's egg while I was a university student.) Only strict hygiene on the farm can protect against Ascaris.

Symptoms of Ascaris infection are abdominal pain, vomiting, nausea and a protruding abdomen. Once ingested, the larvae burrow into tissues where they can cause severe damage. As they grow, they seek out the body's intestinal tract and lodge there to produce more eggs. On occasion, they can even crawl up the throat and out the mouth or nose. It occurs fairly commonly in North America. Many individual cases (although no outbreaks) have been reported. Over 600 million people worldwide are estimated to be infected with Ascaris worms.

Trichinella

Trichinella spiralis causes the disease known as trichinellosis. This disease was first uncovered in England in 1835 during a postmortem examination of a human cadaver. Its significance as a pathogen came to light 25 years later when a death was attributed to eating undercooked, infected pork. This Trichinella parasite is unique in that it lives its entire life cycle within a single host and is freed to continue a new life cycle only upon the death and consumption of its original host.

The process starts by eating undercooked muscle meat containing tiny Trichinella larvae that are enclosed in heavy, walled cysts. The gastric juices dissolve the cyst wall and release the larvae, which then pass down

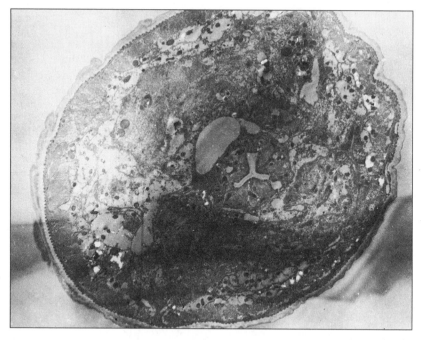

Figure 40. *Trichinella* **Section**
Courtesy Istituto Superiore di Sanità, Rome, Italy.

to the small intestine, grow and mate. The female then sheds her newly born larvae, which find their way into the circulatory system and eventually invade the muscles. They soon become encysted and can survive this way for years.

Most carnivorous animals can harbor *Trichinella* (see figure 40). Humans acquire trichinellosis by eating undercooked meat from infected animals. Pigs are occasionally fed undercooked waste meat from other slaughtered pigs and, if that meat happened to be infected, the cycle continues with an ever greater number of animals. Horse meat has been found infected, because horses occasionally gobble up field mice that may have fed on infected dead animals. The consumption of wild animals is risky and has resulted in many cases of human trichinellosis. Wild boar, bear and even cougar meats have been implicated.[329, 330] The symptoms of trichinellosis include fever and very painful and inflamed muscles, including those that control both breathing and speech.

Trichuris

Trichuris trichiura (whipworm) is quite similar to *Ascaris,* being found in the same foods and causing the same symptoms, and occurs more commonly in Europe. This worm does not migrate through the tissues and therefore does not cause as much damage as ascaris does.

FLUKES

These little creatures are a type of flatworm called trematodes. They are responsible for a wide number of disease conditions in both developed and developing countries. These parasites go through a complicated life cycle involving one or two intermediate hosts and possibly a free-living stage. Our desire for raw or undercooked fish or meat and even certain raw vegetables provide ample opportunity for infections to occur.

Opisthorchis viverrini is a freshwater fish liver fluke that infects millions of people in Asia. Recent reports indicate infection in more than 80 percent of the population in northeastern Thailand.[331] It eventually ends up consumed by freshwater fish whose flesh it promptly invades. If the fish are not properly cooked before eating, the parasite infects consumers. The effects of *Opisthorchis viverrini* are serious and include liver obstruction, fibrosis and jaundice. Other species similar to *Opisthorchis* occur throughout the world.

A North American counterpart is *Nanophyetus salmincola*. The infection is transmitted through the consumption of fish (such as salmon) in whose flesh the parasitic larvae have encysted. The symptoms are characterized by nausea and abdominal pain. It does not occur very commonly.

The sheep liver fluke is called *Fasciola hepatica*. Although uncommon in North America, human infections have been recorded in the rest of the world. Eggs released from the feces of human or animal hosts hatch out and find their way into snails. The larvae develop in the snails and eventually move out to encyst on certain plants. Humans contract the disease simply by eating the uncooked vegetables, particularly watercress.

OTHER PARASITES

Several other parasites cause food-borne illness. The following will discuss six parasites of growing significance.

Cryptosporidium parvum

Cryptosporidium is the unusual name of a tiny, single-celled protozoan parasite that is steadily becoming a greater concern in the food industry (see figure 41). The parasite is transmitted by the ingestion of oocysts (a type of egg), which are excreted in the feces of infected animals or humans. Infection can therefore be spread through drinking contaminated water (tap or swimming pool water), by eating contaminated food, from animals to people and from person to person.[332] All of these types of outbreaks have been documented. The parasite causes severe watery diarrhea that can be fatal if extreme dehydration is allowed to occur.[333] As of yet, no drugs or drug combinations have been developed to which *Cryptosporidium* is sensitive. Consequently, the host of this parasite has no choice and must allow the disease to run its course, the only possible therapy being intravenous rehydration.

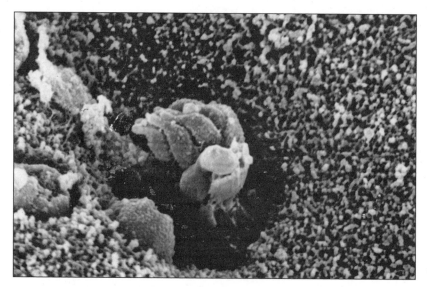

Figure 41. **Cryptosporidium**
Courtesy Istituto Superiore di Sanità, Rome, Italy.

The disease may last for several weeks, and bowel movement frequency can be as high as 25 times per day. Eventually, the immune system kicks in with enough force to halt the infection. In some people, the symptoms may be similar to traveler's diarrhea, but in immunocompromised people such as those with AIDS, it is a life-threatening disease. Recent reports indicate that it is one of the most prevalent parasites.[334] Serological studies have indicated that approximately 80 percent of the North American population have been exposed to some form of cryptosporidiosis at one time or another. Although pasteurized, canned, dried and frozen foods do not appear to be good vehicles for *Cryptosporidium*, no particular preventative measures are in place today to handle this parasite in fresh foods.[335]

In 1993, *Cryptosporidium* was responsible for the largest outbreak of waterborne disease in the United States when more than 400,000 people in Milwaukee, Wisconsin came down with the infection after consuming contaminated drinking water.[336] During the outbreak, many people resorted to drinking bottled water, because the infective organisms were filtered out.[337] Indeed, the Environmental Protection Agency and the Centers for Disease Control and Prevention have advised all immunocompromised people to boil their drinking water, use an appropriate filter or buy bottled water to avoid *Cryptosporidium* exposure.[338] The common occurrence of this parasite in water supplies results in their presence in a wide variety of fruits and vegetables.[339] The parasite has also been recently found in apple cider.[340] Because of the widespread presence of *Cryptosporidium parvum*, it is considered by the Centers for Disease Control and Prevention to be one of the most significant of the newly emerging infective diseases.[341]

Cyclospora cayetanensis

In May and June 1996, hundreds of cases of diarrheal illness were reported throughout the United States and Canada.[342] These incidents occurred in both clusters and sporadic cases. In a relatively short period of time, laboratory analyses revealed that the organism responsible was *Cyclospora cayetanensis*—a tiny, single-celled parasite that is eight to 10 microns in diameter, or about twice the size of *Cryptosporidium*. *Cyclospora* (see figure 42) is a relatively rare infection first diagnosed in 1977. A few incidents were reported in the mid-1980s, but it was not considered to be a serious pathogen. This parasite is transmitted via the fecal-oral route and was thought to be associated with the consumption of strawberries and raspberries. Contamination can arise through the use of unsterilized night soil or contaminated groundwater for irrigation. Originally, the suspected produce was thought to have originated in California but was later deemed to have come from south of the border.

Since it occurred during midsummer, the economic significance of this incident did not go unnoticed. Many states and provinces openly suggested to their consumers that buying local produce would be far safer and healthier than buying the imported kind. This added to the general confusion since no one was quite certain from which area the infected produce originated. The very wide geographic area in which the incidents took place clearly demonstrated how poor practices in one part of the world might negatively affect hundreds of consumers very far away.

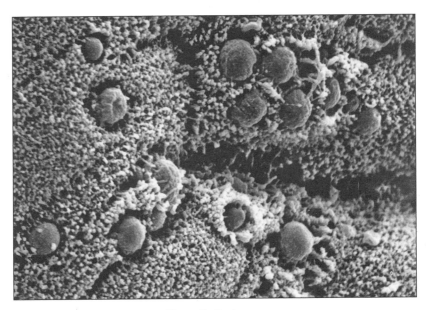

Figure 42. **Cyclospora**
Courtesy Istituto Superiore di Sanità, Rome, Italy.

Cyclospora cayetanensis typically infects the small intestine and causes watery diarrhea often accompanied by loss of appetite, bloating, weight loss, stomach cramps, vomiting and fever. On average, symptoms begin to be noticed about one week after the consumption of infected foods. This parasite is routinely treated with antibiotics for a course of seven days. In some individuals, a relapse may occur at a later date. The infection results in far more serious symptoms and considerable weight loss in AIDS patients.[343]

Entamoeba hystolytica

Entamoeba hystolytica is a single-celled protozoa, which mainly infects humans and, to a lesser extent, monkeys. This organism is perpetuated by the victims, who continually shed cysts containing dormant larvae in their feces. These cysts can easily survive for long periods in both soil and water. When cysts are swallowed, the digestive juices dissolve them, and the larvae are freed to start the process all over again. *Entamoeba hystolytica* causes amebic dysentery, which can be fatal if the parasite migrates to the liver, lungs or brain. The amebiasis infection can last for years and is often accompanied by bloody diarrhea, ulcers and intestinal blockages.

This infection occurs fairly commonly where poor sanitation and inadequate water treatment exist, such as in most developing countries. However, it has also been known to cause outbreaks in developed countries. An example was the Chicago amebiasis epidemic of 1933, which resulted from the accidental contamination of drinking water with untreated sewage.[344] Chlorine treatment alone is not sufficient to kill this parasite in drinking water. In all areas where it is found, filtration and boiling are required. The organism can be transmitted by sexual contact and is often found among homosexual men. Entamoeba can easily be transmitted via foods when handlers fail to observe proper hygiene practices. As in other instances, raw vegetables are very susceptible carriers of this disease, particularly if night soil (unsterilized human feces) is used as a natural fertilizer.

Giardia lamblia (G. intestinalis)

Giardia lamblia (G. intestinalis) is a small, single-celled protozoa that has five flagellae on its body in order to guide its locomotion (see figure 43). It is believed that the first person to describe it was van Leeuwenhoek when he was "troubled with a looseness." This organism exists as cysts and is common throughout nature. When ingested, the cysts dissolve, and the parasite (or trophozite) causes an infection of the small intestine known as giardiasis, which results in diarrhea, cramps and weight loss. It is commonly found in developing countries and to a lesser extent in developed countries.[345] In North America, giardiasis is the most frequently reported cause of nonbacterial diarrhea and is considered to be the most common intestinal parasitic infection worldwide. Although the symptoms normally last one to two weeks, giardiasis can persist for many weeks or even months if it is not diagnosed and treated promptly. Its

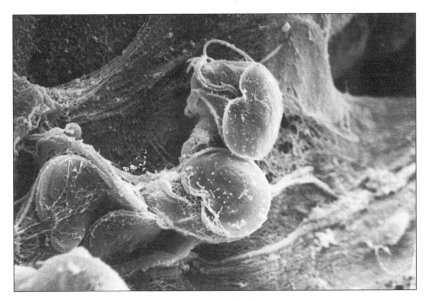

Figure 43. *Giardia*
Courtesy Istituto Superiore di Sanità, Rome, Italy.

spread is very similar to that of entamebiasis, and therefore the preventative hygienic measures required by food handlers are also similar.

Giardiasis is really a major problem for travelers, particularly older people, whose immune system may not function perfectly. Of the more than 75 million people who annually travel to tropical regions, 20 million come from developed countries where this organism does not commonly occur. Aside from infected water supplies, giardiasis can result from the consumption of raw vegetables mishandled by the food preparer.[346] Evidence shows that breast-feeding provides babies with a significant degree of protection against the symptoms of giardiasis but does not prevent infections from occurring.[347] The ubiquitousness of this organism ranks it as one of the emerging pathogens to be reckoned with in the future.

Pfiesteria piscicida

Although this parasitic ameba is not currently considered to be a foodborne disease, it may be an organism to watch. *Pfiesteria* has been responsible for some massive freshwater fish kills. A number of human illnesses have been linked to infections resulting from exposure to mist, vapor or water from infected rivers.[348, 349]

Pfiesteria works by causing lesions and neurological damage to fish through the two types of toxins it produces. The first one, called nogatoxin, is fat-soluble and causes lesions. The second water-soluble one affects the nervous system and causes memory loss. This latter neurological symptom has been found in people who were accidentally exposed to the toxin.

Currently, no evidence shows that this organism poses a food-borne problem simply because the dead fish are not harvested and sold to the public. However, oysters without any disease symptoms have been found containing *Pfiesteria*. Consumers could possibly eat these. The FDA Center for Food Safety and Applied Nutrition is keeping a close watch on this organism.

Toxoplasma gondii

Toxoplasmosis is a disease caused by a tiny protozoan parasite that requires the presence of cats to ensure its proliferation since felines are an integral part of the organism's life cycle. *Toxoplasma gondii* occurs quite commonly all over the world. The incidence of prior infection (as determined by the presence of antibodies in blood samples) in the United States has been estimated to be as high as 50 percent of the population.[350] This disease is serious because it can attack nervous and muscular tissue. On the European continent, toxoplasmosis occurs in almost 5 percent of newborns. In the United States, an estimated more than 3,000 babies are born annually with toxoplasmosis. The rates of death or vital neural disorders are very high among these infants. Of the victims that are born healthy, almost 70 percent soon develop active infections. It is one of the most dangerous pathogens for people infected with human immunode-ficiency virus. In fact, toxoplasmic encephalitis (TE) is the second most common AIDS-related infection of the central nervous system. Research has found that 10–50 percent of AIDS patients show antibodies to *Toxo-plasma gondii*,[351] indicating prior infection.

Cysts of this parasite have been found in pork and lamb. Ingestion of undercooked meat products from these animals potentially causes toxo-plasmosis. It is a particular problem for anyone who regularly eats raw meat dishes such as steak tartare. Of all the meat commonly available to consumers, pork holds the greatest potential for possible toxoplasma infection. Caution must be exercised when consuming wild game as well since 60 percent of deer examined from different regions of the United States tested positive for *Toxoplasma gondii* antibodies.[352, 353]

VIRAL DISEASES

VIRUSES

Viruses are among the strangest organisms in the universe, because they consist simply of genetic material encased in a protective coating. The term virus (which means poison in Latin) was originally coined in the late 1890s to describe things that caused disease but were considerably smaller than bacteria. The existence of viruses was first verified in 1892 when the Russian microbiologist Dimitri Ivanovsky discovered tiny, microscopic particles capable of causing mosaic disease in tobacco plants. Over 40 years later, the American biochemist W. M. Stanley purified the same virus and conclusively demonstrated that it consisted of only the genetic material ribonucleic acid (RNA) and an outer protective protein covering.

Viruses are not a form of life in the traditional sense. They are sophisticated organic chemical complexes that can actually be crystallized like other chemicals. However, they cannot live and grow by themselves. All viruses must have a living host to inhabit before they can spring to "life." In a manner reminiscent of a science fiction horror movie, once a live host becomes available, viruses can rapidly reproduce themselves and seriously harm or even destroy their host in the process. Because viruses do not have the vital metabolic systems necessary for self duplication, they must get these from the living cells that they infect. Viral life, therefore, consists of hijacking their host's reproductive system and completely subjugating it to the task of producing more new viruses. It is an extremely efficient form of parasitism but on a molecular level.

Duplication starts when a virus enters the cell. The host cell goes to work to defend itself by using its powerful enzymes to digest the protective protein coat of the virus in an attempt to destroy it. However, this is exactly what the virus needs in order to free its genetic material (DNA or RNA) into the cell. The newly injected virus's DNA or RNA then takes command over the host cell's protein synthesis machinery (ribosomes) and makes it produce large numbers of protective coat proteins. The enzymes required to break these down cannot be replenished, because they require the very same biological production machinery that was just hijacked. Then, the virus's RNA or DNA uses the cell's genetic machinery to replicate itself over and over again. Shortly thereafter, the DNA or RNA and the protective coat proteins are neatly put together to form lots of new viruses. In this manner, one virus can give rise to hundreds of offspring by using a single host cell. Viruses are then released by bursting the cell they infected or by slipping through the cell membranes without killing the host cells.

Viruses can vary considerably in appearance, ranging from tiny polygons to large, rod-shaped creatures. On average, they are considerably

273

smaller than bacteria and are almost impossible to see with a typical light microscope. Typical viral diseases include the common cold, rabies, poliomyelitis, encephalitis, certain hemorrhagic fevers, measles, mumps, chicken pox and hepatitis. Currently, the most infamous virus is human immunodeficiency virus (HIV), which causes acquired immune deficiency syndrome (AIDS). This virus attacks and destroys the lymphocytes that normally provide us with our natural immunity to disease.

For a long time, the precise role of viruses in food-borne illness was not well known. Yet, certain viruses have been responsible for some of the most extensive outbreaks of food-borne diseases. The terrible polio epidemics that broke out during and after World War I were associated with the consumption of unpasteurized milk. Shellfish raised in waters contaminated with human waste have been implicated in the transmission of hepatitis. The consumption of these shellfish in a raw state is considered to be an unacceptable health hazard in some parts of the United States.[354] A massive outbreak occurred in Shanghai in 1988, with more than 16,000 people estimated to have contracted hepatitis from eating raw shellfish.[355] The ensuing person-to-person transmission of the virus from the original victims ultimately resulted in more than an estimated 300,000 cases of hepatitis. Although it is usually not a fatal disease, hepatitis can be very debilitating, and its symptoms may last for a very long time.

Because foods generally do not contain growing and reproducing cells, they ordinarily cannot support the growth of viruses. However, they do serve to transmit the viruses from their original source to the ultimate consumer. Because the infective dose of virus particles is very small, foods carry the same sort of responsibility in disease transmission of viruses as they do with bacteria and parasites.

HEPATITIS

Hepatitis is a disease whose name is derived from the Greek word for liver (*hepato*). It is characterized by an inflammation of the liver and is usually due to viral infection. Several forms of hepatitis exist. They spread through contaminated food and water or by transmission from infected blood, sexual activity, shared syringes or poorly sterilized dental tools.

The main types of food-borne hepatitis are classified hepatitis A and hepatitis E. Hepatitis A virus (HAV) is very small and comprises a single molecule of RNA surrounded by a small protein coating. It was previously known as infectious hepatitis and has commonly occurred in situations where people were crowded together, such as army camps, prisons and children's nurseries. Hepatitis A is distributed on a worldwide basis and can occur in both a sporadic and epidemic manner. The apparent incidence of this form of hepatitis in developing countries is lower than in the United States as a result of the constant exposure to this virus from a very early age. Once exposed, most individuals develop an immunity that provides lifelong protection against further reinfection. An average of 65 percent of Americans over the age of 50 demonstrate this immunity.

Hepatitis A virus is shed in the stools. As a consequence, it is mainly spread through the fecal-oral route. The virus is found in a variety of contaminated foods, water and shellfish. Frequent contact with infected people, regular employment or attendance at nurseries or day care centers, international travel and careless drug use are the chief risk factors.[356] Food-borne outbreaks of hepatitis have occurred in Arkansas,[357] New York[358] and Colorado.[359] A massive outbreak involving more than a million pounds of infected strawberries from Mexico shipped to school lunch programs occurred in several states throughout the United States.[360]

The hepatitis E virus (HEV) is only slightly larger than the hepatitis A virus and is very susceptible to degradation. This form of hepatitis is clinically indistinguishable from hepatitis A and shares virtually all of the symptoms. Hepatitis E is usually associated with contaminated drinking water, and major outbreaks have occurred in Asia and Africa. No reports of outbreaks have occurred in the United States thus far.

Symptoms for both forms involve fever, weakness, loss of appetite, digestive upsets, abdominal pains and muscle pains. The upper part of the abdomen often becomes painful and tender. Jaundice appears several days after the initial onset and reaches a maximum intensity after about two weeks. This disease may take up to six months to run its course. It is usually a mild disease with low fatality rates but can be far more serious in pregnant women. The incidence of hepatitis A in the United States increased by almost 60 percent from 1983 to 1989.

Because of the relatively long incubation time, having suspected food materials around to test for contamination after an incident has been recorded is virtually impossible. However, some foods and beverages found to be responsible for outbreaks in the United States are imported lettuce, ice-slush beverages, iced tea, raw oysters and strawberries. The ice-slush incident occurred in Alaska in July of 1989 and was attributed to the consumption of products prepared in a convenience store. The cause of contamination was thought to be an employee suspected of having hepatitis while preparing the product.

NORWALK VIRUS (NOROVIRUS)

One of the most common of the food-borne viral pathogens is the Norwalk virus. (*Norovirus* was recently approved as the official genus name for the group of viruses.) It is also known as SRSV (small, round, structured virus) because of its size and shape. Under the electron microscope, these virus particles look like miniature raspberries. Although a number of outbreaks have been associated with the consumption of raw shellfish, other foods such as fresh salads, coleslaw, fruits, eggs and bakery products have also been implicated.

On May 5, 2005, the Kent County Health Department (KCHD) in Michigan was notified of a gastroenteritis outbreak among employees who had attended a school staff luncheon two days earlier. Staff members were served a party-sized submarine sandwich catered by a national franchise restaurant. Eighty percent of the 29 staff members reported becoming ill with fever, abdominal cramps or nausea a day or two later. Other symptoms were severe diarrhea and vomiting. Of the six stool specimens collected, all tested positive for *Norovirus*. A study on exposure to food was conducted and although lettuce was suspected, no specific food item was significantly associated with the illness.

On May 6, 2005, there was another gastroenteritis outbreak at a publishing company staff luncheon. Party-sized submarine sandwiches were served by the same restaurant that catered the luncheon in the first outbreak. In this instance, 55 people became ill. This time the food analysis indicated that eating lettuce was significantly associated with illness. Two other foods were also associated with the illness: jalapeño peppers and onions. Fifteen of 52 ill people for whom data were available reported eating jalapeños, and 21 of 50 reported eating onions. Of the two stool specimens that were tested during this outbreak, one was positive for *norovirus*. The owner of the restaurant was contacted, and a log of other catered events was prepared.

Later the same day, KCHD learned of another outbreak through inquiries to groups identified in the same restaurant's catered event log. A social service organization that held a luncheon the day before reported that employees became sick after eating a party-sized submarine sandwich. Of 18 people who attended the luncheon, nine became ill.

Investigators discovered that a food handler employed by the restaurant had experienced vomiting and diarrhea on May 2. The food handler believed he had acquired his illness from his child, who had vomited on May 1. The child's illness was traced to an ill cousin who had been exposed to *norovirus* at a child care center. The food handler's vomiting ended by the early morning of May 3, and he returned to work at the restaurant later that morning. A stool specimen from the food handler was collected on May 10 and tested positive for *norovirus*. Further analysis was performed on the *norovirus* strains from the food handler and eight customers who had illness. All nine matched the strain identified in the previous outbreaks.[361]

ROTAVIRUS

Under high magnification in the electron microscope, these viruses look a bit like microscopic litchi fruit. They are roughly twice the size of the Norwalk virus and have been divided into three distinct groups. Group A rotavirus is found worldwide and is the leading cause of severe infant diarrhea. In the United States, it is estimated that in excess of 3 million cases of rotavirus gastroenteritis occur annually. It is the most important cause of pediatric gastroenteritis and is responsible for about one-third of all hospitalizations for diarrhea in children under five years old. This disease usually occurs during the winter months, but in the tropics it is found year-round. Group B rotavirus occurs more commonly in adults, and major epidemics have been reported in China. Group C rotavirus occurs fairly rarely and characteristically affects children.

The onset of symptoms occurs between 24 and 72 hours after exposure and usually lasts for three to eight days. It starts with vomiting and is followed by diarrhea. In severe cases, if fluids and electrolytes are not replaced, death can occur. When fatalities occur, they are generally limited to the very young or old. Although childhood mortality is low in the United States (about 100 cases per year), it is estimated that over 1 million infant deaths per year occur around the world due to this virus.

Rotaviruses are commonly transmitted through contaminated hands. Close, social groupings such as family homes, day care centers and pediatric wards serve to spread this virus rapidly. Infected food handlers can contaminate foods. If the foods do not require cooking, the virus remains viable. This is the reason why salads, fruit, sandwiches and appetizers are often implicated.

Human Influenza Virus

Although influenza is not considered a food-borne disease, food animals have been shown to play an integral role in the spread of worldwide influenza epidemics. Most global influenza pandemics are of Asian origin. The viruses responsible for these pandemics originally come from wild and domesticated ducks. Normally, the genetic arrangement of these viruses does not allow them to be freely transmitted between ducks and humans. However, the duck virus has been shown to infect pigs who can turn around and infect the humans with whom they are in contact. In other words, the pigs act as mixing bowls and can rearrange the duck influenza virus so that it can then infect humans. The common ground between pigs and duck are the fish bred through aquaculture.[362] The virus migrates steadily from the ducks to the fish to pigs and finally to humans. The results are the annual flu epidemics that move around the globe at lightning speed and make millions of people everywhere sick.

Aquaculture has a long history in many parts of Asia. In order to make complete use of all resources available, feces from both ducks and pigs are added to the ponds in order to fertilize them and improve the output of fish. Fish offals and residues are then fed back to the pigs. This fully integrated duck-fish-pig culture is extremely efficient at producing much-needed high-protein foods. However, it also dramatically increases the potential to rearrange duck influenza viruses through pigs so that humans can be infected. This form of highly integrated farming system has been very successful and is being spread throughout Asia and other developing countries. As the practice of aquaculture becomes more prevalent in the world, the potential for additional influenza pandemics will likewise increase.

BOVINE SPONGIFORM ENCEPHALOPATHY*

Bovine spongiform encephalopathy (BSE), commonly known as mad cow disease, is a fatal disease of cattle that was discovered in Britain by pathologist Carol Richardson in 1986. It manifests itself as a brain disorder and, after a period, results in death. BSE is unique in that its cause is ascribed to a little-known infectious agent called a prion. Prions are tiny particles consisting solely of protein. American neurologist S. B. Prusiner first identified and named them after he found them in the brains of sheep that had died of a disease called scrapie (from the infected animals' habit of trying to scrape the skin off their backs). Similar protein particles were then observed in other animal diseases, such as bovine spongiform encephalopathy, and in human diseases such as Creutzfeldt-Jakob disease (CJD) and kuru. Prusiner proposed that prion particles worked by coming into close contact with normal proteins of the brain membrane and then inducing them to twist into abnormal conformations. These abnormal proteins would then go on to induce other proteins to do the same and so on. This ultimately results in dramatic pathological changes in the brain leading to severe neurological disorders and death. The groundbreaking research in this field recently earned Prusiner a Nobel Prize.

The rare condition of Creutzfeldt-Jakob disease (CJD) is the human equivalent of this ailment, although no direct evidence shows that it can be transmitted via food. A similar, if not identical, disease in Papua New Guinea is called kuru. In the past, it was proposed that cannibalism and particularly the habit of eating a victim's brain was the means of its transmission. Women, who were primarily affected by kuru, traditionally ate the victims' brains while the men ate the muscle.[363]

It is generally conceded that BSE in cattle originated through a species jump from scrapie in sheep through the British practice of using rendered offals in commercial cattle feed. As a result, the traditional rendering procedures have been modified to eliminate this possibility but not before the infectious agent became very widespread throughout the British cattle herds. This situation erupted into a national disaster on March 20, 1996, when the British Government announced a suspected link between BSE and a new variation of CJD. This new variation appeared to occur in people of much younger ages than was typical for the classical CJD victim and demonstrated several distinct pathological differences from it. Beef prices dropped through the floor, and the British cattle industry faced its greatest disaster in recorded history. Within a week, the European Community declared a worldwide ban on British beef and the sale of beef in Europe dropped by more than 30 percent. The European Community requested that the British destroy millions of cattle.

Two weeks later, the World Health Organization (WHO) convened a meeting of international experts to review the public health issues

---

* Bovine spongiform encephalopathy (BSE) is not classified as a viral disease and is placed in this section simply for convenience.

associated with a possible linkage of BSE to the new variant of Creutzfeldt-Jacob disease (V-CJD). They concluded that whether a direct link occurs between BSE and V-CJD was still scientifically uncertain. However, the established jump of this infective agent between species and other circumstantial evidence suggested that exposure to BSE could be considered a likely explanation. Among the recommendations made was a global ban on the use of ruminant (sheep and cattle) tissues, in any form, for use in ruminant feeds. The total cost of this disaster in monetary terms to the British farming and meat industry soared well into the billions of dollars.

APPENDIX I
DISEASES, CAUSES
AND SYMPTOMS

BACTERIAL DISEASES		
BACTERIAL DISEASE AND RESPONSIBLE ORGANISM	CAUSE OF ILLNESS	ONSET TIMES AND TYPICAL SYMPTOMS
Bacillus cereus poisoning	*Bacillus cereus* Large, heat-sensitive protein toxin	6–15 hours: watery diarrhea, cramps and abdominal pain
	Small, heat-resistant protein toxin	1/2–5 hours: vomiting and abdominal cramps
Botulism (toxin) *Clostridium botulinum*	Botulinum neurotoxin (nerve poison)	4–24 hours: muscle paralysis in head, neck, throat, chest and extremities; death by suffocation
Campylobacteriosis *Campylobacter jejuni*	Gastrointestinal infection	12–36+ hours: diarrhea, cramps, vomiting, fever and headache; possibility of septicemia and serious longer-term sequelae
Enterohemorrhagic colitis *Escherichia coli* (EHEC) e.g., O157:H7	Gastrointestinal infection causing toxin-induced bleeding	8–24+ hours: bloody diarrhea and painful abdominal cramps; hemolytic uremic syndrome (HUS); kidney failure
Enteroinvasive colitis *Escherichia coli* (EIEC)	Infective invasion of surface cells of the colon or small intestine	8–24+ hours: diarrhea, vomiting and fever
Enteropathogenic colitis *Escherichia coli* (EPEC)	Infection damaging inner surface of the intestine	6–24+ hours: diarrhea, cramps and dehydration
Enterotoxigenic colitis *Escherichia coli* (ETEC)	Toxins that interfere with the water- and electrolyte-absorbing mechanisms of the intestine	6–24+ hours: diarrhea, cramps, severe dehydration; a major cause of infant diarrheal deaths in developing countries

BACTERIAL DISEASE AND RESPONSIBLE ORGANISM	CAUSE OF ILLNESS	ONSET TIMES AND TYPICAL SYMPTOMS
Helicobacter stomach ulcers *Helicobacter pylori*	Thought to be an autoimmune response to *Helicobacter* invasion in stomach lining	Long term: stomach ulcers and increased risk of stomach cancer
Listeriosis *Listeria monocyogenes*	Infections in various organs and nervous system	24+ hours: abortions, meningitis, encephalitis and death; strikes at individuals with low immune responses
Perfringens food poisoning *Clostridium perfringens*	Toxicoinfection of intestine	8–12 hours: intense stomachache, diarrhea and dehydration
Salmonellosis *Salmonella* spp.	Gastrointestinal infection	8–24 hours: diarrhea, dehydration, fever, vomiting, headache and abdominal cramps; possibility of septicemia
Shigellosis *Shigella* spp.	Gastrointestinal infection causing toxin-induced bleeding	12–36+ hours: extremely harsh form of bloody diarrhea (dysentery), abdominal cramps and dehydration
Staphylococcus poisoning *Staphylococcus aureus*	Toxin	1/2–6 hours: intense nausea, vomiting, cramps and diarrhea
Streptococcus infection *Streptococcus* spp.	Group A: *Streptococcus pyogenes* infection	24–72 hours: sore throat, swallowing pain, tonsillitis, fever and headache
	Group D: other *Streptococcus* spp. toxiconinfection	2–36 hours: diarrhea, vomiting, abdominal cramps, fever and dizziness
Vibrio infection *Vibrio* spp.	Gastrointestinal infection	1–12 hours: vomiting, severe diarrhea, thirst, cramps, weakness and, if not quickly and properly treated, death
Yersiniosis *Yersinia* spp.	Gastrointestinal infection	6–24 hours: intense abdominal pain, diarrhea, headache and nausea

FUNGAL DISEASES		
BACTERIAL DISEASE AND RESPONSIBLE ORGANISM	CAUSE OF ILLNESS	ONSET TIMES AND TYPICAL SYMPTOMS
MOLDS		
Aflatoxicosis *Aspergillus flavus*	Potent aflatoxin	Acute short term: high fever, jaundice, edema, vomiting, pain and enlarged livers. Chronic long term: cirrhosis and cancer of the liver
Aleukia *Fusarium* spp.	Mold toxin	Long term: alimentary toxic aleukia, vomiting, gastroenteritis and throat inflammation, shrinkage of the bone marrow, pulmonary hemorrhages and death
Ergotism (St. Anthony's Fire) *Claviceps purpurea*	Toxin in infected rye	Long term: intense muscular pain, gangrene and death
MUSHROOMS		
Amatoxicosis *Amanita* spp.	Amatoxin	Long onset time: then sudden severe abdominal pains, vomiting, diarrhea, restricted urine flow and death
Muscimol toxicosis fly agaric and panthercap mushrooms	Muscimol toxin	Rapid onset: tiredness, dizziness, abdominal pain, delirium and occasionally death
Psilocybin toxicosis Psylocybe mushroom	Intentional intoxication for perception alteration	Rapid onset: hallucinations and occasionally death

PARASITIC DISEASES

PARASITIC DISEASE AND RESPONSIBLE ORGANISM	CAUSE OF ILLNESS	ONSET TIMES AND TYPICAL SYMPTOMS
ROUNDWORMS		
Anisakid infection *Anisakis simplex*	Worm infection from consumption of raw, infected fish	Long term: fever and acute abdominal pains; inflamed stomach tissue
Ascaris infection *Ascaris lumbricoides*	Worm infection from consumption of contaminated raw vegetables or meat	Long term: abdominal pain, vomiting, nausea, possibility of severe general tissue damage and occasionally death
Trichinosis *Trichinella spiralis*	Worm infection from consumption of contaminated meat, chiefly pork and wild game	Long term: fever and very painful and inflamed muscles; occasionally death
Trichuris infection *Trichuris trichiura*	Worm infection from consumption of contaminated raw vegetables or meat	Long term: abdominal pain, vomiting and nausea
FLUKES		
Fasciola infection *Fasciola hepatica*	Sheep liver fluke from eating infected uncooked vegetables, particularly watercress	Long term: liver obstruction, fibrosis and other liver complications
Nanophyetus infection *Nanophyetus salmincola*	Fish liver fluke infection in North America (salmon)	Long term: nausea and abdominal pain (quite rare)
Opisthorchis infection *Opisthorchis viverrini*	Freshwater fish liver fluke infection mainly in Asia	Long term: liver obstruction, fibrosis and jaundice
TAPEWORMS		
Fish tapeworm *Diphyllobothrium latum*	Ingestion of larval cysts in undercooked fish	Long term: abdominal discomfort, nervousness, loss of weight and anemia
Beef tapeworm *Taenia saginata*	Ingestion of larval cysts in undercooked beef	Long term: abdominal discomfort, nervousness and loss of weight
Pork tapeworm *Taenia solium*	Ingestion of larval cysts in undercooked pork	Long term: abdominal discomfort, nervousness, loss of weight, serious tissue damage and death

PARASITIC DISEASE AND RESPONSIBLE ORGANISM	CAUSE OF ILLNESS	ONSET TIMES AND TYPICAL SYMPTOMS
OTHER PARASITES		
Amebiasis *Entamoeba hystolytica*	Gastrointestinal infection through ingestion of parasite in raw food, particularly fruit and vegetables; also through sexual contact	48+ hours: amebic dysentery (bloody diarrhea), ulcers and intestinal blockages; can be fatal if the parasite migrates to the liver, lungs or brain
Cryptosporidiosis *Cryptosporidium parvum*	Ingestion of parasite egg cysts in water or raw food	72+ hours: severe watery diarrhea and dehydration
Cyclospora infection *Cyclospora cayetanensis*	Infection of small intestine by ingestion of parasite in raw food, particularly fruits	Longer term: watery diarrhea, loss of appetite, bloating, weight loss, stomach cramps, vomiting and fever
Giardiasis *Giardia lamblia*	Infection of small intestine by ingestion of parasite in raw food, particularly fruits and vegetables	24+ hours: diarrhea, cramps and weight loss; serious problem for travelers
Toxoplasmosis *Toxoplasma gondii*	Infection through ingestion of cysts in undercooked meat, particularly pork and wild game	Long term: attacks nervous and muscular tissue, one of the most dangerous pathogens for people infected with HIV; can be lethal in babies

TOXIC SUBSTANCES

DISEASE AND RESPONSIBLE TOXIN	CAUSE OF ILLNESS	ONSET TIMES AND TYPICAL SYMPTOMS
MARINE SOURCES		
Ciguatera poisoning	Reef fish toxin	1–4 hours: tingling of lips and tongue, numbness, nausea, vomiting and diarrhea; this is followed by headache, vertigo, paralysis, heart palpitations, respiratory paralysis and occasionally death
Puffer fish poisoning *Tetraodontidae* spp.	Tetrodotoxin neurointoxication through ingestion of fugu puffer fish	1/2–4 hours: tingling and numbness of lips, tongue, fingers and toes, as well as a tightness of the chest; sometimes accompanied by nausea, diarrhea and vomiting; death
Scombroid poisoning	Ingestion of histamine from poorly handled fish such as tuna, mackerel and barracuda	1–4 hours: nausea, vomiting, headache, difficulty swallowing and itching of the skin; rarely death
Shellfish poisoning	Ingestion of affected shellfish Amnesic shellfish poisoning (ASP)	Symptoms similar to Alzheimer's disease
	Neurotoxic shellfish poisoning (NSP)	Pallor, drowsiness, slurred speech, breathing difficulty and staring
	Paralytic shellfish poisoning (PSP)	Tingling of lips, tongue and fingertips, vomiting, nausea, paralysis, respiratory failure and death
PLANT SOURCES		
Cyanogenic glycoside poisoning	Cyanide intoxication from ingestion of cassava roots, lima beans, fava beans and the seeds of almonds, peaches and apricots	1/2–4 hours: shortness of breath, inability to absorb oxygen and death

DISEASE AND RESPONSIBLE TOXIN	CAUSE OF ILLNESS	ONSET TIMES AND TYPICAL SYMPTOMS
PLANT SOURCES		
Goitrogen poisoning	Ingestion of goitrogens from cabbages, rutabagas, rapeseed, mustard seed, brussels sprouts and cauliflower; prevents thyroid function	Long term: goiter
Hemagglutinin poisoning	Ingestion of hemagglutinins from legumes such as soybeans, lima beans, lentils, kidney beans and peanuts	Agglutination of red blood cells and death
Oxalate poisoning	Ingestion of rhubarb and sorrel	1–6 hours: ulcers of the mouth or gastrointestinal tract, gastric hemorrhaging and convulsions
Pressor amine intoxication	Ingestion of histamine, tyramine and tryptamine, particularly from cheeses	1–6 hours: nausea, vomiting, headache and itching of the skin
OTHER SOURCES		
Honey intoxication	Ingestion of grayanotoxin from affected honey	1–6 hours: weakness, dizziness, nausea, perspiration and vomiting
Solanine poisoning	Ingestion of green-tinged potatoes	1–12 hours: rare but occasional deaths

VIRUSES		
DISEASE AND RESPONSIBLE ORGANISM	CAUSE OF ILLNESS	ONSET TIMES AND TYPICAL SYMPTOMS
Hepatitis A	Infection through ingestion of a wide variety of foods	24–72 hours: fever, weakness, loss of appetite, digestive upsets and abdominal and muscular pains
Hepatitis E	Infection through ingestion of contaminated water	24–72 hours: fever, weakness, loss of appetite, digestive upsets, abdominal and muscular pains; rare in North America
Norwalk virus	Infection through ingestion of a wide variety of foods	24–72 hours: vomiting, nausea, abdominal pains and diarrhea
Rotavirus	Infection through ingestion of a wide variety of foods	24–72 hours: vomiting, diarrhea and dehydration; the most important cause of pediatric gastroenteritis
Bovine spongiform encephalitis Creutzfeldt-Jakob disease	Prion neural infection through ingestion of contaminated beef	Long term: pathological changes in the brain leading to severe neurological disorders and death

APPENDIX II
SOURCES OF INFORMATION
ABOUT FOOD-BORNE DISEASES

As a result of the growing importance of food-borne diseases, there is no lack of information about the subject. Unfortunately, although many technical texts discuss the issue, very few books are available for the layperson. As a result, the most comprehensive and up-to-date source of information for consumers (and professionals) is the Internet. Literally hundreds of sites carry information related to food and food-borne diseases. However, as most people who have used the Internet know, because no controls are placed upon the material that appears online, the quality and honesty of the information can be a problem. Nevertheless, a sufficient number of reliable and reputable sites is available to ensure that consumers have access to the latest information about the subject of food-borne diseases.

Generally speaking, Internet sites related to food-borne diseases fall into a limited number of categories such as government, university/academic, industrial or professional association, consumer association and private sites. Several well-designed and informative government sites are prepared courtesy of your tax dollars. These include Web sites from the United States Department of Agriculture, the Food and Drug Administration, the Centers for Disease Control and Prevention, the National Agricultural and Medical Libraries and even the United States Department of Commerce. In addition, government agencies have worked together with universities and other institutions to develop joint Web sites that provide an even wider range of coverage. A major advantage of these sites is that consumers can usually communicate with the site for specific inquiries via e-mail. In addition, most of these sites are equipped with excellent subject search capabilities so that consumers can seek out particular information.

University sites take advantage of the wealth of information and academic resources they embody. Since universities were among the very first users of the Internet, their sites are generally well designed and informative. Many of these sites make an effort to reach the public and, as a result, the technical jargon is limited. Few of these sites have subject search capabilities. The limited resources available at universities make reaching anyone to ask specific questions difficult.

Among the most professional-looking and animated Web sites are those of professional or industrial associations. These organizations are usually well funded and very public relations oriented, as their sites demonstrate. Some of these sites have subject search capabilities. They are usually accessible through e-mail to answer specific questions. One of the problems is that these sites cater to professionals as well as to consumers, so the amount of general material for the public may be limited. Another problem is that they generally represent certain industries or professions, so the information presented may have a particular bias or spin.

A number of Internet sites represent consumer advocacy groups. These sites can be very informative and often have links to specific sites so that consumers can get additional information about the issues. The material is generally presented in a lively and animated manner. In fact, the information is occasionally somewhat sensationalist in order to emphasize a particular position. A bonus with these Internet locations is that they usually have links to a very wide range of consumer information and services. Unfortunately, the amount of information they present about the issue of food-borne diseases is rather limited. They seem to have a preference for issues such as additives and labeling and may therefore be omitting a major contemporary consumer concern. These sites usually have subject search capabilities. They almost always have e-mail communication services because, in addition to answering specific questions, advocacy groups can use this facility to increase their membership.

Finally, a great number of private commercial and noncommercial sites are on the Internet. Since these often reflect the particular interests of creative individuals, they can be extraordinarily inventive. In fact, most large corporations can learn much about communication, presentation and public relations from these individuals. However, consumers must treat the information posted on these sites with a certain degree of discrimination because they often represent particular views or opinions. With some sites, the goal is clearly to induce the consumer to buy goods or services of some type. In other cases, the sites may represent a discrete introduction to one religious group or another. These sites can be very informative. However, consumers must be prepared to distinguish between fact and opinion and avoid the traps that these locations can occasionally present.

The following list of sites is far from complete but should provide a solid entry for those seeking additional information about food-borne diseases. For individuals who do not have direct Internet access, many public libraries provide this service free to members. The ratings given for the sites are purely subjective and reflect nothing more than my own opinion about their value in providing consumers with information about food-borne diseases. Don't forget that web addresses change frequently, so be prepared to look up the site in your favorite search engine.

GOVERNMENT-RELATED SITES

The National Food Safety Database (NFSD)

Internet address: http://www.foodsafety.gov
Subject search: √ E-mail: √
Overall rating: *****

This location is a joint venture between the University of Florida and the United States Department of Agriculture. It is one of the most informative food safety sites on the Internet. The goal of the National Food Safety Database is to provide consumers, industry and public health officials with a highly informative, effective and accurate Web site that will provide one-stop shopping for food safety information.

This site provides the latest information about subjects of current controversy in a section called "Critical Issues in Food Safety." This includes recently published disease outbreaks at home and abroad as well as the latest reports about major food safety issues concerning consumers. In order to provide comprehensive coverage about past issues, it includes a link to previous archived reports as well as an important link to accounts of food products recalled because of food safety concerns.

Another section of this excellent site is simply entitled "Other Items of Interest." It features a broader spectrum of issues such as the influence of household pets on health, general food safety in the home, television programs related to health and the latest food safety-related news stories. It also includes a useful link to previously posted archives of this section.

Finally, another section contains direct links to other major sites around the world devoted to the issue of food safety. All the sites listed are trustworthy, and their quality and reliability rate highly. This is important for anyone looking for authoritative information about the subject. This section is divided into two sections, "Other Sites with Critical Issues" and "Other Food Safety Related Sites on the Web." This latter section is extensive and extremely helpful for anyone seeking to search issues in depth.

The Food Safety and Inspection Service of the United States Department of Agriculture (FSIS)

Internet address: http://www.fsis.usda.gov
Subject search: √ E-mail: √ Phone/Fax: √
Overall rating: *****

Food Safety and Inspection Service
Room 1175-South Building
1400 Independence Ave, SW
Washington, D.C. 20250
Tel: (202) 720-7943
Fax: (202) 720-1843

The Food Safety and Inspection Service of the USDA is responsible for ensuring that the nation's commercial food supply is safe. This site represents their comprehensive involvement in the issue of food-borne diseases. Its accessibility by phone or fax reflects that it is one of the best locations for direct follow-up consumer information.

This site is frequently updated with the latest information and features the vast selection of food safety publications about a great many common foods. Several bulletins contain practical hints about food prep-aration and avoiding hazards in the home. It even has a section about coping with food complications that arise from natural disaster situations such as fires, floods, tornadoes and others.

This really is one of the most practical, if not animated, sites on the Internet. It is comprehensive and authoritative and reflects the tremen-dous effort made to provide consumers with information. In the past, this information was there, but it was not as readily accessible as it is now on the Internet. Unfortunately, this location has very limited information about fruits and vegetables and has limited links to other sites. However, for anyone interested in the issue of food safety, this is a prime address.

The Center for Food Safety and Applied Nutrition of the Food and Drug Administration (CFSAN)

Internet address: http://www.cfsan.fda.gov/
Subject search: √ E-mail: √ Phone/Fax: —
Overall rating: *****

CFSAN
200 C St.
Washington, D.C. 20204
Tel: 1-800-FDA-4010
Fax: (301) 443-9057

The Center for Food Safety and Applied Nutrition is another excellent government site. It is a product of the Food and Drug Administration and, in addition to food-borne disease, has an extensive range of other food safety-related topics. This site has extensive subject search capabilities and an excellent section of food safety questions and answers of greatest interest to consumers. In addition, consumers may contact them directly by e-mail for any information not specifically available on the site.

In the area about "Food-borne Illness," sections are devoted to con-sumer information, food-borne pathogens and natural toxins (the superb Bad Bug Book), specific product safety and links to other sources of food safety and regulatory information. It also contains a very comprehensive list of links to other government sites and non-U.S. government sources of information about food safety and nutrition at home and around the world.

An important area entitled "Food Safety Advice for Persons with AIDS" is very useful for all individuals who are permanently or tem-porarily immunocompromised. It provides information about the rela-tionship between pathogenic bacteria and food poisoning, what to look for when shopping for foods, how to prepare foods in the home and the precautions to take while traveling. There is even an area on the CFSAN site with a complete quiz for safe kitchen practices. Finally, it includes a list of links to other related sites that are trustworthy and reliable.

The Centers for Disease Control and Prevention (CDC)

Internet address: http://www.cdc.gov/
Subject search: √ E-mail: √ Phone/Fax: √
Overall rating: *****

Centers for Disease Control and Prevention
1600 Clifton Rd., NE
Atlanta, GA 30333 USA
Tel: (404) 639-3311

As the title of this homepage indicates, the Centers for Disease Control
and Prevention is the nation's official disease prevention agency. With little doubt, this Web site offers the most comprehensive information about
the subject of food-borne diseases in the world. However, much of this
data is designed for professionals rather than for consumers. Nevertheless, consumers cannot find a better source of in-depth information about
food-borne diseases, and a great deal of it is easily understandable.

This site has links to the CDC's major publication series, the *Morbidity
and Mortality Weekly Report* or *MMWR,* which lists a wide range of disease
outbreaks including those of food-borne origin. The site also has sections
about *MMWR Recommendations and Reports, Summaries of Notifiable Diseases*
and other publications. The site also contains excellent sections about
general health information and travelers' health.

Most importantly, this location includes an area for The National
Center for Infectious Diseases located at http://www.cdc.gov/ncidod/dis
eases/food/index.htm. This site is devoted to food-borne diseases—few
sites are better than this for anyone interested in food-borne diseases.

"The Division of Bacterial and Mycotic Diseases" is almost exclusively
devoted to food-borne diseases and has many links to outside institutions dealing with this issue. The range of information about infectious
diseases available on this site is extraordinary. All in all, this is one of the
most useful sites about food-borne disease on the Internet.

The Food and Nutrition Information Center

Internet address: http://fnic.nal.usda.gov/
Subject search: √ E-mail: √ Phone/Fax: √
Overall rating: ***

Food and Nutrition Information Center
Agricultural Research Service, USDA
National Agricultural Library, Room 304
10301 Baltimore Avenue
Beltsville, MD 20705-2351
Tel: (301) 504-5719
Fax: (301) 504-6409

This site is the product of the National Agricultural Library of the United States Department of Agriculture. It really specializes in nutrition information but can be of some value for those seeking information about foodborne diseases. Of greater interest is the "USDA/FDA Foodborne Illness Education Information Center" located at http://www.nal.usda.gov/fnic/foodborne/fbindex/. This site has links to its various publications and to other related national and international sites.

The Medical Matrix

Internet address: http://www.medmatrix.org/
Subject search: √ E-mail: — Phone/Fax: —
Overall rating: **

This site is not really designed for consumers but rather for physicians and health care workers. This is a well-edited and reviewed site that categorizes its information resources according to specific technical criteria. Despite its professional bias, this site does contain material of interest to the layperson, because it does access articles from a wide range of sources including newspapers. A great many useful links are accessible from this page.

The National Technical Information Service
Health and Safety Page

Internet address: http://www.ntis.gov
Subject search: √ E-mail: √ Phone/Fax: —
Overall rating: *

This site is prepared by the U.S. Department of Commerce Technology Administration. It provides up-to-date information about federal publications pertaining to a range of health-related issues. It is of limited use to the average consumer but does contain references to health legislation materials.

Department for Environment, Food and Rural Affairs, U.K.

Internet address: http://www.defra.gov.uk
Subject search: √ E-mail: — Phone/Fax: —
Overall rating: *

United Kingdom
Tel: 011(645)33-55-77

Defra is the British equivalent of the USDA. Naturally, this site highlights issues of particular interest to the United Kingdom, such as bovine spongiform encephalopathy (BSE) and *Salmonella enteritidis* in eggs.

The World Health Organization (WHO)

Internet address: http://www.who.int/en/
Subject search: √ E-mail: √ Phone/Fax: —
Overall rating: ***

WHO
Avenue Appia, 20
1211 Geneva 27, Switzerland
Tel: 011(4122) 791-2111
Fax: 011(4122) 791-0746

This is the Web site of the Geneva-based World Health Organization. Despite its priority role in international public health and its close link to national health institutions, the WHO Food Safety Unit has managed to prepare a site of value and interest to consumers around the world. It contains general articles about food safety, a guide for travelers and the "WHO Golden Rules for Safe Food Preparation." This site has an extensive range of links to food safety sites around the world, which allows the searcher to become aware of a much broader range of international opinions about this subject. This site is well worth a visit.

Other international sites well worth a visit are Canada's FoodNet (http://foodnet.fic.ca) and Australia's Commonwealth Scientific and Industrial Research Organization (http://www.dfst.csiro.au/) Web pages.

UNIVERSITY-RELATED SITES

The number of university-related sites are unlimited because every university with a department of food science has a page on the Internet. These sites usually do not have unique information regarding food-borne diseases but can be valuable because they have become quite responsive to the need for public education in this area. Only one site has been listed as an example. No doubt, many more comprehensive and larger university sites are on the Internet. It is best to use your favorite search engine with keywords such as "food-borne," "foodborne," "food poisoning," "toxins," and so forth.

Utah State University Extension

Internet address: http://extension.usu.edu/
Subject search: √ E-mail: √ Phone/Fax: —
Overall rating: ***

This is a rather simple Web site that has links to a great many practical publications available through its http://extension.usu.edu/htm/publications Web page. It also has links to other useful sites.

INDUSTRIAL AND PROFESSIONAL ASSOCIATION SITES

The Partnership for Food Safety Education (Fight BAC!)

Internet address: http://www.fightbac.org
Subject search: — E-mail: — Phone/Fax: —
Overall rating: ****

Partnership for Food Safety Education
800 Connecticut Avenue, NW, Suite 500
Washington, D.C. 20006-2701
Tel: (202) 429-8273

The Partnership for Food Safety Education is a partnership organization composed of leading food and beverage associations, the federal
government and consumer-oriented groups to promote the circulation of
educational information about food safety. This is a very interesting and
comprehensive site, which has very many links to other key Web pages.
It also provides considerable information about hygiene and sanitation
on-site and is regularly updated.

The Food Marketing Institute (FMI)

Internet address: http://www.fmi.org
Subject search: √ E-mail: √ Phone/Fax: √
Overall rating: ****

Food Marketing Institute
2345 Crysta Drive, Suite 800
Arlington, VA 22202
Tel: (202) 452-8444

An excellent site representing the supermarket industry. A lot of interesting information and the very best information available for routine home
storage and handling of a wide variety of foods. It is regularly updated.

The International Food Information Council

Internet address: http://ific.org
Subject search: √ E-mail: √
Overall rating: **

International Food Information Council
1100 Connecticut Ave., NW, Suite 430
Washington, D.C. 20036

The International Food Information Council is an organization supported
by leading food and beverage corporations to promote the dissemination
of technical information about food safety and nutrition. In addition to

food safety and food-borne illness, areas are devoted to labeling, food regulations, additives, biotechnology, nutrition and other issues. This is a comprehensive site but provides little in addition to the above-mentioned Web pages.

The Institute of Food Science and Technology (IFST) U.K.

Internet address: http://www.ifst.org
Subject search: √ E-mail: √ Phone/Fax: —
Overall rating: ****

Institute of Food Science and Technology
5 Cambridgecourt
210 Shepherd's Bush Road
London W6 7NJ, United Kingdom
Tel: 011(44)171-603-6316
Fax: 011(44)171-602-9936

Although this is the site of a professional association, it has much useful information for consumers, particularly in the area of food-borne diseases. It also has an excellent section entitled "Current Hot Topics" written in a manner to attract journalists. This may be a site specifically designed for British audiences, but it is certainly worth a visit.

Other sites in this category include the Web pages of the American Medical Association (http://www.ama-assn.org/) and Science Online from the American Association for the Advancement of Science (http://www. sciencemag.org/).

CONSUMER ADVOCATE SITES

The Center for Science in the Public Interest

Internet address: http://www.cspinet.org/
Subject search: √ E-mail: √ Phone/Fax: —
Overall rating: ***

CSPI
1875 Connecticut Ave., NW, Suite 300
Washington, D.C. 20009
Tel: (202) 332-9110
Fax: (202) 265-4954

Although this consumer organization focuses on the subjects of food safety and nutrition, food-borne diseases do not appear to be a major preoccupation. This site has a tendency to concentrate on food additives and to sensationalize certain aspects of diet and nutrition. It is unfortunate that an organization with close to 1 million subscribers does not place more stress on the issue of food-borne diseases.

The Consumer World Site

Internet address: http://www.consumerworld.org/
Subject search: √ E-mail: √ Phone/Fax: —
Overall rating: *

Actually, I have not found any information about food-borne diseases on this page. However, it has so many other consumer-related connections that it is worth anyone's time to pay a short visit.

PRIVATE COMMERCIAL AND NONCOMMERCIAL SITES

Infectious Disease News

Internet address: http://www.infectiousdiseasenews.com
Subject search: — E-mail: — Phone/Fax: —
Overall rating: **

This Web site features publications by experts in the field of infectious diseases as well as proceedings from medical conferences and other research reports. The site is prepared by Slack Incorporated, a long-established publisher of health care information.

Food Science and Food Safety

Internet address: http://www.foodscience.csiro.au/food-safety.htm
Subject search: — E-mail: —
Overall rating: **

Although no original information is available on this Web site, it makes an admirable effort by establishing links to a very wide range of topics related to the subject of food science and safety. It is definitely worth a visit.

VISUAL MICROBIOLOGY SITES

These sites are not directly related to food-borne diseases per se. However, they do provide a fascinating insight into the microscopic world.

The Digital Learning Center for Microbial Ecology

Internet address: http://commtechlab.msu.edu/sites/dlc-mel/
Overall rating: **** (Great for kids—including the microbe zoo!)
Tel: (804) 296-8994

Cells Alive!

Internet address: http://www.cellsalive.com/
Overall rating: ***** (Some animated material is astonishing!)

The Nanoworld Home Page

Internet address: http://www.uq.edu.au/nanoworld/
Overall rating: ** (Excellent photographs of all things microscopic.)

Microbiology Web Sites

Internet address: http://www.accessexcellence.org/RC/microbiology.html
Overall rating: **

In conclusion, the Internet provides a wealth of information about all subjects, including food-borne diseases. However, it is incumbent upon the searcher/consumer to distinguish between reliable and deceptive information. Caveat emptor!

APPENDIX III
STORAGE CONDITIONS
FOR SELECTED FOODS

STORAGE CONDITIONS FOR SELECTED FOODS				
FOOD	PANTRY	REFRIGERATOR	FREEZER	SPECIAL COMMENTS
FRUITS AND VEGETABLES				
Apples		2–3 weeks		Best stored in crisper; wash thoroughly just before eating
Asparagus		2–3 days		Best stored in crisper
Bananas	Until almost ripe	Only after they are ripe 2 days		Protect from flies
Beans and peas, dried	1 year			Keep sealed and check occasionally for insects
Beans and peas, fresh		1–3 days		Best stored in crisper
Beets		1–2 weeks		Best stored in crisper; remove tops
Berries, fresh		1–2 days	10 months	
Cabbage		1–2 weeks		
Canned fruit, after opening		5 days		Store in sealed glass or plastic containers before placing in refrigerator
Canned tomato sauce		5 days		Store in sealed glass or plastic containers before placing into refrigerator; check for mold
Canned vegetables		2–3 days		Store in sealed glass or plastic containers before placing into refrigerator

FOOD	PANTRY	REFRIGERATOR	FREEZER	SPECIAL COMMENTS
Carrots, celery		1–2 weeks		Best stored in crisper
Cherries		2–3 days		Best stored in crisper, wash thoroughly just before eating
Corn, on cob		2–4 days		
Flour, wheat	8 months			Store in sealed containers; check occasionally for insects
Citrus fruit		1 week		
Citrus juice		5 days		
Lettuce, iceberg type		5 days		If washed and dried in spinner, 4 days; keep in crisper
Melons		1 week		
Onions		3 weeks		Keep away from moisture and light
Peaches	Until ripe	After ripe up to 1 week		
Pears		After ripe up to 1 week		
Pineapple	Until ripe	After ripe up to 1 week		
Potatoes	2 months			Keep very cool and away from moisture and light
Rice	12–24 months			Store in sealed containers; check occasionally for insects
Spices, whole and dry	12–24 months			Store in sealed containers; check occasionally for insects
Spices, ground	6–12 months			Store in sealed containers
Spinach	3–4 days			
Vegetables, frozen			10 months	

FOOD	PANTRY	REFRIGERATOR	FREEZER	SPECIAL COMMENTS
		FISH, MEAT AND POULTRY		
Bacon, opened		5 days		Keep cold (in meat keeper) and sealed
Bacon, unopened		2 weeks	2–3 months	Keep cold (in meat keeper)
Beef, steaks		2–3 days	2–4 months	Wrap thoroughly in plastic wrap before freezing
Beef, ground		1–2 days	2–3 months	Wrap thoroughly in plastic wrap before freezing
Beef, roast		3–4 days	6 months	Wrap thoroughly in plastic before freezing
Chicken		2–3 days	10 months	Should be thoroughly sealed in plastic wrap before freezing
Clams, shelled		1 day	3 months	Wrap thoroughly in plastic wrap before freezing
Clams, in shell		2 days		Check carefully before eating
Crab, in shell		2 days	8–10 months	Should be thoroughly sealed in plastic wrap before freezing
Duck		2–3 days	6 months	Should be thoroughly sealed in plastic wrap before freezing
Fish, lean (cod, flounder, sole and so on)		1–2 days	6 months	Should be thoroughly sealed in plastic wrap before freezing
Fish, fat (mackerel, salmon and bluefish)		1–2 days	3 months	Should be thoroughly sealed in plastic wrap before freezing
Ham, whole		6 days		Check color and aroma carefully before eating
Lamb		2–3 days	4 months	Should be thoroughly sealed in plastic wrap before freezing

FOOD	PANTRY	REFRIGERATOR	FREEZER	SPECIAL COMMENTS
Lobster, in shell		2 days	3 months	Should be thoroughly sealed in plastic wrap before freezing
Oysters		1–2 days		Check carefully before eating
Pork, chops		2–3 days	3–4 months	Should be thoroughly sealed in plastic wrap before freezing
Pork, ground		1–2 days	1–2 months	Should be thoroughly sealed in plastic wrap before freezing
Pork, roast		2–4 days	4–6 months	Should be thoroughly sealed in plastic wrap before freezing
Scallops		1 day	2–3 months	Should be thoroughly sealed in plastic wrap before freezing
Shrimp, fresh		1 day		Check for black shell edges
Shrimp, frozen			12 months	
Turkey		2–3 days	6–8 months	Should be thoroughly sealed in plastic wrap before freezing
Veal, chops		2–3 days	3–4 months	Should be thoroughly sealed in plastic wrap before freezing
Veal, ground		1–2 days	2–3 months	Should be thoroughly sealed in plastic wrap before freezing
Venison and game			8–12 months	Check for arrowheads, bullets and buckshot

GLOSSARY

abdomen The part of the body that extends between the thorax and the pelvis and encloses the stomach, intestines and other internal organs.

abscess A localized collection of pus in part of the body, formed by tissue damage and usually inflamed.

aerobic organism An organism that can live or occur only in the presence of oxygen.

aflatoxin A toxic compound produced by the mold *Aspergillus flavus*. It contaminates stored foods such as grains and nuts.

AIDS Acquired immune deficiency syndrome. A severe immunologic disorder caused by the HIV virus. It results in a defective immune response and increased susceptibility to infections and cancers.

aleukia A toxic and often fatal mold disease caused by *Fusarium fungus,* which attacks grain. See ALIMENTARY TOXIC ALEUKIA.

alimentary toxic aleukia Pathological changes in the blood production and maintenance system reflected by a complete shrinkage of the bone marrow caused by the toxic mold *Fusarium.*

amatoxin A toxin produced by various mushrooms of the genus *Amanita,* many of which are extremely poisonous.

amebiasis An intestinal infection caused by amebas, in particular *Entamoeba histolytica.*

anaerobic organism An organism that can live or occur in the absence of atmospheric oxygen.

aneurysm A localized dilation of a blood vessel caused by a weakening of the vessel's wall.

animalcules Name given by van Leeuwenhoek to the living microscopic organisms he observed.

anisakid A parasitic roundworm that originates in fish.

ankylosing spondylitis The stiffening and immobility of joints as the result of disease, surgery or abnormal bone fusion.

anthrax A fatal disease of cattle and sheep caused by the anthrax bacillus.

antibiotic A metabolic substance, usually produced by microorganisms, that can inhibit the growth and infection of other microorganisms.

antibody A protein substance produced in response to a specific antigen, such as a bacterium or a toxin.

antigen A substance such as toxins, bacteria, foreign cells and cells of transplanted organs that, when introduced into the body, stimulates the production of an antibody.

antitoxin An agent capable of neutralizing a specific toxin (usually of biological origin).

appendicitis A severe inflammation of the appendix.

arthritis A chronic condition characterized by stiffness and inflammation of the bone joints, pain, loss of mobility and flexibility, weakness and deformity.

arthritis (reactive type) An inflammatory arthritic condition that occurs in the joints in response to the presence of bacterial antigens even though the bacteria themselves are not present.

Ascaris   A nematode roundworm of the family Ascaridae, exemplified by the intestinal parasite, *Ascaris lumbricoides.*

bacillus   A bacterium characterized by a rod-like shape.

Bacillus cereus   A large, rod-shaped Gram-positive, spore-forming bacteria.

Bacillus enteritidis   The original name for salmonella.

bacteria   Unicellular microorganisms that vary in terms of structure, nutritional requirements and mobility. They may be capable of causing diseases in plants and animals.

bacteria—Gram-negative Bacteria that cannot absorb a deep blue dye (gentian violet) when stained.

bacteria—Gram-positive Bacteria that can absorb a deep blue dye (gentian violet) when stained.

black plague   A variety of bubonic plague characterized by the dark splotches it causes on the skin of its victims. It was caused by the bacteria *Pasturella* (or *Yersinia*) *pestis* and was prevalent throughout Europe and Asia in the 14th century.

blood poisoning   A disease caused by pathogenic microorganisms in the circulatory system (septicemia).

botulism   A lethal form of food poisoning due to the ingestion of a food or beverage contaminated with botulinum toxin produced by *Clostridium botulinum.*

botulism toxin   A powerful bacterial toxin that affects the central nervous system and causes difficulty in swallowing and paralysis of the respiratory muscles, suffocation and death.

bovine spongiform encephalopathy (BSE)   A degenerative brain disease of cattle characterized by a spongelike development of brain tissue (similar to Creutzfeldt-Jakob disease in humans).

bubonic plague   See BLACK PLAGUE.

Campylobacter   A bacterium commonly found in food-borne diarrhea and gastroenteritis incidents.

cephalopods   A class of marine mollusks containing the octopus, squid and cuttlefish.

cestodes   Parasitic flatworms, including the tapeworms.

cholecystitis   A gallbladder inflammation.

ciguatera toxin   A toxin found in reef fish, such as parrot fish and other species that routinely feed on poisonous algae (dinoflagellates).

cirrhosis   A chronic liver disease characterized by destruction of normal liver cells. It is caused by alcohol abuse or hepatitis infections.

claviceps   The toxin-producing mold of rye responsible for ergotism.

Clostridium botulinum   An anaerobic, rod-shaped bacterium that inhabits soils and secretes a potent neurotoxin.

Clostridium perfringens   An anaerobic, rod-shaped bacterium that causes a common toxicoinfection.

cocci   Spherical or spheroidal-shaped bacteria.

cold pasteurization   Any cold process (such as irradiation or microfiltration) that reduces the level of pathogenic or spoilage bacteria in a food product to the same degree that conventional pasteurization would in beverages.

colon   See INTESTINE, LARGE.

commensal   An organism that lives harmlessly and symbiotically with another organism.

cramps A sudden, spasmodic contraction of the intestine usually causing pain.

Creutzfeldt-Jakob disease (CJD) A degenerative brain disease characterized by a spongelike development of brain tissue. (Similar to bovine spongiform encephalopathy.)

Crohn's disease Chronic inflammation of the intestine.

crustaceans A variety of mainly aquatic arthropods, including lobsters, shrimps and crabs.

Cryptosporidium A tiny, single-celled protozoan parasite pathogenic to humans.

cyanogenic glycosides Natural compounds containing cyanide found in cassava roots, lima beans, fava beans as well as in the seeds of almonds, peaches and apricots.

Cyclospora A tiny, single-celled protozoan parasite pathogenic to humans.

cysticercosis An infection with tapeworm larvae.

dehydration An excessive loss of water from the body.

diarrhea The frequent evacuation of watery feces, usually associated with some acute form of gastrointestinal illness.

digestive enzymes The biological catalysts secreted into the digestive tract to aid in the breakdown of foods into simpler substances that could then be assimilated and used by the body.

digestive tract The conduit through which food passes where digestion and absorption take place and from which wastes are eventually eliminated. Stretching from the mouth to the anus, the tract includes the pharynx, esophagus, stomach and intestines.

dinoflagellates Mainly marine protozoans characteristically having two flagella. A chief constituent of plankton, some forms of which are responsible for toxic red tides.

Diphyllobothrium Fish tapeworm genus.

DNA The self-replicating nucleic acid that carries the cell's genetic information.

domoic acid A dinoflagellate toxin responsible for amnesic shellfish poisoning, which is very serious in elderly people and is characterized by symptoms similar to Alzheimer's disease.

duodenum See INTESTINE, SMALL.

dysentery Bloody diarrhea usually caused by microbial infection.

dysphagia Difficulty in swallowing.

edema Excessive accumulation of fluids in body tissues.

edible vaccines An antigen component biogenetically incorporated into a food to stimulate antibody production against a particular pathogen once the food is consumed.

emerging infectious diseases Infectious diseases that have greatly proliferated during the last two decades and threaten to increase in severity in the future.

encephalitis Brain and spinal chord inflammation.

encephalomyelitis See ENCEPHALITIS.

entamoeba A parasitic ameba often responsible for causing severe diarrhea or dysentery.

enteric viruses Viruses that affect the gastrointestinal system.

enterotoxin A toxin produced by a pathogenic organism that acutely affects tissues of the gastrointestinal tract.

ergotism   A toxin-induced (ergot) disease characterized by severely inflamed muscles and death. Also known as St. Anthony's Fire.

ergot toxin   A toxin produced by the mold *Claviceps purpurea*, which often infects rye and other cereals.

Escherichia coli   A common intestinal bacteria, some strains of which have recently become very virulent.

esophagus   That section of the gastrointestinal tract that stretches from the throat to the stomach.

Fasciola   A parasitic fluke usually affecting the liver.

flagella   Long, threadlike appendages usually attached to the surface of small organisms and used for locomotion.

flatworms   A variety of worms (platyhelminths), some of which are parasitic, such as tapeworms.

fluke   A variety of parasitic flatworm called trematodes.

food-borne disease   A disease resulting from a causative agent, such as a microorganism or toxin, present in consumed food.

food infection   An infection caused when pathogenic microorganisms ingested with food multiply in the gastrointestinal tract and attack tissues, resulting in disease.

food intoxication   A condition arising when a toxin present in food results in intoxication when consumed.

food irradiation   The process of preserving food through exposure to ionizing radiation.

food poisoning   A general term that includes almost all forms of serious food injury resulting in irritation and inflammation of the digestive tract.

food service industry   The restaurant and food-catering trade.

fugu fish   A variety of puffer fish whose skin and organs contain the potent poison tetrodotoxin.

fumigation   The employment of volatile sprays or fumes to control insect proliferation.

fungi   A group of primitive organisms that lack chlorophyll and vary in form from a single cell to a filamentous mass that produces spores. The group includes the molds, yeasts and mushrooms.

Fusarium   A contaminating mold in grain that can cause fatal disease (alimentary toxic aleukia).

gastric juice   The digestive fluid secreted by the stomach that consists chiefly of hydrochloric acid and digestive enzymes.

gastroenteritis   An inflammation of the stomach and/or intestines.

gastrointestinal tract   See DIGESTIVE TRACT.

geonosis   A disease resulting from a causative agent present in all natural sources, such as soil and water as well as animals.

Giardia   A flagellated pathogenic protozoan that affects the intestines of vertebrates, including humans.

goitrogens   Plant toxins found in cabbages, rutabagas, rapeseed, mustard seed, brussels sprouts and cauliflower. They act by preventing the thyroid gland from using iodine and, consequently, inhibit production of the thyroid hormones necessary for normal growth and metabolism.

grayanotoxin   A toxin found in honey derived from rhododendron nectar.

Guillain-Barré syndrome   A neural inflammation causing pain, weakness and paralysis in the extremities. It has been associated with food-borne *Campylobacter* bacteria.

HACCP   Hazard analysis of critical control points system of food control.

hantavirus   A form of virus transmitted by rodents and that causes severe enterohemorrhagic symptoms including kidney failure, internal bleeding and death.

Helicobacter pylori   The microorganism responsible for the majority of stomach ulcers found.

hemolytic uremic syndrome (HUS)   A condition where mature red blood cells are broken down faster than new ones can be produced by the bone marrow. HUS often requires kidney dialysis and blood transfusions and can result in death.

hepatitis   An inflammation of the liver usually caused by an infectious agent or a toxin and manifested by symptoms of liver enlargement, jaundice and abdominal pain.

histamine   A natural metabolite originating from the amino acid histidine. When tissues are injured or come under stress from antibodies, histamine is released from certain cells and causes edema (swelling of tissue), hives and itching.

histidine   An essential amino acid.

honey intoxication   See GRAYANOTOXIN.

immune system   The body's complex system of organs, tissues, specialized cells and metabolites that has evolved to combat intrusive challenges such as allergens, toxic substances and pathogenic microorganisms.

immunocompromised   The condition that results when the body's immune system has a reduced effectiveness.

infection   Multiplication of pathogenic organisms in the body leading to fever and disease.

infective dose   The number of organisms required to cause a disease incident.

intestine, large   Also referred to as the colon. This section of the intestine follows the small intestine and is considerably wider but much shorter. This is whereall of the excess water and salts used in the digestion process are absorbed so they can be recycled for the body's reuse.

intestine, small   Also referred to as the duodenum. The narrow but long (20-foot) section of the intestine running from the stomach to the cecum. Here is where the liver, the pancreas and the gallbladder combine to inject digestive fluid (bile and pancreatic juice) that neutralizes the stomach acid and breaks down all those components of the food that the stomach was unable to digest. Nutrient absorption begins here.

irradiation   See FOOD IRRADIATION.

kuru   A neurological disorder, similar to Creutzfeldt-Jakob disease, found in certain tribes of New Guinea and originally thought to be transmitted by cannibalism.

lactobacilli   Bacteria capable of actively fermenting the sugar lactose.

Listeria monocytogenes   A food-borne bacteria particularly dangerous to people with weakened immune systems.

macrophages   Any of the large phagocytic cells of the immune system.

mad cow disease   See BOVINE SPONGIFORM ENCEPHALOPATHY (BSE).

mastitis   An inflammation of a cow's udder usually arising from a bacterial infection.

meningitis   An inflammation of the meninges (membranes) of the brain and the spinal cord caused by a bacterial or viral infection.

microorganism   An organism of microscopic or submicroscopic size such as a bacterium or a protozoan.

minimally processed foods   Foods processed by a variety of mild techniques designed to keep highest product eating quality.

mold   See FUNGI.

mollusks   Invertebrates (usually marine) having a soft body protected by a hard shell, such as edible shellfish and snails.

mucosal immunity   The production of antibodies in the saliva and the other secretions that coat the surfaces of the respiratory, gastrointestinal and urinary tracts in order to defend against organisms invading through open surfaces.

muscimol toxin   A potent neurotoxin produced by mushrooms.

mutations   A genetic change in an organism that results in the creation of a new feature or trait.

mycotoxin   Any toxin produced by a fungus.

nausea   A sensation of sickness in the stomach and chest accompanied by the urge to vomit.

necrotic enteritis   Inflammation of the intestinal tract accompanied by significant tissue injury.

nematode   A roundworm having an unsegmented, cylindrical body, including parasitic forms such as ascaris and the hookworm.

neurocysticercosis   A condition where pork tapeworm embryos burrow their way into neural tissue.

neurotoxic shellfish poisoning   Shellfish poisoning originating from dinoflagellate planktonic blooms and resulting in severe neurological disorders.

neurotoxin   Any toxin that damages nervous tissue.

night soil   A euphemism for human feces used as fertilizer.

norepinephrine   A natural substance secreted by the adrenal gland that causes blood vessel constriction and increases blood pressure.

Norwalk virus   A common food-borne virus, also known as SRSV (small, round,structured virus) because of its size and shape.

nucleus   A membrane-bound, central structure within a cell that contains the cell's DNA and plays a dominant role controlling metabolic functions.

ohmic heating   A process where an electric current is passed through the food product, and the solid materials heat up faster than the surrounding fluid so that the final temperatures required to kill or inhibit bacteria are reached with less heat treatment.

oocysts   A type of parasite egg.

Opisthorchis   A trematode parasite that infects fish.

pandemic   An epidemic spread over a very wide geographic area.

paralytic shellfish poisoning   Shellfish poisoning originating from dinoflagellate planktonic blooms resulting in severe disorders including tingling of lips, vomiting, nausea, paralysis, respiratory failure and death.

parasites   Any organism that infects another host organism without contributing to the host's survival.

pasteurization   The process of destroying most spoilage and pathogenic micro-organisms in certain beverages or foods without changing the basic nature of the food. This process may or may not require heat treatment.

pathogen   A disease-causing microorganism.

phocanema   A parasitic roundworm that infects fish and can be transmitted to humans.

plague   An epidemic outbreak of disease.

plasmids   Bacterial cell components that contain nonchromosomal DNA capable of coding for virulence or resistance characteristics. Bacteria are able to transfer plasmids among one another.

pressor amines   Compounds found in certain cheeses, animal tissues and plants. They include potent biochemicals such as histamine, tyramine and tryptamine. They cause nausea, vomiting, headaches and increases in blood pressure.

prion   Tiny protein particles considered responsible for the spongiform enceph-alopathies, such as BSE and Creutzfeldt-Jakob disease.

protozoa   Single-celled organisms with a clearly defined nucleus, such as an ameba.

psilocybin toxin   A hallucinogenic toxin from the psylocybe species of mushroom.

psoriasis   An inflammatory skin condition with unsightly red patches on the skin.

ricin   A poisonous toxin from castor beans.

risk assessment   Evaluating relative degrees of risk.

rotavirus   A spherical virus that is a common cause of gastroenteritis.

roundworm   See NEMATODE.

St. Anthony's Fire   See ERGOTISM.

salmonella   Gram-negative, rod-shaped microorganisms of the genus *Salmonella* that generally have flagella. A very common cause of food-borne disease outbreaks.

scombroid poisoning   A poison that develops in tuna and mackerel that have not been quickly refrigerated or cooked right after being caught. It is due to the bacterial breakdown of the amino acid histidine.

scrapie   A degenerative brain disease of sheep characterized by their habit of scraping themselves against fences (similar to BSE in cattle).

sepsis   The occurrence of pathogenic organisms in the blood.

septicemia   Blood infection.

sequelae   Long-term secondary sequences of a disease incident.

shigella   A small, Gram-negative bacillus that is highly virulent and often asso-ciated with dysentery.

spontaneous generation   The theory describing the spontaneous generation of life from inanimate matter.

staphylococcal enterotoxin   A heat-resistant toxin of staphylococcus bacteria and responsible for acute food poisoning.

streptococcus   A small, round, Gram-positive bacteria of the genus *Steptococcus* that usually appears like a chain of miniature beads under the microscope. Some species are responsible for food-borne illness.

superantigens   Toxins that can trigger massive immune or autoimmune responses.

symbiosis A mutually beneficial close association between two or more different organisms.

Taenia A genus of flatworm including tapeworms.

Tapeworm A parasitic ribbon-like flatworm that inhabits the intestinal tract.

tetrodotoxin A very toxic poison concentrated in the liver, gonads, skin and intestines of certain varieties of puffer fish.

toxin Poison.

toxoplasma A tiny food-borne protozoan parasite that can attack nervous and muscular tissue.

transduction The exchange of bacterial genetic material that employs viruses to interchange DNA between bacteria.

transformation The exchange of DNA among bacterial chromosomes.

transposons Specific sections of chromosomal DNA that can jump into plasmids or other chromosomes.

traveler's diarrhea The most common syndrome faced by tourists. This is typically characterized by frequent loose bowel movements often accompanied by cramps, urgency, bloating, nausea and prostration. It can result from any number of infectious organisms to which insufficient resistance has been developed.

trematode Flatworms.

Trichinella A genus of small, parasitic roundworms whose larvae can become encysted in muscles.

Trichuris An intestinal roundworm.

tyramine A potent biochemical found in some cheeses. It can have a strong effect on blood pressure.

ulcers Lesions of the lining of the stomach.

ultrahigh temperature (UHT) A modern method of pasteurization employing higher processing temperatures for shorter periods of treatment.

Vibrio Small, curved or comma-shaped Gram-negative rods responsible for several serious food-borne diseases.

virus A submicroscopic parasite that usually consists of DNA (or RNA) surrounded by a protein layer.

vomiting The sudden and powerful expelling of stomach and intestinal contents up through the mouth.

Yersinia enterocolitica A small, rod-shaped, Gram-negative bacterium that can cause severe abdominal pain, diarrhea, headaches and nausea.

REFERENCES

1. Grivetti, L. E., and R. M. Pangborn, "Origin of Selected Old Testament Dietary Prohibitions," *Journal of the American Dietary Association,* 65, no. 12 (1974): 634.

2. Morrey, C. B., *The Fundamentals of Bacteriology* (Philadelphia: Lea and Febiger, 1921).

3. Fracastoro, G., *De Contagione et Contagiosis Morbis et eorurn Curatione* (1546).

4. Bacon, F., *The First Book of Francis Bacon of the Proficiency and Advancement of Learning, Divine and Human, to the King* (London: A. Millar, 1753).

5. De Kruif, P., *Microbe Hunters* (New York: Blue Ribbon Books, 1926).

6. Löhnis, F., *Vorrlesungen über Landwirtschaftliche Bakteriologie* (Berlin: Verlag von Gebrüder Borntraeger, 1913).

7. Thanks to Larry ten Harmsel, University of Western Michigan, "Vermeer's Letter to Anton van Leewenhoek" (1997).

8. Ford, B. J., "Found—Van Leeuwenhoek's Original Specimens," *New Scientist* 91 (July 30, 1981): 301.

9. Rogers, J., "What Leeuwenhoek Saw," *Scientific American* 246, no. 1 (1982): 79–80.

10. Vallery-Radot, R., *The Life of Pasteur* (New York: Doubleday, Page and Co., 1924).

11. Pasteur, L., *Études sur le Vin* (Paris: L'Imprimerie Impériale, 1866).

12. Rosenau, M. J., *Preventative Medicine and Hygiene* (New York: D. Appleton and Co., 1921).

13. Cutter, C., *First Book on Anatomy, Physiology, and Hygiene* (New York: Clark, Austin, Maynard & Co., 1861).

14. Council for Agricultural Science and Technology, "Foodborne Pathogens: Risks and Consequences," *CAST Task Force Report* 122 (Ames, Ia., 1994).

15. Zottola, E. A., and L. B. Smith, "The Microbiology of Foodborne Disease Outbreaks: An Update," *Journal of Food Safety* 11 (1990): 13.

16. Bean, N. H., and P. M. Griffin, "Foodborne Disease Outbreaks in the United States, 1973–1987: Pathogens, Vehicles, and Trends," *Journal of Food Protection* 53, no. 9 (1990): 804.

17. Jones. T. F., and D. E. Gerber, "Perceived Etiology of Foodborne Illness among Public Health Personnel," *Emerging Infectious Diseases* 7, no. 5 (2001).

18. Garthwright, W. E., D. L. Archer and L. E. Kvenberg, "Estimates of Incidence and Costs of Intestinal Infectious Disease in the United States," *Public Health Reports* 103, no. 2 (1988): 107.

19. Collins, J. E., "Impact of Changing Consumer Lifestyles on the Emergence/Reemergence of Foodborne. Pathogens," *Emerging Infectious Diseases* 3, no. 4 (1997): 471–479.

20. Schmidt, A. M., "Food and Drug Law: A 200 Year Perspective," *Nutrition Today* 10, no. 4 (1975): 32.

21. European Commission, "Risk Issues—Executive Summary on Food Safety," *Special Eurobarometer* (February 2006).

22. Jackson, G. J., C. F. Langford and D. L. Archer, "Control of Salmonellosis and Similar Foodborne Infections," *Food Protection* 2, no. 1 (1991): 26.
23. Hennessy, T. W., C. W. Hedberg, L. Slutsker, et al., "A National Outbreak of *Salmonella Enteritidis* Infections from Ice Cream," *New England Journal of Medicine* 334, no. 20 (1996): 1,281–1,286.
24. D'Aoust, J. Y., "*Salmonella*" in *Foodborne Bacterial Pathogens,* ed. by M. P. Doyle. (New York: Marcel Dekker, 1989): 327–445.
25. Palmer, S. R., J. E. M. Watkeys, I. Zamiri, et al., "Outbreak of Salmonella Food Poisoning Amongst Delegates at a Medical Conference," *Journal of the Royal College of Physicians of London* 24, no. 1 (1990): 26.
26. Unpublished data.
27. Blackman, M. A., and D. L. Woodland, "*In Vivo* Effects of Superantigens," *Life Sciences* 57, no. 19 (1995): 1,717–1,735.
28. Schiffenbauer, J., H. M. Johnson, E. J. Butfiloski, L. Wegrzyn and J. M. Soos, "Staphylococcal Enterotoxins Can Reactivate Experimental Allergic Encephalomyelitis," *Proceedings of the National Academy of Sciences of the United States of America* 90, no. 18 (1993): 8,543–8,546.
29. Baca-Estrada, M. E., D. K. H. Wong and K. Croitoru, "Cytotoxic Activity of V-Beta-8+ T Cells in Crohn's Disease: The Role of Bacterial Superantigens," *Clinical and Experimental Immunology* 99, no. 3 (1995): 398–403.
30. Achong, M. R., et al., *Lancet,* 2 (1977): 118.
31. Stooley, P. D., et al. *Annals of Internal Medicine* 76 (1972): 537.
32. Moss, F., et al. *Lancet* 2 (1981): 349, 407, 461.
33. Liss, R. H., and F. R. Batchelor, "Economic Evaluations of Antibiotic Use and Resistance—A Perspective: Report of Task Force 6," *Reviews of Infectious Diseases* 9, no. 3 (1987): S297–S312.
34. Yamamoto, T., P. Echeverria, P. and T. Yokota, *Journal of Infectious Diseases* 165 (1992): 744.
35. Levy, S. B., G. B. FitzGerald and A. B. Macone, "Spread of Antibiotic Resistant Plasmids from Chicken to Chicken and from Chicken to Man," *Nature* 260 (1976): 40–42.
36. Holmberg, S. D., M. T. Osterholm, K. A. Senger and M. D. Cohen, "Drug-Resistant Salmonella from Animals Fed Antimicrobials," *The New England Journal of Medicine* 311, no. 10 (1984): 617–622.
37. Spika, J. S., S. H. Waterman, G. W. Soo Hoo, et al., "Chloramphenicol Resistant Salmonella Newport Traced through Hamburger to Dairy Farm," *New England Journal of Medicine* 316, no. 10 (1987): 565–570.
38. O'Brien, T. F., J. D. Hopkins, E. S. Gilleece, et al., "Molecular Epidemiology of Antibiotic Resistance in Salmonella from Animals and Human Beings in the United States," *New England Journal of Medicine* 307, no. 1 (1982): 1–6.
39. WHO Working Group, "Antimicrobial Resistance," *Bulletin of the World Health Organization* 61, no. 3 (1983): 383–394.
40. Marshall, B. D. Petrowski, and S. B. Levy, "Inter- and Intraspecies Spread of Escherichia coli in a Farm Environment in the Absence of Antibiotic Usage," *Proceedings of the National Academy of Sciences* 87 (1990): 6,609–6,613.
41. Williams, R. D., L. D. Rollins, D. W. Pocurull, et al., *Antimicrobial Agents and Chemotherapy* 14 (1978): 710.
42. Levy, S. B., "The Challenge of Antibiotic Resistance," *Scientific American* 278, no. 3 (1998): 32–39.

43. Tacket, C. O., H. S. Mason,G. Losonsky, et al., "Human Immune Responses to a Novel Norwalk Virus Vaccine Delivered in Transgenic Potatoes," *Journal of Infectious Diseases* 182 (2000): 302–305.

44. *Science Daily,* August 19, 2004 © 1995–2007 ScienceDaily LLC. Available online. URL: http://www.sciencedaily.com/releases/2004/08/0408160015 48.htm. Accessed on January 13, 2007.

45. Garrett, L., *The Coming Plague* (New York: Penguin Books, 1994).

46. *Emerging Infectious Diseases* 1, no. 1 (Jan–March 1995).

47. World Health Organization, "Communicable Disease Prevention and Control: New, Emerging, and Re-Emerging Infectious Diseases," WHO Doc. A48/15 (February 1995): 22.

48. Käferstein, F. K., Y. Motarjermi and D. W. Bettcher, "Foodborne Disease Control: A Transnational Challenge," *Emerging Infectious Diseases* 3, no. 4 (1997): 503–510.

49. Amit X. Garg, MD, MA; Rita S. Suri, MD; Nick Barrowman, PhD; et al. "Long-term Renal Prognosis of Diarrhea-Associated Hemolytic Uremic Syndrome, a Systematic Review, Meta-analysis, and Meta-regression." *JAMA* 290 (2003): 1,360–1,370.

50. Bentham G., and I. Langford, "Climate change and the incidence of food poisoning in England and Wales," *J Biometeorol.* 39 (1995): 81–86.

51. U.S. Food and Drug Administration Center for Food Safety and Applied Nutrition, "The Food Defect Action Levels, levels of natural or unavoidable defects in foods that present no health hazards for humans." Available online. URL: http://www.cfsan.fda.gov/~dms/dalbook.html#CHPTA. Accessed January 14, 2007. See also Food, Drug, and Cosmetics Act § 402(a) (3).

52. Buchtmann, L. "Hand washing understanding and behavior by Australian consumers," *Food Safety Information Council,* © 2003. Available online. URL: http://www.foodsafety.asn.au/publications/articlesandsurveys/handwashingsurvey.cfm. Accessed January 14, 2006.

53. Daniels, R. W., "Home Food Safety," *Food Technology* 52, no. 2 (1998): 54–56.

54. NRA, "ServSafe Serving Safe Food Certification Coursebook," Education Foundation (Washington, D.C.: National Restaurant Association, 1995).

55. Palmer, S. R., J. E. M. Watkeys, I. Zamiri, et al., "Outbreak of Salmonella Food Poisoning Amongst Delegates at a Medical Conference," *Journal of the Royal College of Physicians of London* 24, no. 1 (1990): 26–29.

56. Anonymous, "Staphylococcal Food Poisoning from Turkey at a Country Club Buffet—New Mexico," *Morbidity and Mortality Weekly Report* 35, no. 46 (1986): 715–716, 721–722.

57. Anonymous, "Salmonella hadar Associated with Pet Ducklings—Connecticut, Maryland, and Pennsylvania, 1991," *Morbidity and Mortality Weekly Report* 41, no. 11 (1992): 185–187.

58. Holt, P., "Older Hens: Fasting, Eggs, and *Salmonella*," *Agricultural Research* (November 23, 1996).

59. Notermans, S., and E. H. Kampelmacher, "Attachment of Some Bacterial Strains to the Skin of Broiler Chickens," *British Poultry Science* 15 (1974): 573.

60. Lillard, H. S., "Incidence and Recovery of Salmonellae and Other Bacteria from Commercially Processed Poultry Carcasses at Selected Pre- and Post-Evisceration Steps," *Journal of Food Protection* 52, no. 2 (1989): 89.

61. Public Health Laboratory Service, "Memorandum of Evidence to the Agriculture Committee Inquiry on Salmonella in Eggs," Public Health Laboratory Service, *Microbiological Digest* 6 (1989): 1, quoted in Roberts, D., "Sources of Infection: Food," *The Lancet* 336 (1990): 859.

62. Bailey, J. S., A. C. Nelson and L. C. Blankenship, "A Comparison of an Enzyme Immunoassay, DNA Hybridization, Antibody Immobilization, and Conventional Methods for Recovery of Naturally Occurring *Salmonellae* from Processed Broiler Carcasses," *Journal of Food Protection* 54, no. 5 (1991): 354.

63. USDA Food Safety and Inspection Service, "Analysis of Salmonella Serotype Profiles, 2006." Available online. URL: http://www.fsis.usda.gov/PDF/Serotypes_Profile_Salmonella_Tables_&_Figures.pdf. Accesed January 21, 2007.

64. Altekruse S., N. Bauer, A. Chanlongbutra, et al., "*Salmonella* Enteritidis in broiler chickens, United States, 2000–2005," *Emerg. Infect. Dis.* [serial on the Internetl Dec. 2006. Available online. URL: http://www.cdc.gov/ncidod/EID/vol12no12/06-0653.htm. Accessed January 21, 2007.

65. USDA Agricultural Research Service, "Finding Solutions to *Campylobacter* in Poultry Production," *Agricultural Research Magazine*, 54, no. 2 (February, 2006). Available online. URL: http://www.ars.usda.gov/is/AR/archive/feb06/. Accessed January 21, 2007.

66. Logue, C. M., J. S. Sherwood, L. M. Elijah, et al., "The incidence of Campylobacter spp. on processed turkey from processing plants in the midwestern United States," *Journal of Applied Microbiology* 95 (2003): 234–241.

67. Nde, C. W., J. M. McEvoy, J. S. Sherwood, et al., "Cross Contamination of Turkey Carcasses by *Salmonella* Species During Defeathering," *Poult Sci* 86, no. 1, (2007): 162–167.

68. Schnepf, M., and W. E. Barbeau, "Survival of *Salmonella Typhimurium* in Roasting Chickens Cooked in a Microwave Convention Microwave and Conventional Electric Oven," *Journal of Food Safety* 9 (1989): 45–52.

69. Genigeorgis, C. A., P. Oanca and D. Dutulescu, "Prevalence of *Listeria Spp.* In Turkey Meat at the Supermarket and Slaughterhouse Level," *Journal of Food Protection* 53, no. 4 (1990): 282–288.

70. Genigeorgis, C. A., D. Dutulescu and J. F. Garayzabal, "Prevalence of *Listeria Spp.* In Poultry Meat at the Supermarket and Slaughterhouse Level," *Journal of Food Protection* 52, no. 9 (1989): 618–624, 630.

71. Reilly, W. J., G. I. Forbes, J. C. M. Sharp, et al., "Poultry-Borne Salmonellosis in Scotland," *Epidemiology and Infection* 101 (1988): 115.

72. Lapidot, M., I. Klinger, E. Eisenberg, et al., "Application of Ionizing Radiation in Israel to Produce Safe Foods and Reduce Foodborne Infections," presented at the Agricultural Research Institute Conference on Safeguarding the Food Supply Through Irradiation Processing Techniques (Orlando, Fla.: October 1992): 25–31.

73. Thayer, D. W., S. Songprasertchai and G. Boyd, "Effects of Heat and Ionizing Radiation on *Salmonella typhimuruim* in Mechanically Deboned Chicken Meat," *Journal of Food Protection* 54, no. 9 (1991): 718–724.

74. Anonymous, "Trichinosis—Maine, Alaska," *Morbidity and Mortality Weekly Report* 35, no. 3 (1986): 33–35.

75. "Bovine Spongiform Encephalopathy (BSE)," *World Health Organization Fact Sheet*, No. 113 (Geneva: WHO, March 1996).

76. Anonymous, "Epidemiological Notes and Reports Common Source Outbreaks of Trichinosis—New York City, Rhode Island," *Morbidity and Mortality Weekly Report* 31, no. 13 (1984): 161–164.

77. Anonymous, "Outbreaks of Trichinellosis Associated with Eating Cougar Jerky—Idaho, 1995," *Morbidity and Mortality Weekly Report* 45, no. 10 (1996): 205–206.

78. Carlson, G. S., "House Subcommittees Told of Effort to Improve Meat Inspection System," *Feedstuffs* 65, no. 12 (1993): 1.

79. Brody, J. E., "Why the Food You Eat May Be Hazardous to Your Health: Flaws Are Seen in Food Inspection," *New York Times* (October 5, 1993): C11.

80. Burros, M., "Agriculture Dept. Unveils Cooking Labels for Meat," *New York Times* (August 12, 1993): A 18.

81. FAO Newsroom, September 4, 2006, "Nearly half of all fish eaten today farmed, not caught." Available online. URL: http://www.fao.org/newsroom/en/news/2006/1000383/index.html. Accessed March 23. 2007.

82. Peréz-Arellano J.-L., O. P. Luzardo, A. P. Brito, et al., "Ciguatera fish poisoning, Canary Islands." *Emerg Infect Dis* (Dec. 2005). Available online. URL: http://0-www.cdc.gov.mill1.sjlibrary.org:80/ncidod/EID/vol11no 12/05-0393.htm. Accessed March 30, 2007.

83. Anonymous, "Outbreak of Type E Botulism Associated with an Uneviscerated, Salt-Cured Fish Product—New Jersey, 1992," *Morbidity and Mortality Weekly Report* 41, no. 29 (1992): 521–522.

84. Anonymous, "Epidemiologic Notes and Reports Paralytic Shellfish Poisoning—Massachusetts and Alaska, 1990," *Morbidity and Mortality Weekly Report* 40, no. 10 (1991): 157–161.

85. Anonymous, "Epidemiologic Notes and Reports Scombroid Fish Poisoning—Illinois, South Carolina," *Morbidity and Mortality Weekly Report* 38, no. 9 (1989): 140–142, 147.

86. Holt, J., D. Propes, C. Patterson, et al., "Multistate Outbreak of *Salmonella* Serotype Typhimurium Infections Associated with Drinking Unpasteurized Milk—Illinois, Indiana, Ohio, and Tennessee, 2002–2003," *Morbidity and Mortality Weekly Report* 52, no. 26 (July 4, 2003): 613–615.

87. Anonymous, "Epidemiologic Notes and Reports Multi-State Outbreak of Yersiniosis," *Morbidity and Mortality Weekly Report* 31, no. 37 (1982): 505–506.

88. Anonymous, "Epidemiologic Notes and Reports Campylobacter Outbreak Associated with Raw Milk Provided on a Dairy Tour—California," *Morbidity and Mortality Weekly Report* 35, no. 19 (1986): 311–312.

89. Olsen, S. J., M. Ying, M. F. Davis, et al., "Multidrug-resistant Salmonella Typhimurium infection from milk contaminated after pasteurization," *Emerg Infect Dis* (May 2004). Available online. URL: http://www.cdc.gov/ncidod/EID/vol10no5/03-0484.htm. Accessed March 30, 2007.

90. Anonymous, "Epidemiologic Notes and Reports Update: Milk-borne Salmonellosis—Illinois," *Morbidity and Mortality Weekly Report* 34, no. 15 (1985): 215–216.

91. Anonymous, "Epidemiologic Notes and Reports Listeriosis Outbreak Associated with Mexican-Style Cheese—California," *Morbidity and Mortality Weekly Report* 34, no. 24 (1985): 357–359.

92. Hall, C. W., and G. M. Trout, *Milk Pasteurization* (Westport, Connecticut: Avi Publishing Company, 1968).

93. Wiley, H. W., *Foods and Their Adulteration*, 3rd edition (Philadelphia: P. Blakiston's Son and Co., 1917).

94. Nduati, R. W., G. C. John, B. A. Richardson, et al., "Human Immunodeficiency Virus Type I-Infected Cells in Breast Milk: Association with Immunosuppression and Vitamin A Deficiency," *Journal of Infectious Diseases* 172, no. 6 (1995): 1,461–1,468.

95. Van De Perre, P., "Postnatal Transmission of Human Immunodeficiency Virus Type 1: The Breast-Feeding Dilemma," *American Journal of Obstetrics and Gynecology* 173, no. 2 (1995): 483–487.

96. Read, J. S., "Human Milk, Breastfeeding, and Transmission of Human Immunodeficiency Virus Type 1 in the United States," *Pediatrics* 112, no. 5 (2003): 1,196–1,205.

97. Datta, P., J. E. Embree, J. K. Kreiss, et al., "Mother-to-child transmission of human immunodeficiency virus type 1: report from the Nairobi Study," *J. Infect. Dis.* 170 (1994): 1,134–1,140.

98. Bertolli, J., M. E. St Louis, R. J. Simonds, et al., "Estimating the timing of mother-to-child transmission of human immunodeficiency virus in a breast-feeding population in Kinshasa, Zaire," *J. Infect. Dis.* 174 (1996): 722–726.

99. UNAIDS/UNICEF/WHO. "HIV and infant feeding. A review of HIV transmission through breastfeeding," Geneva, Switzerland: WHO/UNAIDS (1998). Available online. URL: http://data.unaids.org/Publications/IRC-pub03/hivmod3_en.pdf?preview=true. Accessed January 21, 2007.

100. CDC, "Possible West Nile Virus Transmission to an Infant Through Breast-Feeding—Michigan, 2002," *Morbidity and Mortality Weekly Report* 51, no. 879 (2002).

101. Riedo, F. X., R. W. Pinner, M. D. L. Tosca, et al., "A Point-Source Foodborne Listeriosis Outbreak: Documented Incubation Period and Possible Mild Illness," *Journal of Infectious Diseases* 170, no. 3 (1994): 693–696.

102. Bula, C. J., J. Bille and M. P. Glauser, "An Epidemic of Foodborne Listeriosis in Western Switzerland: Description of 57 Cases Involving Adults," *Clinical Infectious Diseases* 20, no. 1 (1995): 66–72.

103. Jensen, A., W. Frederiksen, and P. Gerner-Smidt, "Risk Factors for Listeriosis in Denmark, 1989–1990," *Scandinavian Journal of Infectious Diseases* 26, no. 2 (1994): 171–178.

104. Anonymous, "Update: Salmonella enteritidis Infections and Grade A Shell Eggs—United States," *Morbidity and Mortality Weekly Report* 37, no. 32 (1988): 490, 495–498.

105. Mishu, B., J. Koehler, L. A. Lee, et al., "Outbreaks of *Salmonella enteritidis* Infections in the United States, 1985–1991," *Journal of Infectious Diseases* 169, no. 3 (1994): 547–552.

106. Hedberg, C. W., M. J. David, K. E. White, et al., "Role of Egg Consumption in Sporadic *Salmonella Enteritidis* and *Salmonella Typhimurium* Infections in Minnesota," *Journal of Infectious Diseases,* 167, no. 1 (1993): 107–111.

107. Jones, D. R., M. T. Musgrove, A. B. Caudill, and P. A. Curtis, "Frequency of Salmonella, Campylobacter, Listeria and Enterobacteriaceae Detection in Commercially Cool Water-Washed Shell Eggs," *Journal of Food Safety* 26, no. 4, (2006): 264–274.

108. Claesson, B. E. B., N. G. Svensson, L. Gotthardsson, et al., "A Foodborne Outbreak of Group A Streptococcal Disease at a Birthday Party," *Scandinavian Journal of Infectious Diseases* 24, no. 5 (1992): 577–586.

109. Anonymous, "CDC Official Urges Consumer Advisories on Safe Produce Handling," *Food Chemical News* 38, no. 30 (1996): 22–24.

110. "Final Verdict on 2006 Spinach E. Coli Outbreak: Unknown." Available online. URL: http://www.consumeraffairs.com/news04/2007/03/e_coli_verdict.html. Accessed April 7, 2007.

111. Anonymous, "Epidemiologic Notes and Reports Multistate Outbreak of *Salmonella poona* Infections—United States and Canada, 1991," *Morbidity and Mortality Weekly Report* 40, no. 32 (1991): 549–552.

112. Anonymous, "Epidemiologic Notes and Reports Common-Source Outbreak of Giardiasis—New Mexico," *Morbidity and Mortality Weekly Report* 38, no. 23 (1989): 405–407.

113. Anonymous, "Intestinal Myiasis—Washington," *Morbidity and Mortality Weekly Report* 34, no. 10 (1985): 141–142.

114. Anonymous, "Poisoning from Elderberry Juice—California," *Morbidity and Mortality Weekly Report* 33, no. 13 (1984): 173–174.

115. Worth, R. M., "Health in Rural China: From Village to Commune," *American Journal of Hygiene* 77 (1963): 228–239.

116. Mintz, E. D., M. Hudson-Wragg, P. Mshar, et al., "Foodborne Giardiasis in a Corporate Office Setting," *Journal of Infectious Diseases* 167, no. 1 (1993): 250–253.

117. Kilgore, P. E., E. D. Belay, D. M. Hamlin, et al., "A University Outbreak of Gastroenteritis Due to a Small Round-Structured Virus: Application of Molecular Diagnostics to Identify the Etiologic Agent and Patterns of Transmission," *Journal of Infectious Diseases* 173, no. 4 (1996): 787–793.

118. Levine, W. C., R. W. Bennett, Y. Choi, et al., "Staphylococcal Food Poisoning Caused by imported Canned Mushrooms," *Journal of Infectious Diseases*, 173, no. 5 (1996): 1,263–1,267.

119. Satin, M., "The Gory That Was Greece," *Death in the Pot* (Prometheus Books, 2007).

120. The Internet Classics Archive © 1994–2000 by Daniel C. Stevenson, *The History of the Peloponnesian War by Thucydides*, translated by Richard Crawley. Available online. URL: http://classics.mit.edu/Thucydides/pelopwar.html. Accessed July 28, 2005.

121. R. Kobert, "Ueber die Pest des Thukydides," *Janus* 4 (1899): 244–299.

122. Anonymous, "Niacin Intoxication from Pumpernickel Bagels—New York," *Morbidity and Mortality Weekly Report* 32, no. 23 (1983): 305.

123. Anonymous, "Bacillus cereus—Maine," *Morbidity and Mortality Weekly Report* 35, no. 25 (1986): 408–410.

124. Anonymous, "Paprika Recall," *International Food Safety News* 2, no. 9 (1993): 99.

125. Lehmacher, A., J. Bockemühl, and S. Aleksic, "Nationwide Outbreak of Human Salmonellosis in Germany due to Contaminated Paprika and Paprika-Powdered Potato Chips," *Epidemiology and Infection* 115 (1995): 501–511.

126. Narvaiz, P., G. Lescano, E. Kairiyama, and N. Kaupert, "Decontamination of Spices by Irradiation," *Journal of Food Safety* 10 (1989): 49.

127. Anonymous, "Outbreak of Salmonella Enteritidis Infection Associated with Consumption of Raw Shell Eggs, 1991," *Morbidity and Mortality Weekly Report* 41, no. 21 (1992): 369–372.

128. Muirhead, S., "Most Recent *E. coli* Outbreak Traced to Mayonnaise," *Feedstuffs* 65, no. 16 (1993): 29.

129. Hocken, J. C., J. Y. D'Aoust, D. Bowering, et al., "An International Outbreak of *Salmonella Nima* from Imported Chocolate," *Journal of Food Protection* 52, no. 1 (1989): 51–54.

130. D'Aoust, J. Y. "*Salmonella* and the Chocolate Industry," *Journal of Food Protection* 40 (1977): 718–727.

131. *Eurosurveillance Weekly* 3, no. 17 (2002).

132. Anonymous, "Foodborne Hepatitis A—Oklahoma, Texas," *Morbidity amid Mortality Weekly Report* 32, no. 50 (1983): 652–654, 659.

133. Anonymous, "Epidemiologic Notes and Reports Mass Sociogenic Illness in a Day-Care Center—Florida," *Morbidity and Mortality Weekly Report* 39, no. 18 (1990): 301–304.

134. "Restaurant foodhandler-associated outbreak of Salmonella Heidelberg gastroenteritis identified by calls to a local telehealth service, Edmonton, Alberta, 2004," *Canada Communicable Disease Report* 31, no. 10 (2005).

135. Hedberg, C. W., K. L. MacDonald, and M. T. Osterholm, "Changing Epidemiology of Foodborne Disease: A Minnesota perspective," *Clinical Infectious Diseases* 18 (1994): 671–682.

136. Mathias, R. G., P. D. Riben, E. Campbell, et al., "The Evaluation of the Effectiveness of Routine Restaurant Inspections and Education of Food Handlers: Restaurant Inspection Survey," *Canadian Journal of Public Health* 85, sup. 1 (1994): S61–S66.

137. Mathias, R. G., R. Sizto, A. Hazelwood and W. Cocksedge, "The Effects of Inspection Frequency and Food Handler Education on Restaurant Inspection Violations," *Canadian Journal of Public Health* 86, no. 1 (1995): 46–50.

138. Wood, D. B. "Grading Eateries: ABCs of Food Safety," *Christian Science Monitor* 90, no. 51 (1998): 1, 4.

139. Simon, P. A., P. Leslie, G. Run, et al., "Impact of Restaurant Hygiene Grade Cards on Foodborne-Disease Hospitalizations in Los Angeles County," *Journal of Environmental Health* 67, no. 7 (2005): 32–36.

140. WSJ Online/Harris Interactive Health-Care Poll, "Few Americans Report Food-Related Illnesses, Health-Care Poll Shows," *The Wall Street Journal Online*, December 18, 2006. Available online. URL: http://online.wsj.com/article/SB116647589900953683.html. Accessed May 3, 2007.

141. Hargrove, T., "Many states fail to identify food-borne illnesses," *The Albuquerque Tribune*, December 21, 2006. Available online. URL: http://www.abqtrib.com/news/2006/dec/21/many-states-fail-identify-food-borne-illnesses/. Accessed May 3, 2007.

142. Archer, D. L., and J. E. Kvenberg, "Incidence and Cost of Foodborne Diarrheal Disease in the United States," *Journal of Food Protection* 48, no. 10 (1985): 887.

143. Todd, E. C. D., "Preliminary Estimates of Costs of Foodborne Disease in the United States," *Journal of Food Protection* 52, no. 8 (1989): 595.

144. ———. "Preliminary Costs of Foodborne Disease in Canada and Costs to Reduce Salmonellosis," *Journal of Food Protection* 52, no. 8 (1989): 586.

145. Buzby, J. C., Roberts, T., Jordan Lin, C. T., and MacDonald, J. M. "Bacterial Foodborne Disease: Medical Costs and Productivity Losses." *Agricultural Economics Report,* no. AER741, USDA-ERS, August 1996.

146. Jackson, J. J., C. F. Langford, and D. L. Archer, "Control of Salmonellosis and Similar Foodborne Infections," *Food Control* 2, no. 1 (1991): 26.

147. Todd, E. C. D., "Preliminary Estimates of Cost of Foodborne Disease in the United States," *Journal of Food Protection* 52, no. 8 (1989): 595.

148. CDC Update. "Multistate Outbreak of *E. coli* O157 Infections Linked to Topps Brand Ground Beef Patties." Available online. URL: http://www. pritzkerlaw.com/toppshamburger-ecoli. Accessed January 30, 2008.

149. MSNBC, "Salmonella outbreak still a sticky mystery," February 19, 2007. Available online. URL: http://www.msnbc.msn.com/id/17155561. Accessed May 3, 2007.

150. "FDA Warns Consumers to Avoid Drinking Raw Milk." FDA News Release. Available online. URL: http://www.fda.gov/bbs/topics/NEWS/2005/ NEW01278.html. Accessed on January 30, 2008.

151. Smith, J. L., "Arthritis, Guillain-Barré Syndrome and Other Seguellae of *Campylobacter jejuni* Enteritis," *Journal of Food Protection* 58, no. 10 (1995): 1,153–1,170.

152. Bula, C. J., J. Bille, and M. P. Glauser, "An Epidemic of Foodborne Listeriosis in Western Switzerland: Description of 57 Cases Involving Adults," *Clinical Infectious Diseases* 20, no. 1 (1995): 66–72.

153. Ponka, A., T. Pitkanen, S. Sarna and T. U. Kosunen, "Infection Due to *Campylobacter jejuni:* A Report of 524 Outpatients," *Infection* 12, no. 3 (1984): 175–178.

154. Samuel, M. P., S. H. Zwillich, G. T. D. Thomson, et al., "Fast Food Arthritis—A Clinico-Pathologic Study of Post-*Salmonella* Reactive Arthritis," *Journal of Rheumatology* 22, no. 10 (1995): 1,947–1,952.

155. Finch, M., G. Rodey, D. Lawrence, and P. Blake, "Epidemic Reiter's Syndrome Following an Outbreak of Shigellosis," *European Journal of Epidemiology* 2, no. 1 (1986): 26–30.

156. Kapperud, G., "Yersinia enterocolitica Infection: Epidemiology, Risk Factors and Preventative Measures," *Tidsskrift for den Norske Laegeforening* 114, no. 14 (1994): 1,606–1,608.

157. Al-Rawi, Z. S., N. Al-Khateeb and S. J. Khalifa, "*Brucella* Arthritis among Iraqi Patients," *British Journal of Rheumatology* 26, no. 1 (1987): 24–27.

158. Claesson, B. E. B., N. G. Svensson, L. Gotthardsson, et al., "A Foodborne Outbreak of Group A Streptococcal Disease at a Birthday Party," *Scandinavian Journal of Infectious Diseases* 24, no. 5 (1992): 577–586.

159. Stanley, D., "Arthritis from Foodborne Bacteria?" *Agricultural Research* (October 1996): 16.

160. Rennie, R. P., D. Strong, D. E. Taylor, et al., "*Campylobacter fetus* Diarrhea in a Hutterite Colony: Epidemiological Observations and Typing of the Causative Organism," *Journal of Clinical Microbiology* 32, no. 3 (1994): 721–724.

161. Olsvik, O., Y. Wasteson, A. Lund, and E. Hornes, "Pathogenic *Escherichia coli* Found in Food," *International Journal of Food Microbiology* 12, no. 1 (1991): 103–114.

162. Edwards, A. T., M. Roulson, and M. J. Ironside, "A Milk-borne Outbreak of Serious Infection Due to *Streptococcus zooepidemicus* (Lancefield Group c)," *Epidemiology and Infection* 101, no. 1 (1988): 43–51.

163. Challoner, K. R., K. B. Riley and R. A. Larsen, *"Brucella* meningitis," *American Journal of Emergency Medicine* 8, no. 1 (1990): 40–42.

164. Goldblith, S. A., "The Science and Technology of Thermal Processing," *Food Technology* 25 (1971): 1,256–1,262.

165. Farrer, K. T. H., "Who Invented the Brine Bath?," *Food Technology* 33, no. 2 (1979): 75–77.

166. Fryer, P., and L. Zhang, "Electrical Resistance Heating of Food," *Trends in Food Science and Technology* 4 (1993): 364–369.

167. Knorr, D., M. Gielen, T. Grahl, and W. Sitzmann, "Food Application of High Electric Field Pulses," *Trends in Food Science and Technology* 5 (1994): 71–75.

168. Ohshima, T., H. Ushio, and C. Koizumi, "High Pressure Processing of Fish and Fish Products," *Trends in Food Science and Technology* 4 (1993): 370–375.

169. Gould, G. W., "Methods for the Preservation and Extension of Shelf Life," *International Journal of Microbiology* 33 (1996): 51–64.

170. Ohlsson, T., "Minimal Processing—Preservation Methods of the Future: An Overview," *Trends in Food Science and Technology* 5 (1994): 341–344.

171. Archer, D. L., "Preservation Microbiology and Safety: Evidence That Stress Enhances Virulence and Triggers Adaptive Mutations," *Trends in Food Science and Technology* 7, no. 3 (1996).

172. Darwin, C., *On the Origin of Species,* 6th edition (London: John Murray, 1906).

173. Bauman, H. E., "The HACCP Concept and Microbiological Hazard Categories," *Food Technology* 28, no. 9 (1974): 30–34.

174. Kauffmann, L. F., "How FDA Uses HACCP" *Food Technology* 28, no. 9 (1974): 51, 84.

175. Purdum, T. S., "Meat Inspections Facing Overhaul, First in 90 Years: Scientific Testing Will Replace 'Sniff and Poke' Inspections," *New York Times* (July 7, 1996): 1.

176. Anonymous, "Emerging Pathogens Seen Needing Military-Style Thinking," *Food Chemical News* 38, no. 32 (1996): 7.

177. Klima, R. A., and T. J. Montville, "The Regulatory and Industrial Responses to Listeriosis in the USA: A Paradigm for Dealing with Emerging Foodborne Pathogens," *Trends in Food Science and Technology* 6, no. 3 (1995): 87–93.

178. Foster, A., "Consumer Attitudes to Irradiation," *Food Control* 2, no. 1 (1991): 12.

179. Taylor, J., "Consumer Views on Acceptance of Irradiated Food," Keynote address at the Joint FAO/IAEA/WHO/ITC-UNCTAD/GATT International Conference on the Acceptance, Control of and Trade in Irradiated Food (Geneva, Switzerland: WHO, December 12–16, 1988).

180. Council for Agricultural Science and Technology (CAST), "Foodborne Pathogens: Risks and Consequences," *Task Force Report* no. 122 (Washington, D.C., September 1994).

181. Archer, D. L., and J. E. Kvenberg, "Incidence and Cost of Foodborne Diarrheal Disease in the United States," *Journal of Food Protection* 48 (1985): 887–894.

182. Maurice, J., "The Rise and Rise of Food Poisoning," *New Scientist* 144, no. 1,956 (1994): 28–33.

183. Altekruse, S. F., D. A. Street, S. B. Fein, and A. S. Levy, "Consumer Knowledge of Foodborne Microbial Hazards and Food-handling Practices" *Journal of Food Protection,* 59, no. 3 (1996): 287–294.

184. Bean, N. H., and P. M. Griffin, "Foodborne Disease Outbreaks in the United States, 1973–1987: Pathogens, Vehicles and Trends," *Journal of Food Protection* 53 (1990): 804–817.

185. Michanie, S., F. L. Bryan, P. Alvarez, et al., "Critical Control Points for Foods Prepared in Households Whose Members Had Either Alleged Typhoid Fever or Diarrhea," *International Journal of Food Microbiology* 7, no. 2 (1988): 123–134.

186. Humphrey, T. J., "Heat Resistance in *Salmonella Enteritidis* Phage Type 4: The Influence of Storage Temperatures before Heating," *Journal of Applied Bacteriology* 69, no. 4 (1990): 493–497.

187. Humphrey, T. J., M. Greenwood, R. J. Gilbert, et al., "The Survival of *Salmonellas* in Shell Eggs Cooked under Simulated Domestic Conditions," *Epidemiology and Infection* 103, no. 1 (1989): 35–45.

188. Pless, P., "Effects of Storage and Heating Methods on *Salmonella Enteritidis* in Eggs," *Ernaehrung* 17, no. 2 (1993): 87–91.

189. Lighton, L., and L. Greenwood, "Raw Eggs in Recipes in Magazines Should Go," *British Medical Journal* 308, no. 6,928 (1994): 595–596.

190. Lee, M. B., "The Reliability of Pop-Up Timers in Turkeys," *Dairy, Food and Environmental Sanitation* 13, no. 11 (1993): 626–630.

191. Powers, E. M., M. Cioffi, A. Hiokala, and C. Lee, "Waterless (Towelette) Emergency Sanitation System for Food-Serving Utensils and Equipment," *Dairy Food and Environmental Sanitation* 15, no. 4 (1995): 215–221.

192. Teuber, M., O. Guillaume-Gentil, M. Eggmann, et al., "Hygienic Safety of Microwave-Heated Food," *Mitteilungen aus dem Gebiete der Lebensmitteluntersuchung und Hygiene* 86, no. 2 (1995): 140–156.

193. Heddleson, R. A., and S. Doores, "Factors Affecting Microwave Heating of Foods and Microwave Induced Destruction of Foodborne Pathogens: A Review," *Journal of Food Protection* 57, no. 11 (1994): 1,025–1,037.

194. Badeka, A. B., and M. G. Kontominas, "Effect of Microwave Heating on the Migration of Dioctyladipate and Acetyltributylcitrate Plasticizers from Food-Grade PVC and PVDC/PVC Films into Olive Oil and Water," *Zeitschrift fuer Lebensmittel-Untersuchung und Forschung,"* 202, no. 4 (1996): 313–317.

195. Fleckinger, S., A. Roulin, and P. Mafart, "Effect of Sodium Chloride on the Microwave Heating of Mashed Potatoes," *Sciences des Aliments* 15, no. 5 (1995): 445–454.

196. Kingsland, J., "Salty Food Stays Cool to Its Core in Microwaves," *New Scientist* 126, no. 1,713 (April 1990): 21, 28.

197. Sigman-Grant, M., G. Bush, and R. Anantheswaran, "Microwave Heating of Infant Formula: A Dilemma Resolved," *Pediatrics* 90, no. 3/1 (1992): 412–415.

198. Schnepf, M., and W. E. Barbeau, "Survival of *Salmonella Typhimurium* in Roasting Chickens Cooked in a Microwave, Convection-Microwave and a Conventional Electric Oven," *Journal of Food Safety* 9, no. 4 (1989): 245–252.

199. Gessner, B. D., and M. Beller, "Protective Effect of Conventional Cooking Versus Use of Microwave Ovens in an Outbreak of *Salmonellosis,"* *American Journal of Epidemiology* 139, no. 9 (1994): 903–909.

200. Anonymous, "Making Products That Kids Can Cook," *Chilton's Food Engineering International* 14 (June 1989): 13–14.

201. Donahue, C., "Kid's Kitchen May Face Safety Backlash," *Adweek's Marketing Week* 30, no. 30 (1989) 25, 27.

202. Anonymous, "Microwaved Bacon Safer," *Microwave World* 11, no. 4 (1990): 7.

203. Hashim, I. B., A. V. A. Resurrection, and K. H. McWatters, "Consumer Acceptance of Irradiated Poultry," *Poultry Science* 74, no. 8 (1995): 1,287–1,294.

204. Bussewitz, W., "Restaurant Request Rise for Food Poisoning Cover," *National Underwriter Property & Casualty-risk & Benefits Management Edition* 97, no. 40 (1993): 13.

205. Smith, R., "Beef Has Stake in 'Heating Up' Fast Food Competition," *Feedstuffs* 68, no. 3 (1996): 9, 17.

206. Adams, A. M., L. L. Leja, K. Jinneman, et al., "Anisakid Parasites, *Staphylococcus aureus* and *Bacillus cereus* in Sushi and Sashimi from Seattle Area Restaurants," *Journal of Food Protection* 57, no. 4 (1994): 311–317.

207. De Sylva, D. P., "Distribution and Ecology of Ciguatera Fish Poisoning in Florida, with Emphasis on the Florida Keys," *Bulletin of Marine Science* 54, no. 3 (1994): 944–954.

208. Hoge, C. W., D. R. Shlim, P. Echeverria, et al., "Epidemiology of Diarrhea among Expatriate Residents Living in a Highly Endemic Environment," *Journal of the American Medical Association* 275, no. 7 (1996): 533–538.

209. Bryan, F. L., "Hazard Analysis of Street Foods and Considerations for Food Safety," *Dairy Food and Environmental Sanitation* 15, no. 2 (1995): 64–69.

210. Bryan, F. L., S. C. Michanie, P. Alvarez, and A. Paniagua, "Critical Control Points of Street-Vended Foods in the Dominican Republic," *Journal of Food Protection* 51, no. 5 (1988): 373–383.

211. Koo, D., K. Maloney, and R. Tauxe, "Epidemiology of Diarrheal Disease Outbreaks on Cruise Ships," *Journal of the American Medical Association* 275, no. 7 (1996): 545–547.

212. Brucha, R. F., A. J. Howard, G. R, Thomas, et al., "Chaos Under Canvas: A Salmonella Enteritidis PT 6B Outbreak," *Epidemiology and Infection* 115, no. 3 (1995): 513–517.

213. Ming, X. T., J. W. Ayres, and W. E. Sandine, "Effect of Yogurt Bacteria on Enteric Pathogens," In *Yogurt: Nutritional and Health Properties* by R. C. Chandan (McLean, Va.: National Yogurt Association, 1989).

214. Rosenau, M. J., *Preventative Medicine and Hygiene* (New York: D. Appleton and Company, 1921).

215. Anonymous, "Travel to Surge in 21st Century," *WTO Newsletter* (Madrid: World Tourist Organization, November 1997).

216. Hilton, E., P. Kolakowski, C. Singer, and M. Smith, "Efficacy of Lactobacillus GG as a Diarrheal Preventive in Travelers," *Journal of Travel Medicine* 4, no. 1 (March 1997).

217. Calvin, L. "Outbreak Linked to Spinach Forces Reassessment of Food Safety Practices." *AmberWaves.* (June 2007). Available online. URL: http://www.ers.usda.gov/AmberWaves/June07/Features/Spinach.htm. Accessed January 31, 2008.

218. FEMA Web site. *General Information about Terrorism.* Available online. URL: http://www.fema.gov/hazard/terrorism/info.shtm. Accessed on January 31, 2008.

219. Seth Cams, *Bioterrorism and Biocrimes: The Illicit Use of Biological Agents Since 1900* (Washington, D.C.: Center for Counterproliferation Research, National Defense University, August 1998–February 2001 Revision).

220. T. J. Torok et al., "A Large Community Outbreak of Salmonellosis Caused by Intentional Contamination of Restaurant Salad Bars," *J. Amer. Med. Assoc.* (August 6, 1997): 389–395.

221. Frances Fitzgerald, "A Reporter at Large; Rajneeshpuram—I," *New Yorker,* September 22 and 29, 1986.

222. Barboza, D., and A. Barrionuevo, "Filler in Animal Feed Is Open Secret in China," *New York Times,* April 30, 2007. Available online. URL: http://www.nytimes.com/2007/04/30/business/worldbusiness/30food.html?ex=1181534400&en=e25f2d4b529dcd34&ei=5070. Accessed May 30, 2007.

223. *ABC News Turning Point,* "Deadly Meat: When a Hamburger Can Kill," transcript #134 (October 20, 1994).

224. DeWaal, C. S., "Letter to Committee on Agriculture," May 8, 2007. Available online. URL: http://cspinet.org/new/pdf/usda_testimony.pdf. Accessed June 9, 2007.

225. International Agency for Research on Cancer, WHO IARU Monographs on the Evaluation of Carcinogenic Risks to Humans 52, *Chlorinated Drinking Water; Chlorination By-Products; Some Other Halogenated Compounds; Cobalt And Cobalt Compound* (Lyon, France, 1991).

226. Fischhoff, B., and J. S. Downs, "Communicating Foodborne Disease Risk," *Emerging Infectious Diseases* 3, no. 4 (1997).

227. Neill, M. A., "E. coli O157:H7 Time Capsule: What Do We Know and When Did We Know It?" *Daily, Food and Environmental Sanitation* 14, no. 7 (1994): 374–377.

228. Levy, A. J., "A Gastroenteritis Outbreak Probably Due to a Bovine Strain of Vibrio," *Yale Journal of Biological Medicine* 18 (1946): 243.

229. Skirrow, M. B., "Epidemiology of *Campylobacter* Enteritis," *International Journal of Food Microbiology* 12 (1991): 9.

230. Reed, R. P., I. R. Friedland, F. O. Wegerhoff, and M. Khoosal, "*Campylobacter* Bacteremia in Children," *Pediatric Infectious Disease Journal* 15, no. 4 (1996): 345–348.

231. Anonymous, "Campylobacter Appears to Be Major Cause of Guillain-Barré Syndrome," *Food Chemical News* 38, no. 15 (1996): 2–5.

232. Hudson, S. J., A. O. Sobo, K. Russel, and N. F. Lightfoot, "Jackdaws as Potential Source of Milk-Borne *Campylobacter jejuni* Infection," *The Lancet* 335 (1990): 1,160.

233. Courtesy of the Istituto Superiore di Sanità, Rome, Italy.

234. Lund, B. M., "Foodborne Disease Due to *Bacillus* and *Clostridium* Species," *The Lancet* 336 (1990): 982–986.

235. De Guzman, A. M. S., B. Micalizzi, C. E. T. Pagano, and D. Giménez, "Incidence of *C. perfringens* in Fresh Sausages in Argentina," *Journal of Food Protection* 53, (1990): 173.

236. Centers for Disease Control, "*Clostridium perfringens* Gastroenteritis Associated with Corned Beef Served at St. Patrick's Day Meals—Ohio and Virginia, 1993," *Morbidity and Mortality Weekly Report* 48, no. 8 (March 4, 1994).

237. Miyazawa, F., K. Eto, M. Kanai, et al., "Microbial contaminants in foods prepared by vacuum-packed pouch cooking (sous-vide)," *Journal of the Food Hygienic Society of Japan* 35, no. 5 (1994): 530–537.

238. Regan, C. M., O. Syed, and P. J. Tunstall, "A Hospital Outbreak of *Clostridium Perfringens* Food Poisoning-Implications for Food Hygiene Review in Hospitals," *Journal of Hospital Infection* 29, no. 1 (1995): 69–73.

239. Juneja, V. K., P. O. Snyder, Jr., M. Cygnarowicz-Provost, "Influence of Cooling Rate on Outgrowth of *Clostridium Perfringens* Spores in Cooked Ground Beef," *Journal of Food Protection* 57, no. 12 (1994): 1,063–1,067.

240. Escherich, T., "Die Darmbakterien des Neugeborenen und Säuglings," *Fortschr. Med.* 3 (1885): 515–522, 547–554.

241. Courtesy of the Istituto Superiore di Sanità, Rome, Italy.

242. Riley, L. W., R. S. Remis, S. D. Helgerson, et al., "Hemorrhagic Colitis Associated with a Rare *Escherichia Coli* Serotype," *New England Journal of Medicine* 308, no. 12 (1983): 681–685.

243. "Safeguarding the Food Supply Through Irradiation Processing Techniques: An International Conference." Agricultural Research Institute, Orlando, Florida (October 25–31, 1992).

244. Whitman, T. S., M. L. Wolfe, K. Wachsmuth, et al., "Clonal Relationship among Escherichia Coli Strains That Cause Hemorrhagic Colitis and Infantile Diarrhea," *Infectious Immunology* 61 (1993): 1,619–1,629.

245. American Gastroenterological Society, Consensus Conference Statement, *E. coli O157:H7 Infections: An Emerging National Health Crisis* (July 11–13, 1994).

246. Cieslak, P. R., T. J. Barret, P. M. Griffin, et al., "*Escherichia coli O157:H7* Infection from a Manured Garden," *The Lancet* 342 (1993): 367.

247. Besser, R. E., S. M. Lett, J. T. Weber, et al., "An Outbreak of Diarrhea and Hemolytic Uremic Syndrome from *Escherichia coli* O157:H7 in Fresh-Pressed Apple Cider," *Journal of the American Medical Association* 269, no. 17 (1993): 2,217–2,220.

248. Renwick, S. A., J. B. Wilson, R. C. Clarke, et al., "Evidence of Direct Transmission of *Escherichia coli O157:H7* Infection between Calves and a Human," *Journal of Infectious Diseases* 168 (1993): 793ff.

249. Anonymous, "Food Safety—Enterohemorrhagic *Escherichia coli* Infection," *Weekly Epidemiological Record* (World Health Organization) 71 (1996): 267–268.

250. Reuters, "Japan Aide Kills Self Over Food Scare," *International Herald Tribune* (November 4, 1996): 4.

251. Nataro, J. P., T. Steiner, and R. L. Guerrant, "Enteroaggregative *Escherichia coli*," *Emerging Infectious Diseases* 4, no. 2 (1998): 251–261.

252. Van der Wouden, E. J., A. A. van Zwet, J. C. Thijs, et al., "Rapid Increase in the Prevalence of Metronidazole-Resistant Helicobacter pylori in the Netherlands," *Emerging Infectious Diseases* 3, no. 3 (1997): 385–389.

253. Anonymous, "*H. Pylori* Prior Infection Strongest Stomach Cancer Link Among Japanese Men in Hawaii," *Food Chemical News* 37, no. 39 (1995): 5.

254. Rocourt, J., "Listeria monocytogenes: the State of the Science," *Dairy, Food and Environmental Sanitation* 14, no. 2 (1994): 70–82.

255. Saxbe, W. B. Jr., "*Listeria monocytogenes* and the Queen Anne," *Pediatrics* 49 (1972): 97–101.

256. Lovett, J., "*Listeria monocytogenes*," in *Foodborne Bacterial Pathogens*, edited by M. P. Doyle (New York: Marcel Dekker, 1989): 283–310.

257. Silliker, J. H., "*Listeria monocytogenes*, Bacteria in the News," *Food Technology* 24 (August 1986).

258. Harwig, J., Mayers, P. R., Brown, B., and Farber, J. M., "*Listeria monocytogenes* in Foods," *Food Control* 4 (1991): 66.

259. Schlech, W. F. III, P. M. Lavigne, R. A. Bortolussi, et al., "Epidemic Listeriosis—Evidence for Transmission by Food," *New England Journal of Medicine* 308 (1983): 203.

260. Tilney, L. G., and D. A. Portnov, "Actin Filaments and the Growth, Movement, and Spread of the Intercellular Bacterial Parasite, *Listenia monocytogenes, Journal of Cellular Biology* 109 (1989): 1,597–1,608.

261. Gallagher, R. B., "Enter *Listeria,* Unruffled," *Science* 271 (March 29, 1996): 1,825.

262. U.S. Department of Commerce, *Statistical Abstracts of the United States* (Washington, D.C.: National Databook, Bureau of Census, U.S. Department of Commerce, 1991).

263. U.S. Department of Health and Human Services. "HIV/AIDS Surveillance Report," 3rd-quarter edition, October 1993, vol. 5, no. 3 (Atlanta: Centers for Disease Control and Prevention, 1993).

264. Gellen, B. G., and C. V. Broome, "Listeriosis," *Journal of the American Medical Association,* 261 (1989): 1,313–1,320.

265. Stamm, A. M., W. E. Dismukes, B. P. Simmons, et al., "Listeriosis in Penal Transplant Recipients: Report of an Outbreak and Review," *Review of Infectious Diseases* (1982): 665–682.

266. Johnson, J. L., M. P. Doyle, and R. G. Cassens, *Listeria monocytogenes* and Other *Listeria spp* in Meat and Meat Products—A Review," *Journal of Food Protection* 53, no. 1 (1990): 81.

267. Breer, C., and K. Schopfer, "Listerien in Nahrungsmitteln," *Schweizerische Medizinische Wochenschrift* 119, no. 10 (1989): 306.

268. Vanderlinde, P. B., and F. H. Grau, "Detection of Listeria spp. in Meat and Environmental Samples by an Enzyme-Linked Immunosorbent Assay (ELISA)," *Journal of Food Protection* 54, no. 3 (1991): 230.

269. Goulet, V., C. Jacquet, V. Vaillant, et al., "*Listeriosis* from Consumption of Raw-Milk Cheese," *The Lancet* 345, no. 8,964 (1995): 1,581–1,582.

270. Hollywood, N. W., Y. Varabioff and G. E. Mitchell, "The Effect of Microwave and Conventional Cooking on the Temperature Profiles and Microbial Flora of Minced Beef," *international Journal of Food Microbiology* 14 (1991): 67.

271. Schlech, W. F. III, P. M. Lavigne, R. A. Bortolussi, et al., "Epidemic *Listeriosis*: Evidence for Transmission by Food," *New England Journal of Medicine* 308 (1983): 203–206.

272. Bailey, J. S., D. L. Fletcher, and N. A. Cox, "Recovery and Serotype Distribution of *Listeria monocytogenes* from Broiler Chickens in the South-Eastern United States," *Journal of Food Protection* 53 (1989): 148–150.

273. Anonymous, "U.S. Zero Tolerance *Listeria Monocytogenes* Policy Should Be Changed for Low Risk Consumers, NFPA Says," *Food Chemical News* 38, no. 8 (1996): 12–13.

274. Lay, J., J. Varma, R. Marcus, et al., and EIP FoodNet Working Group. "Higher incidence of Listeria infections among Hispanics": FoodNet, 1996–2000. International Conference on Emerging Infectious Diseases. Atlanta, GA. (March 2002).

275. J. Rocourt, Personal Communication (1996).

276. Council for Agricultural Science and Technology, "Foodborne Pathogens: Risks and Consequences," *CAST Task Force Report* no. 122 (Ames, IA, 1994).

277. Enloe, C. F., Jr., "A Salmonella by Any Other Name," *Nutrition Today* 2, no. 3 (1967): 11.

278. Courtesy of the Istituto Superiore di Sanità, Rome, Italy.

279. Rosenau, M. J., *Preventative Medicine and Hygiene* (New York: D. Appleton and Company, 1921).

280. D'Aoust, J. Y., "Pathogenicity of Foodborne *Salmonella,*" *International Journal of Food Microbiology* 12 (1991): 17.

281. Soper, G. A., *Military Surgery* 45 (1919): 1.

282. Usera, M. A., A. Aladuena, A. Echeita, et al., "Investigation of an Outbreak of Salmonella Typhi in a Public School in Madrid," *European Journal of Epidemiology* 9, no. 3 (1993): 251–254.

283. Mandal, B. K., "Salmonella Typhi and Other Salmonellas," *Gut* 35, no. 6 (1994): 726–728.

284. Edel, W., M. van Schothorst, and E. H. Kampelmacher, "Epidemiological Studies on Salmonella in a Certain Area ("Walcherin Project"), 1. The Presence of Salmonella in Man, Pigs, Insects, Seagulls and in Foods and Effluents," *Zbl. Bakt. Hyg. L. Abt. Orig. A* (National Institute of Health, Bilthoven, Netherlands) 325 (1976): 476.

285. Fain, A. R., *Scope* (Silliker Laboratories) 5, no. 1 (1990): 1.

286. Anonymous, "About Half of Feed Meals, 16% of Complete Feeds Found Positive for Salmonella in CVM Survey," *Food Chemical News* (November 20, 1995): 8.

287. Hennessy, T. W., C. W. Hedberg, L. Slutsker, et al., "A National Outbreak of *Salmonella Enteritidis* Infections from Ice Cream," *New England Journal of Medicine* 334, no. 20 (1996): 1,281–1,286.

288. Centers for Disease Control, "Outbreaks of Salmonella Infections Associated with Eating Roma Tomatoes—United States and Canada, 2004," *Morbidity and Mortality Weekly Report* 54, no. 13 (2005): 325–328.

289. Goma Epidemiology Group, "Public Health Impact of Rwandan Refugee Crisis: What Happened in Goma, Zaire, in July, 1994?" *The Lancet* (North American edition) 345, no. 8,946 (1995): 339–344.

290. Koo, D., K. Maloney, and R. Tauxe, "Epidemiology of Diarrheal Disease Outbreaks on Cruise Ships, 1986–1993: What Is the Preventable Fraction?" *Abstracts of the Interscience Conference on Antimicrobial Agents and Chemotherapy* 35 (1995): 321.

291. Courtesy of the Istituto Superiore di Sanità, Rome, Italy.

292. Centers for Disease Control, "Two Cases of Toxigenic Vibrio cholerae O1 Infection after Hurricanes Katrina and Rita—Louisiana, October 2005," *Morbidity and Mortality Weekly Report* 55, no. 02 (2006): 31–32.

293. Centers for Disease Control, "*Vibrio vulnificus* Infections Associated with Raw Oyster Consumption—Florida, 1981–1992," *Morbidity and Mortality Weekly Report* 42, no. 21 (June 4, 1993).

294. Anonymous, "Hot Sauce Provides No Protection Against *V. vulnificus* in Oysters," *Food Chemical News* 37, no. 32 (1995): 9.

295. Doyle, M. P., "The Emergence of New Agents of Foodborne Disease in the 1980s," *Food Research International* 27, no. 3 (1994): 219–226.

296. Centers for Disease Control, "Two Cases of Toxigenic Vibrio cholera O1 Infection after Hurricanes Katrina and Rita—Louisiana, October 2005," MMWR, 55(02), 31–32, (2006).

297. Centers for Disease Control, *"Bacillus Cereus* Food Poisoning Associated with Fried Rice at Two Child Day Care Centers—Virginia, 1993," *Morbidity and Mortality Weekly Report* 43, no. 10 (March 18, 1994).

298. MacDonald, K. L., R. F. Spengler, C. L. Hatheway, et al., "Type Botulism from Sauteed Onions; Clinical and Epidemiological Observations," *Journal of the American Medical Association* 253 (1985): 1,275–1,278.

299. Sakaguchi, G., "Botulism," in Reimann, H., and F. L. Bryan, eds. *Food-Borne Infections and Intoxications,* 2nd edition (New York: Academic Press, 1979).

300. Centers for Disease Control, "International Outbreak of Type E Botulism Associated With Ungutted, Salted Whitefish," *Morbidity and Mortality Weekly Report* 36, no. 49 (December 18, 1987).

301. Centers for Disease Control, "Foodborne Botulism—Oklahoma, 1994," *Morbidity and Mortality Weekly Report* 44, no. 11 (March 24, 1995).

302. Sugiyama, H., "Botulism," in *Foodborne Diseases,* Cliver, D. O., ed. (San Diego: Academic Press, 1990).

303. Fenicia, L., A. M. Ferrini, P. Aureli, and T. Padovan, "Botulism Outbreak from Black Olives," *Industrie Alimentari* 31, no. 303 (1992): 307–308.

304. Conner, D. E., V. N. Scott, D. T. Bernard, and D. A. Kautter, "Potential *Clostridium Botulinum* Hazards Associated with Extended Shelf-Life Refrigerated Foods: A Review," *Journal of Food Safety* 10 (1989): 131.

305. Centers for Disease Control and Prevention. "Update: International Outbreak of Restaurant-Associated Botulism—Vancouver, British Columbia, Canada," *Morbidity and Mortality Weekly Report* 34, no. 41, 643, (1985).

306. Morse, D. L., Pickard, L. K., Guzewich, J. J., et al., "Garlic-in-oil Associated Botulism: Episode Leads to Product Modification," *Am J Public Health* 80, 1,372–1,373.

307. Courtesy of the Istituto Superiore di Sanità, Rome, Italy.

308. Bergdoll, M. S., *"Staphylococcus Aureus,"* in *Foodborne Bacterial Pathogens,* ed. M. P. Doyle (New York: Marcel Dekker, 1989): 463–523.

309. Tranter, H. S., "Foodborne Staphylococcal Illness," *The Lancet* 336 (1990): 1,044.

310. U.S. Food and Drug Administration Center for Food Safety and Applied Nutrition, *Foodborne Pathogenic Microorganisms and Natural Toxins* (1992).

311. Lowy, F. "Staphylococcus aureus infections." *N. Engl. J. Med.* 339 (1998): 520–532.

312. Herold, B. C., Immergluck, L. C., Maranen, M. C., et al., "Community-acquired methicillin-resistant Staphylococcus aureus in children with no identified predisposing risk." *JAMA* 279 (1998): 593–598.

313. Jones, T. F., Kellum, M. E., Porter, S. S., Bell, M., and W. Schaffner. "An Outbreak of Community-Acquired Foodborne Illness Caused by Methicillin-Resistant Staphylococcus aureus." *Emerging Infectious Diseases Journal* 8, no. 1 (2002): 82–84.

314. Eng, K., "Poison Plants Can Be Major Problem for Beef Cattle Industry," *Feedstuffs* 66, no. 29 (1995): 11, 25.

315. Hlywka, J. J., G. R. Stephenson, M. K. Sears, and R. Y. Yada, "Effects of Insect Damage on Glycoalkaloid Content in Potatoes *(Solanum tuberosum),"* *Journal of Agricultural and Food Chemistry* 42, no. 11 (1994): 2,545–2,550.

316. Speijers, G. J. A., "Toxicological Data Needed for Safety Evaluation and Regulation on Inherent Plant Toxins," *Natural Toxins* 3, no. 4 (1995): 222–226.

317. Y. Ogura, "Fugu (puffer fish) poisoning and the Pharmacology of crystalline tetrodotoxin in poisoning," in L. L. Simpson, ed. *Neuropoisons*, vol. I., pp. 139–159 (Plenum Press, New York, 1971).

318. Cendes, F., F. Andermann, S. Carpenter, R. J. Zatorre and N. R. Cashman, "Temporal Lobe Epilepsy Caused by Domoic Acid Intoxication: Evidence for Glutamate Receptor-Mediate Excitotoxicity in Humans," *Annals of Neurology* 37, no. 1 (1995): 123–126.

319. Lampe, F., "Rhododendrons, Mountain Laurel, and Mad Honey," *Journal of the American Medical Association* 259, no. 13 (1988): 2,009.

320. Sugimura, T., M. Nagao, T. Kawachi, et al., "Mutagen-Carcinogens in Foods with Special Reference to Highly Mutagenic Pyrolytic Products in Broiled Foods," in *Origins of Human Cancer*, H. H. Hiatt, J. D. Watson and J. A. Winsten, eds. (New York: Cold Spring Harbor Laboratory Press, 1977): Book C 1,561–1,576.

321. Sugimura, T., "The Formation of Mutagens and Carcinogens During Food Processing," in *Proceedings of the XIII International Congress of Nutrition*, Taylor, T. G., and N. K. Jenkins eds. (London: John Libbey and Company Ltd., 1986): 833–837.

322. Sato, S., "Carcinogenicity of Mutagens Formed During Cooking," in *Proceedings of the XIII International Congress of Nutrition*, T. G. Taylor and N. K. Jenkins, eds. (London: John Libbey and Company Ltd., 1986): 561–564.

323. Feng, J. N., and Z. G. Wang, "Food Poisoning Caused by Mouldy Rice Contaminated with Fusarium and T-2 Toxin," *Chinese Journal of Preventive Medicine* 26, no. 5 (1992): 284–286.

324. Anonymous, "FDA to Monitor Vomitoxin Levels in Consumer Wheat Products," *Food Chemical News* 38, no. 9 (1996): 14–15.

325. O'Brien, B. L., and L. Khuu, "A Fatal Sunday Brunch: Amanita Mushroom Poisoning in a Gulf Coast Family," *American Journal of Gastroenterology* 91, no. 3 (1996): 581–583.

326. Bauer, T. M., J. Bruehwiler, M. Aschwanden, et al., "Neurocysticercosis" *Deutsche Medizinische Wochenschrift* 119, no. 6 (1994): 175–179.

327. Smith, J. L., "*Taenia solium* Neurocysticercosis," *Journal of Food Protection* 57, no. 9 (1994): 831–844.

328. Adams, A. M., L. L. Leja, K. Jinneman, et al., *Anisakid parasites, Staphylococcus aureus and Bacillus cereus in Sushi and Sashimi from Seattle Area Restaurants*," *Journal of Food Protection* 57, no. 4 (1994): 311–317.

329. Pozio, E., P. Varese, M. A. Gomez-Morales, et al., "Comparison of Human Trichinellosis Caused by *Trichinella spiralis* and by *Trichinella britovi*," *American Journal of Tropical Medicine and Hygiene* 48, no. 4 (1993): 568–575.

330. Anonymous, "Outbreak of *Trichinellosis* Associated with Eating Cougar Jerky—Idaho, 1995," *Morbidity and Mortality Weekly Report* 45, no. 10 (1996): 205–206.

331. Maleewong, W., P. Intapan, S. Wongwajana, et al., "Prevalence and Intensity of *Opisthorchis viverrini* in Rural Community Near the Mekong River on the Thai-Laos Border in Northeast Thailand," *Journal of the Medical Association of Thailand* 75, no. 4 (1992): 231–235.

332. Juranek, D. D., "Cryptosporidiosis: Sources of Infection and Guidelines for Prevention," *Clinical Infectious Diseases* 21, Sup 1 (1995): S57–S61.

333. Courtesy of the Istituto Superiore di Sanità, Rome, Italy.

334. Holley, H. P., and C. Dover, "Cryptosporidium: A Common Cause of Parasitic Diarrhea in Otherwise Healthy Individuals," *Journal of Infectious Diseases* 153 (1986): 365.

335. Hoskin, J. C., and R. E. Wright, "Cryptosporidium: An Emerging Concern for the Food Industry," *Journal of Food Protection* 54, no. 1 (1991): 53.

336. MacKenzie, W. R., W. L. Schell, K. A. Blair, et al., "Massive Outbreak of Waterborne *Cryptosporidium* Infection in Milwaukee, Wisconsin: Recurrence of Illness and Risk of Secondary Transmission," *Clinical Infectious Diseases* 21, no. 1 (1995): 57–62.

337. Anonymous, "Milwaukee Water Scare Spells Beverage Business Bonanza," *Beverage Industry* 84, no. 5 (1993): 13–14.

338. Anonymous, "*Cryptosporidium*: Guidance for People with Severely Weakened Immune Systems," *Dairy Food and Environmental Sanitation* 15, no. 10 (1995): 622–623.

339. Monge, R., and M. Chinchilla, "Presence of *Cryptosporidium* Oocysts in Fresh Vegetables," *Journal of Food Protection* 59, no. 2 (1996): 202–203.

340. Millard, P. S., K. F. Gensheimer, D. G. Addiss, et al., "An Outbreak of *Cryptosporidiosis* from Fresh-Pressed Apple Cider," *Journal of the American Medical Association* 272, no. 20 (1994): 1,592–1,596.

341. Berkelman, R. L., "Emerging Infectious Diseases in the United States, 1993," *Journal of Infectious Diseases* 170, no. 2 (1994): 272–277.

342. Anonymous, *Morbidity and Mortality Weekly Report* 45, no. 25 (June 28, 1996): 549–551.

343. Sifuentes-Osornio, J., G. Porras-Cortes, R. P. Bendall, et al., "*Cyclospora cayetanensis* Infection in Patients with and without AIDS: Biliary Disease as Another Clinical Manifestation," *Clinical Infectious Diseases* 21, no. 5 (1995): 1,092–1,097.

344. Tartakow, I. J., and J. H. Vorperian, *Foodborne and Waterborne Diseases* (Westport, Conn.: Avi Publishing Co., 1981).

345. Casemore, D. P., "Foodborne Protozoal Infection," *The Lancet* 336 (1990): 1,427.

346. Mintz, E. D., M. Hudson-Wragg, P. Mshar, et al., "Foodborne *Giardiasis* in a Corporate Office Setting," *Journal of Infectious Diseases* 167, no. 1 (1993): 250–253.

347. Walterspiel, J. N., A. L. Morrow, M. L. Guerrero, et al., "Secretory Anti-*Giardia-lamblia* Antibodies in Human Milk: Protective Effect against Diarrhea," *Pediatrics* 93, no. 1 (1994): 28–31.

348. Anonymous, "FDA Watching East Coast *Pfiesteria* Fish Kills with Interest and Doing Limited Research," *Food Chemical News* 39, no. 31 (1997): 25–26.

349. Anonymous, "NIH Project Set to Characterize *Pfiesteria* Toxin and Assess Human Health Risk," *Food Chemical News* 39, no. 34 (1997): 6–8.

350. Kirk, J. A., and J. S. Remington, "*Toxoplasmosis* in the Adult—An Overview," *New England Medical Journal* 298 (1978): 550.

351. Richards, F. O., Jr., J. A. Kovacs, and B. J. Luft, "Preventing Toxoplasmic Encephalitis in Persons Infected with Human Immunodeficiency Virus," *Clinical Infectious Diseases* 21, Sup. 1 (1995): S49–S56.

352. Humphreys, J. G., R. L. Stewart, and J. P. Dubey, "Prevalence of *Toxoplasma gondii* Antibodies in Sera of Hunter-Killed White-Tailed Deer in Pennsylvania," *American Journal of Veterinary Research* 56, no. 2 (1995): 172–173.

353. Vanek, J. A., J. P. Dubey, P. Thulliez, et al., "Prevalence of *Toxoplasma gondii* Antibodies in Hunter-Killed White-Tailed Deer *(Odocoileus virginianus)* in Four Regions of Minnesota," *Journal of Parasitology* 82, no. 1 (1996): 41–44.

354. Dupont, H. L., "Consumption of Raw Shellfish—Is the Risk Now Unacceptable?," *New England Journal of Medicine* 314 (1986): 707.

355. Jianxiang, W., et al., "Seroepidemiological Survey of Viral Hepatitis A During an Epidemic in Shanghai," *Acta Academiæ Medicinæ Shanghai* 15 (1988): 379.

356. Koff, R. S., "Seroepidemiology of Hepatitis A in the United States," *Journal of Infectious Diseases* 171, sup. 1 (1995): S19–S23.

357. Williams, I. T., B. Bell, D. Berry, and C. Shapiro, "Foodborne Outbreak of Hepatitis A, Arkansas, 1994," *Abstracts of the Interscience Conference on Antimicrobial Agents and Chemotherapy* 35, no. 0 (1995): 315.

358. Weltman, A. C., N. M. Bennett, J. H. Misage, et al., "Multi-County Outbreak of Hepatitis A, New York State," *American Journal of Epidemiology* 139, Sup. 11 (1994): S80.

359. Morris, B. K., "Colorado Food Workers Blamed for Outbreak of Hepatitis A," *Occupational Health & Safety News* 9, no. 3 (1993): 11.

360. Smith, S., "Toss Strawberries Out, Some Florida Schools Told," *Miami Herald,* April 3, 8A (1997).

361. Centers for Disease Control, "Multisite Outbreak of Norovirus Associated with a Franchise Restaurant—Kent County, Michigan, May 2005," *Morbidity and Mortality Weekly Report,* 55, no. 14 (2006): 395–397.

362. Scholtissek, C., and E. Naylor, "Fish Farming and Influenza Pandemics," *Nature* 331 (January 21, 1988): 215.

363. Colee, J. G., "Bovine Spongiform Encephalopathy," *The Lancet* 336 (1990): 1,300–1,303.

INDEX

Note: Page numbers followed by *f* and *t* indicate figures and tables, respectively. Abbreviated names of genera are filed as if spelled in full.

A

absorbents, for traveler's diarrhea 175
accuracy, of Internet information 145
acetylsalicylic acid 105
acidity 103, 136, 240, 242
activated charcoal 175
aerobic bacteria 207
Aeromonas hydrophilia 235
aerosol dispersal 26
aflatoxins 254, 255
  in dried fruit 91
  in grain products 98
  in nuts 94
  symptoms from 254, 282*t*
agendas, information and 150
Alaska, hepatitis outbreak in 275
aleukia 255–256, 282*t*
alimentary toxic aleukia (ATA) 97, 98, 255–256, 282*t*
Amanita mushroom 258–259, 258*f*
amatoxins 164*t*, 258–259, 282*t*
amberjack 63
amebic dysentery 270
anaerobic bacteria 207, 212, 238
Anaximander 4
animalcules 8, 9*f*
animal feed
  aflatoxin in 94, 255
  antibiotics used in 25
  bovine spongiform encephalopathy in 278
  fecal matter in 36, 277, 278
  influenza virus in 277
  for poultry, contamination of 48
  Salmonella in 228
animal heat 5
animal products, antibiotic resistance and 24
anisakids 62, 264–265, 283*f*
ankylosing spondylitis 125–126
Anne (queen of Great Britain) 220
Antelope, Oregon 182–183
anthrax *(Bacillus anthracis)* 12, 181
antibiotic resistance 22–32
  agricultural practices and 25–26
  evolution of 23, 208
  forms of 23–24
  of *H. pylori* 219

of *L. monocytogenes* 224
  in plasmid DNA 208
  of *S. typhi* 227
  of *S. aureus* 244
antibiotics
  agricultural use of 25
  costs of 26
  course of treatment with, resistance and 24
  early use of 22
  justification of misuse 24–25
  overprescription of 24
  preventative use of 24
  subtherapeutic doses of 25
  for traveler's diarrhea 172, 176
antidiarrheals 162, 175–176
antigens 214, 226, 226*f*
antinuclear protests, of irradiation 136
antipasto, botulism from 240
appendicitis, *Y. enterocolitica* and 234
Appert, Nicholas 74, 130–131
apple juice, unpasteurized 91
Aristotle 4–6
arthritis 125–126
Ascaris lumbricoides 264*f*
Ascaris spp. 48, 265, 283*f*
Aspergillus flavus 91, 94, 255. *See also* aflatoxins
assassination, with hemagglutinins 246–248
Association of Food and Drug Officials 191
Athens, plague of 96–97
auction houses, for fish 65
Australian agricultural exports 187
Australian Food Safety Information Council (FSIC) 40
availability of foods, decisions on 142, 144
avian influenza 45–46
Azerbaijan, avian influenza in 45–46

B

bacillary dysentery 229
bacilli 207, 207*f*
Bacillus anthracis (anthrax) 12, 181
Bacillus cereus 97–98, 165*t*, 236–237, 280*t*
Bacillus enteritidis. See Salmonella

331